Trauma and Racial Minority Immigrants

CULTURAL, RACIAL, AND ETHNIC PSYCHOLOGY BOOK SERIES

Trauma and Racial Minority Immigrants

TURMOIL,

UNCERTAINTY,

AND RESISTANCE

Edited by Pratyusha Tummala-Narra

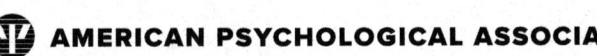 AMERICAN PSYCHOLOGICAL ASSOCIATION

Published by
American Psychological Association
750 First Street, NE
Washington, DC 20002
https://www.apa.org

Order Department
https://www.apa.org/pubs/books
order@apa.org

In the U.K., Europe, Africa, and the Middle East, copies may be ordered from Eurospan
https://www.eurospanbookstore.com/apa
info@eurospangroup.com

Typeset in Meridien and Ortodoxa by Circle Graphics, Inc., Reisterstown, MD

Printer: Gasch Printing, Odenton, MD
Cover Designer: Nicci Falcone, Potomac, MD

Library of Congress Cataloging-in-Publication Data

Names: Tummala-Narra, Pratyusha, editor.
Title: Trauma and racial minority immigrants : turmoil, uncertainty, and resistance / edited by Pratyusha Tummala-Narra.
Description: Washington, DC : American Psychological Association, [2021] | Series: Cultural, racial, and ethnic psychology book series | Includes bibliographical references and index.
Identifiers: LCCN 2020027768 (print) | LCCN 2020027769 (ebook) | ISBN 9781433833694 (paperback) | ISBN 9781433834714 (ebook)
Subjects: LCSH: Immigrants—Mental health.
Classification: LCC RC451.4.E45 T73 2021 (print) | LCC RC451.4.E45 (ebook) | DDC 616.890086/912—dc23
LC record available at https://lccn.loc.gov/2020027768
LC ebook record available at https://lccn.loc.gov/2020027769

https://doi.org/10.1037/0000214-000

Printed in the United States of America

10 9 8 7 6 5 4 3 2 1

*For all those who have lived or continue to live an uncertain,
precarious journey, and for the next generations
&
For Vinod, Keshav, and Ishan*

CONTENTS

CONTRIBUTORS

Ricardo C. Ainslie, PhD, Department of Counseling Psychology,
The University of Texas at Austin

Miriam J. Alvarez, PhD, Department of Psychology, The University of Texas
at El Paso

Angel D. Armenta, MA, Department of Psychology, The University of Texas
at El Paso

Kavita Atwal, PhD, East Side Union High School District, San Jose, CA

Germine H. Awad, PhD, Department of Educational Psychology,
The University of Texas at Austin

Thema Bryant-Davis, PhD, Graduate School of Education and Psychology,
Pepperdine University, Los Angeles, CA

Patricia Cabral, MA, Department of Human Development and Psychology,
University of California at Los Angeles

Flor Castellanos, MEd, Department of Educational Psychology,
The University of Texas at Austin

Lillian Comas-Díaz, PhD, Department of Psychiatry and Behavioral
Sciences, The George Washington University; independent practice,
Washington, DC

Jendayi B. Dillard, BA, BS, Department of Educational Psychology,
The University of Texas at Austin

Kieu Anh Do, PhD, CFLE, Department of Human Ecology, University of
Maryland Eastern Shore, Princess Anne

Diya Kallivayalil, PhD, Department of Psychiatry, Harvard Medical School/
Cambridge Health Alliance, Cambridge, MA

Esprene Liddell-Quintyn, MA, Community Psychology, Department of
Educational and Psychological Studies, University of Miami, Coral Gables, FL

Jia Li Liu, PhD, Asian American Studies Program, University of Maryland, College Park

Guadalupe López Hernández, Department of Human Development and Psychology, University of California at Los Angeles

Amy K. Marks, PhD, Department of Psychology, Suffolk University, Boston, MA

Robert P. Marlin, MD, PhD, MPH, Metta Health Center, Lowell Community Health Center, Lowell, MA

Hannah W. McDermott, PhD, Department of Counseling Psychology, The University of Texas at Austin

Monique C. McKenny, MSEd, Counseling Psychology, Department of Educational and Psychological Studies, University of Miami, Coral Gables, FL

Marisol L. Meyer, Counseling Psychology, Department of Educational and Psychological Studies, University of Miami, Coral Gables, FL

Marit D. Murry, Department of Psychology, Suffolk University, Boston, MA

Kevin L. Nadal, PhD, Department of Psychology, John Jay College of Criminal Justice—City University of New York

Donna K. Nagata, PhD, Department of Psychology, University of Michigan at Ann Arbor

Nadine Nakamura, PhD, Department of Psychology, University of La Verne, La Verne, CA

Guerda Nicolas, PhD, Counseling Psychology, Department of Educational and Psychological Studies, University of Miami, Coral Gables, FL

Reeya A. Patel, MS, Department of Psychology, University of Michigan at Ann Arbor; current affiliation: Social and Behavioral Sciences Branch, Division of Intramural Population Health Research, Eunice Kennedy Shriver National Institute of Child Health and Human Development, National Institutes of Health, Bethesda, MD

Taylor Payne, MS, Department of Educational Psychology, The University of Texas at Austin

Indhushree Rajan, PhD, Founder/CEO, Project Satori; Faculty, Pacifica Graduate Institute, Alameda, CA

Leilani Salvo Crane, PsyD, independent practice, New York, NY

Anmol Satiani, PhD, University Counseling Services, DePaul University, Chicago, IL

Lara Sheehi, PsyD, Professional Psychology Program, The George Washington University, Washington, DC

Sindhu Singh, MA, Chicago School of Professional Psychology, Chicago, IL

D. R. Gina Sissoko, BA, The Graduate Center/John Jay College of Criminal Justice—City University of New York

Matthew D. Skinta, PhD, ABPP, Department of Psychology, Roosevelt University, Chicago, IL

Gemima St. Louis, PhD, Clinical Psychology Department, William James College, Newton, MA

Carola Suárez-Orozco, PhD, Department of Counseling and School Psychology, University of Massachusetts Boston

Pratyusha Tummala-Narra, PhD, Department of Counseling, Developmental and Educational Psychology, Boston College, Boston, MA

Cixin Wang, PhD, Department of Counseling, Higher Education, and Special Education, Faculty Affiliate Asian American Studies Program, University of Maryland, College Park

G. Alice Woolverton, MS, Department of Psychology, Suffolk University, Boston, MA.

Michael A. Zárate, PhD, Department of Psychology, The University of Texas at El Paso

SERIES FOREWORD

As series editor of the American Psychological Association's (APA's) Division 45 (Society for the Psychological Study of Culture, Ethnicity and Race) Cultural, Racial, and Ethnic Psychology Book Series, it is my pleasure to introduce the latest volume in the series: *Trauma and Racial Minority Immigrants: Turmoil, Uncertainty, and Resistance*, edited by Pratyusha Tummala-Narra.

The impetus for the series came from my presidential theme for Division 45, which focused on "Strengthening Our Science to Improve Our Practice." Given the increasing attention to racial and ethnic minority issues within the discipline of psychology, I argued that we needed to both generate more research and get the existing research known. From the *Supplement to the Surgeon General's Report on Mental Health* to the *Unequal Treatment* report from the Institute of Medicine—both of which documented extensive racial and ethnic disparities in our health care system—the complex of culture, race, and ethnicity was becoming a major challenge in both research and practice within the field of psychology.[1]

To meet that challenge, Division 45 acquired its own journal devoted to ethnic minority issues in psychology (*Cultural Diversity and Ethnic Minority Psychology*). At the same time, a series of handbooks on the topic were published, including Bernal, Trimble, Burlew, and Leong's *Handbook of Racial and*

---

[1]U.S. Department of Health and Human Services. (2001). *Mental health: Culture, race, and ethnicity—A supplement to mental health: A report of the Surgeon General.* U.S. Department of Health and Human Services, Substance Abuse and Mental Health Services Administration, Center for Mental Health Services.

Ethnic Minority Psychology.[2] Yet, we felt that more coverage of this subdiscipline was imperative—coverage that would match the substantive direction of the handbooks but would come from a variety of research and practice perspectives. Hence, the Division 45 book series was launched.

The Cultural, Racial, and Ethnic Psychology Book Series was designed to advance our theories, research, and practice regarding this increasingly crucial subdiscipline. It will focus on, but not be limited to, the major racial and ethnic groups in the United States (i.e., African Americans, Hispanic Americans, Asian Americans, and American Indians) and will include books that examine a single racial or ethnic group as well as books that undertake a comparative approach. The series will also address the full spectrum of related methodological, substantive, and theoretical issues, including topics in behavioral neuroscience, cognitive and developmental psychology, and personality and social psychology. Other volumes in the series will be devoted to cross-disciplinary explorations in the applied realms of clinical psychology and counseling as well as educational, community, and industrial–organizational psychology. Our goal is to commission state-of-the art volumes in cultural, racial, and ethnic psychology that will be of interest to both practitioners and researchers.

According to the office of the United Nations High Commissioner for Refugees, there are over 70 million forcibly displaced persons around the world. Many of these individuals come to the United States as immigrants. The Pew Center estimates that 40 million people living in the United States were born in another country, accounting for about one fifth of the world's migrants in 2017. The psychological adaptation of immigrants has long been an interest in our field. Dating as far back as 1926, Emory Bogardus[3] had studied "social distance" from majority groups to racial immigrant groups, where he found that there were different levels of acceptance for different groups. In 2011, APA president Melba Vasquez's presidential initiative included a task force on immigration which was charged with

> developing an evidence-based report that addresses the psychological factors related to the experience of immigration, with particular attention to the mental and behavioral health needs of immigrants across the lifespan, and the effects of acculturation, prejudice/discrimination and immigration policy on individuals, families and society. (https://www.apa.org/topics/immigration/immigration-report.pdf)

From the Chinese Exclusion Act of 1912 to the recent Zero Tolerance policy that led to family separation, the U.S. government has subjected immigrants to some traumatic experiences. The current volume edited by Pratyusha Tummala-Narra is therefore very timely in the focus on the trauma experienced by racial minority immigrants. She has convened a group of national experts to address these issues ranging from xenophobia to microaggressions,

[2]Bernal, G., Trimble, J. E., Burlew, A. K., & Leong, F. T. L. (2003). *Handbook of racial and ethnic minority psychology.* Sage.
[3]Bogardus, E. S. (1926). Social distance in the city. *Proceedings and Publications of the American Sociological Society, 20,* 40–46.

from racial profiling to historical racial trauma. In addition to delineating the problems, the volume also offers strategies for intervention.

Finally, I would like to end by thanking the members of the editorial board who do the work of recruiting and reviewing proposals for the series: Guillermo Bernal, University of Puerto Rico, Rio Piedras Campus; Beth Boyd, University of South Dakota; Lillian Comas-Díaz, private practice, Washington, DC; Sandra Graham, UCLA; Gordon Nagayama Hall, University of Oregon; Helen Neville, University of Illinois at Champaign–Urbana; Teresa LaFromboise, Stanford University; Richard Lee, University of Minnesota; Robert M. Sellers, University of Michigan; Stanley Sue, Palo Alto University; Joseph Trimble, Western Washington University; and Michael Zárate, University of Texas at El Paso. They represent leading scholars in psychology who have graciously donated their time to help advance the field.

—*Frederick T. L. Leong*
Series Editor

ACKNOWLEDGMENTS

I begin with my deep appreciation for my fellow authors. I am sincerely grateful for their expertise and commitment to meaningful inquiry into the experiences of racial minority immigrants. I also thank the many people who, through their own stories, have made it possible for us to learn more about trauma and immigration, including clients, research participants, mentors, colleagues, students, friends, and family.

This volume was made possible through the helpful recommendations provided by Beth Hatch at the American Psychological Association (APA), and I convey my sincere thanks for all of her guidance. Additionally, two critical figures who have brought this volume to fruition are Fred Leong and Susan Reynolds. I am grateful to Fred Leong, editor of the APA Division 45 Book Series, who patiently encouraged me to compile this volume and provided invaluable feedback. Finally, I thank Susan Reynolds at APA, for all of her brilliant feedback, support, and guidance for this book and beyond.

As this volume reached its final stages, Dr. Jean Lau Chin passed away due to complications from COVID-19, a deeply sad loss for all of us. Since her passing, I came to learn that Dr. Chin served as one of the peer reviewers of this volume. With a heavy heart, I regret that we are unable to personally thank her for her recommendations. I am most grateful for her presence in this volume and for her tremendous scholarship and leadership in psychology.

Trauma and Racial Minority Immigrants

Introduction

Challenges Facing Racial Minority Immigrants

Pratyusha Tummala-Narra

In the United States, few issues are more polarizing than immigration. We live in a time of heated debates surrounding immigration policies, such as those affecting Dreamers, migrant families, and refugees and asylum seekers. We also face controversy concerning building a wall at the U.S.–Mexico border and whether the United States should open its borders to people fleeing persecution, poverty, and natural disasters. Immigration policy continues to be in significant flux as political polarization within the United States has escalated, contributing to new forms of oppression and human rights violations.

Political ideologies on immigration are fueled by a growing anti-immigrant sentiment, particularly directed at racial minorities, within the United States and globally. This sentiment has been further heightened in the midst of the COVID-19 pandemic, as racial minorities are both victimized by the virus at disproportionate rates and blamed for causing and spreading the virus in the United States. In fact, the COVID-19 outbreak has brought to the foreground fundamental disparities in health and access to health care among racial minorities. Racial minorities, particularly African Americans, Latinx Americans, and Native Americans (e.g., Navajo Nation) from low-income backgrounds, have been facing alarmingly high levels of infections and deaths due to COVID-19. Public health guidelines requiring social distancing typically do not consider the lack of resources such as clean water, health care, and health insurance, higher density housing, and greater exposure to the coronavirus in the workplace among many racial minority communities. The inadequacy of

https://doi.org/10.1037/0000214-001
Trauma and Racial Minority Immigrants: Turmoil, Uncertainty, and Resistance,
P. Tummala-Narra (Editor)

these structures is also evident in prisons and detention centers, underscoring racial and economic disparities and race- and class-based oppression in the United States (Centers for Disease Control and Prevention, 2020). Despite the rise in xenophobia and racism in recent years and long-standing structural inequality and race-based violence within U.S. society, many Americans are engaged in resisting hate and discrimination directed against immigrants and racial minorities. In fact, the call to address structural violence and discrimination against these communities has been reawakened.

To situate the context of racial minority immigrants, it is important to consider the growth of immigrant populations in the United States. In 2017, approximately 44.4 million immigrants resided in the United States, composing 13.6% of the population. This number reflects an increase of more than 4 times the number of immigrants as in 1960. U.S.-born children of immigrants (i.e., second generation) compose an additional 12% of the population, and it is projected that by 2050, first-generation immigrants will account for 19% of the overall population and the second generation will account for 18%. Additionally, approximately one fourth of the foreign-born population is unauthorized or undocumented (Pew Research Center, 2019).

Since the passage of the 1965 Immigration and Naturalization Act, increasing numbers of immigrants have arrived to the United States from Latin America, Asia, Caribbean, and Africa; in contrast, immigration prior to 1965 was dominated by immigrants from Europe and Canada (American Psychological Association [APA] Presidential Task Force on Immigration, 2012). The growing presence of non-White immigrants has not only marked increasing cultural diversity and pluralism in the United States but has also been met with significant anti-immigrant sentiment. Throughout U.S. history, people considered to be non-White have become racialized upon arriving and, therefore, negotiate their social position within the context of the American racial hierarchy. Racism and race-based violence directed against racial minority immigrants stand alongside the longstanding history of genocide and slavery in the United States and ongoing racism directed against Native Americans and African Americans. Prior to leaving their countries of origin, many immigrants are unaware of the entrenched nature of American racial injustice. Nevertheless, immigrants and their children are socialized into American notions of race and inevitably are exposed to stereotypes and discrimination based on race, religion, gender, and other social locations.

Although xenophobia and discrimination are pervasive within various regions of the world, they take unique forms in U.S. society. In more recent history, the terrorist attacks on September 11, 2001, sparked a rise in Islamophobia, and subsequently, the profiling of people perceived to be Muslim has become normalized. Since 2016, the country has seen a rise in explicit forms of racism and stereotyping that have become increasingly normalized in public discourse, bearing important implications for the physical and psychological safety and well-being of immigrants and their children. The term "Trump effect" has been coined by psychologists to describe the notable increase in racialized, xenophobic, misogynistic, homophobic, and transphobic bullying in schools since the presidential election of Donald Trump (Zimbardo & Sword, 2017). At the time we are completing this volume, the COVID-19 outbreak is rife with racist sentiment and attacks against Chinese Americans and those who are perceived to be of Chinese or East Asian descent. Amidst the pandemic, race-based violence, particularly police brutality, against Black men and women persists.

The real struggles that many immigrants face when leaving behind loved ones and a familiar cultural, religious, and linguistic context, and their resilience in the face of these losses and separations, remain largely invisible in public discourse in the current xenophobic state. Anti-immigrant policies and actions, such as threats to ending the Deferred Action for Childhood Arrivals (DACA) and Temporary Protected Status (TPS), separation of migrant children and parents, and a ban on entry of Syrian refugees and individuals from predominantly Muslim countries, have created profound fear and helplessness among many immigrant families. As such, there is a dire need for psychologists and other mental health practitioners and researchers to engage in deeper inquiry into the experiences of racial minority immigrants and in resisting policies that threaten their basic sense of safety and humanity.

AIMS OF THE BOOK

The literature in psychology concerning immigration has grown significantly over the past 20 years and has spanned issues of education, mental health, and policy (APA Presidential Task Force on Immigration, 2012). Additionally, a number of books focused on immigration have made important advances that have sparked an expansion of research and clinical theory. For example, some books have addressed specific types of discrimination (e.g., racism), the diagnosis and treatment of posttraumatic stress disorder from a global perspective, acculturation among immigrants, and the experiences of specific immigrant communities (e.g., Asian American, Latinx American, women). In 2012, the American Psychological Association published its Presidential Task Force on Immigration Report, which provides a broad and comprehensive review of the literature on the psychology of immigration, particularly that related to mental health and education. The report identified various gaps in the empirical and clinical literature that must be filled to broaden and deepen existing understandings of the immigrant experience within a broader socio-ecological framework. For example, the report calls for the use of multiple research methodologies (e.g., quantitative, qualitative, mixed methods), increased attention to the development of culturally informed interventions (e.g., psychotherapy, community- and school-based interventions), and improved training for psychologists in conducting research with and providing services with immigrant-origin individuals. The report also calls for more research focused on the experiences of vulnerable groups of immigrants, such as undocumented immigrants and victims of trafficking.

Currently, clinicians are contending with how best to help their clients cope with racism, xenophobia, and other forms of oppression within an uncertain and unpredictable social and political climate. Relatedly, multicultural researchers are examining the effects of the current political climate on individuals, families, and communities. Many of us who are racial minority psychologists also bear the burden of examining the effects of this climate on our personal lives and our professional work. For example, I am keenly aware that the research that I have been conducting is focused on the current crises facing immigrants. I am also aware of the ways in which I have modified my clinical practice since the 2016 presidential election, as I work with clients who are in crisis due to the terrifying circumstances created by overtly anti-immigrant and racist rhetoric and policies. Most recently, I have observed the profound impact of illness and death related to COVID-19 and stay-at-home orders on clients' anxiety, depression, and isolation and have observed the challenges of accessing adequate mental health care among individuals who are uninsured or hold undocumented status. This book is an effort to document what we, as multicultural researchers, scholars, and practitioners, are learning about the impact of the sociopolitical climate on racial minority immigrants from the various contexts in which we engage (e.g., research, clinical practice, community-based intervention). Another primary aim of the book is to highlight theory, research, and practice concerning various types of trauma and oppression faced by racial minority immigrants, such as racial profiling, deportation, trafficking, interpersonal violence, and intersectional discrimination. A third purpose of the book is to underscore the link between historical trauma and ongoing trauma faced by racial minority immigrants in the United States as way of understanding the precipitants and processes that underlie oppression of immigrants and of identifying strategies for reducing harm and resisting oppression in our work.

I am truly grateful to the authors of this volume, as they are dedicated to this line of inquiry that is so critically important, especially in this historical moment. The authors of this book are expert researchers, scholars, and clinicians, each with a unique focus on trauma and the immigration experience. Their expertise includes areas such as the psychology of xenophobia and prejudice, profiling, racial and political trauma, historical trauma, trafficking, deportation trauma, interpersonal violence, developmental processes such as identity and intersectionality, clinical and community-based interventions, and human rights.

Because the psychological literature contains a number of classifications concerning immigrants, it is necessary to clarify the terminology in this book. *Racial minority immigrants* and *racial minority immigrant-origin individuals* refer to individuals who either migrated to the United States from another country or are the children or descendants of these immigrants and who are classified or perceived as racial minorities in the United States. *First-generation immigrants* refers to those who arrive to the United States as adults, *1.5-generation immigrants* refers to those who arrive to the United States by age 12 years, and the *second generation* and *later generations* refer to individuals who are born and raised in the United States. *Identity* refers to various aspects of individual and collective identity, such as ethnic identity, bicultural identity, and racial identity, and it refers to intersections of experiences based on age, gender, race, ethnicity, religion, national origin, sexual orientation, social class, authorization or documentation status, and dis/ability, among other factors. Additionally, authors in the book provide specific definitions that guide their perspectives on immigration and trauma.

This book is not designed to be a comprehensive guide to the psychology of trauma or to the psychology of immigration. Rather, it is a necessary step in examining the growing complexity of trauma and traumatic stress experienced by racial minority immigrants. This book makes a unique contribution to the field in that it provides nuanced perspectives on how the historical and current sociopolitical climate in the United States affects traumatic experiences of racial minority immigrants and extends literature concerning the impact of multiple marginalization and traumas occurring both within and outside of immigrant communities. The book approaches trauma with serious attention to rising nationalism and xenophobia, shifting economic and political structures, controversy over immigration policy, alarming rates of displacement within nations, war, trafficking, terrorism, and deportation. As such, there is an emphasis on both crisis states of the immigrant experience (e.g., deportation, fear of deportation, racial and religious-based violence) and complex traumatic experiences rooted in repeated violence and discrimination.

Although the implications of the current sociopolitical climate for the well-being of immigrants and their families are considered herein, the issues raised are not just pertinent to the present context. Rather, the topics reflect historical and ongoing trauma faced by immigrants, and they are relevant to contexts outside of the United States. It is important to note that different racial minority subgroups in the United States face shared and distinct forms of racial, ethnic, and religious discrimination, profiling, and violence, based in historical and contemporary perceptions of specific racial minority groups. For example, a Moroccan immigrant may become racialized and be perceived as African American by people in mainstream context; subsequently, that person's ethnicity and heritage culture may be dismissed in service of maintaining racialized hierarchies and perceptions in the United States.

The book does not aim to address social injustice faced by every racial minority immigrant group or that faced by every subgroup within any particular immigrant community. However, it emphasizes the importance of intersectionality and heterogeneity of experiences across and within different racial minority immigrant groups. With that being said, I want to recognize that some areas of great importance are not covered in depth, such as the experiences of immigrants with disabilities, older adults, multiracial immigrants, and transnational adoptees. This omission, at least in part, reflects the limited attention to these aspects of immigrant experience in theory and research. I further recognize that this book was largely written prior to the global spread of COVID-19 and is therefore limited in scope with regard to discussion of the impact of the virus outbreak on immigrant communities. It is my hope that future work will expand into all these areas, particularly when considering the vulnerability to victimization among some subgroups of immigrants.

The authors in these pages address the following key questions: (a) What are the traumatic experiences of racial minority immigrants in the present-day United States? (b) What are the implications of these experiences for mental health and identity? (c) What does resilience look like among racial minority immigrants coping with and resisting oppression? (d) How can psychologists help in coping with the traumatic effects of oppression and resist further oppression in the face of crisis and ongoing uncertainty? The chapters explore both stress and resilience experienced by racial minority immigrants, and they include clinical and community-based illustrations that bring deeper understanding to theoretical perspectives and empirical findings. It is worth noting that the clinical illustrations have been anonymized and that they are not intended to reflect comprehensive experiences of people who are affiliated with or identify with any particular racial, ethnic, or religious group.

The theoretical perspectives driving the chapters are diverse, reflecting the multifaceted experiences of racial minority immigrants. Specifically, the chapters reflect various perspectives, such as multicultural, feminist, womanist, minority stress, biopsychosocial, psychodynamic, cognitive-behavioral, complex trauma, liberation psychology, human rights, and integrative frameworks. Developing a clear understanding of the experiences of racial minority immigrants requires multiple theoretical lenses, and therefore, authors with diverse theoretical knowledge were invited to contribute to this volume. An overarching framework that underlies these various approaches is the socio-ecological perspective, described in prior reports concerning immigrant and racial minority populations (APA Presidential Task Force on Immigration, 2012; Clauss-Ehlers et al., 2019). For example, the *APA Presidential Task Force Report on Immigration* and the *APA Revised Multicultural Guidelines* (Clauss-Ehlers et al., 2019) integrated Bronfenbrenner and Ceci's (1994) bioecological frame-work to guide understanding stress and resilience among immigrants and racial minorities. Bronfenbrenner's model emphasizes the interaction of multiple layers of a person's ecological context, including the microsystem, mesosystem, exosystem, macrosystem, and chronosystem in determining outcomes regarding one's development and psychological well-being. The ecological perspective has been expanded more recently by García Coll and Marks (2012) to an integrative contextual framework, in which social position factors such as race, ethnicity, gender, and social class contribute to the promotion or inhibition of positive growth among minority youth. These overarching socioecological approaches consider active forms of racism and discriminatory policies directed against immigrants and the impact of this stress on mental health and on intersectional experiences of context and identity. The authors provide their own theoretical perspectives, which guide their empirical and clinical work, bearing in mind the various social position factors and layers of ecological context that shape immigrants' experiences (APA Presidential Task Force on Immigration, 2012; García Coll & Marks, 2012).

ORGANIZATION OF THE BOOK

The book is organized into four separate but overlapping sections: (a) context of xenophobia and racism in the United States, (b) specific forms of trauma in immigrant communities, (c) resilience and identity, and (d) key strategies for intervention. Some important general themes are evident across these sections, including trauma as rooted in systemic injustice and oppression; bridging historical racial and political trauma with contemporary oppression; multiple contexts of trauma in the migration process (pre- and postmigration, in transit to the United States); rise in explicit racism and other forms of bias and discrimination; heterogeneity of sociocultural and intersectional experiences across and within different immigrant groups; unique experiences of immigrants across different developmental periods (e.g., children, adolescents, emerging adults); multiple marginalization occurring within and outside of one's ethnic and religious communities; role of cultural beliefs, acculturation, discrimination, and policy in shaping the experience of and strategies for coping with trauma; and finally, strength and resilience of racial minority immigrants. These themes, while wide in scope, reflect the complexity of immigrants' experiences in the contemporary United States. Each chapter takes on at least one of these themes, aiming to provide a more in-depth analysis of a particular type of traumatic experience, traumatic stress within a specific immigrant community, or a key approach to intervention.

Part I, Context of Xenophobia and Racism in the United States, consists of five chapters that present the problems of explicit and more subtle forms of xenophobia and racism as manifested within the broader sociopolitical climate and policy and within specific developmental and interpersonal contexts pertaining to racial minority immigrant youth and adults. Armenta, Alvarez, and Zárate (Chapter 1) provide an inquiry into contemporary prejudice in the United States and some important factors contributing to White perceptions of immigrants as a threat to American society, such as the fear of social and cultural change and a sense of national nostalgia. McDermott and Ainslie (Chapter 2) explore profiling of Mexican and Central American migrants and specifically complex traumatic stress rooted in four distinct sources of violence directed against these migrants, including violence in the premigration context, during the migration journey, in the postmigration context, and within U.S. immigration policies. Marks, Woolverton, and Murry (Chapter 3) use an integrative risk-and-resilience model of immigrant youth development to examine how interactions within different contexts, such as families and schools, and messages regarding immigrants in broader society shape children's and adolescents' mental health, academic outcomes, and sense of resilience. Satiani and Singh (Chapter 4) present compelling clinical evidence from their practice in a university counseling center showing a rise in anti-immigrant sentiment and racism on U.S. college campuses. They explore the effects on racial minority immigrant students' and international students' safety and well-being and on students' efforts to resist oppression. In the final chapter of this section, Sissoko and Nadal (Chapter 5) present a taxonomy of microaggressions (i.e., eight themes) experienced specifically by racial minority immigrants, underscoring the prevalence of everyday microassaults, microinsults, and microinvalidations that affect individuals' mental health and identity.

Part II, Specific Forms of Trauma in Immigrant Communities, focuses in depth on different contexts of exposure to trauma, highlighting distinct types of traumatic stress faced by racial minority immigrants and their resilience in the face of this stress. The six chapters in this section address historical and ongoing trauma such as the incarceration of Japanese Americans, racial and political violence against Latinx immigrants, and racialized violence against Black immigrants. They also address specific types of explicit traumas such as trafficking, deportation, and interpersonal violence. Nagata and Patel (Chapter 6) provide an important lens into historical trauma, specifically the incarceration of Japanese Americans during World War II, a series of traumatic events with important implications for subsequent generations of Japanese Americans and for current U.S. policies concerning separation of migrant families and placement in detention centers. They remind us of the cyclical and repetitive nature of anti-immigrant sentiment and policies and why it is critical to recognize and resist longstanding national and global patterns of propagating xenophobia and racism. Comas-Díaz (Chapter 7) presents a new theoretical understanding of sociopolitical trauma as distinct from posttraumatic stress disorder and as directly caused by social, political, and systemic factors such as racial oppression, coloniality, and cultural imperialism. She further presents a decolonizing approach to resisting oppression and emphasizes the resilience of immigrant communities. Meyer, McKenny, Liddell-Quintyn, Nicolas, and St. Louis (Chapter 8) examine trauma faced by Black immigrants in the United States while underscoring the diversity of experiences within and across different Black immigrant communities. They provide a model that recognizes racialized violence as a form of complex trauma and places at its core the interaction between individual, interpersonal, and systemic factors in the experience of traumatic stress and resilience.

Part II proceeds with a chapter authored by Rajan and Bryant-Davis (Chapter 9), who examine local and global race-based and gender-based discrimination within human trafficking, with a special focus on Asian and South Asian survivors of trafficking. Suárez-Orozco, López Hernández, and Cabral (Chapter 10) focus on traumatic stress rooted in family separations and threats and realities of deportation and its implications for youth growing up in unauthorized homes. They underscore the problem that these youth face in accessing structural and social belonging. My chapter on interpersonal violence (Chapter 11) completes this section of the book, exploring the complexity of conceptualizing interpersonal violence, such as sexual violence, within different immigrant communities. I also explore immigrants' experiences of multiple marginalization, occurring within and outside of their ethnic and religious communities.

Part III, Resilience and Identity, consists of two chapters that focus on how racial minority immigrants negotiate resilience and identity in the face of individual and systemic oppression. Awad, Castellanos, Dillard, and Payne (Chapter 12) use a model of cumulative racial/ethnic trauma for Americans of Descent to discuss protective and resilience factors among racial minority immigrants, in particular Middle Eastern and North African (MENA) Americans. They draw attention to the importance of understanding legal protections, cultural strengths, ethnic identity, religious faith, and social supports in coping with and resisting oppression. Skinta and Nakamura (Chapter 13) explore how the global persecution of LGBTQ people shapes intersectional identities and traumatic experience prior to, during, and after migration and how resilience plays a significant role in lives of LGBTQ immigrants and asylum seekers. They provide a compelling analysis of the complexity of navigating stress across and within multiple communities and contexts.

Part IV, Key Strategies for Intervention, includes three chapters that present culturally informed approaches to community-based intervention, assessment and clinical practice, and advocacy. Wang, Liu, Atwal, and Do (Chapter 14) describe an innovative community-based intervention focused on preventing bullying of racial minority immigrant youth, in particular, Chinese American and Sikh American children and adolescents. Their work underscores the importance of researchers collaborating with schools and specific immigrant communities to address race-, ethnicity-, and religious-based bullying. Sheehi and Crane (Chapter 15) challenge Eurocentric conceptualizations of trauma that underlie diagnosis and clinical practice with immigrants. They use a liberation psychology framework to guide recommendations for clinicians, shifting away from the notion of trauma as an individual disorder. Kallivayalil and Marlin (Chapter 16) provide an important case for adopting a human-rights framework in conducting research, practice, and teaching within psychology and other mental health professions. While focusing on legal advocacy and community-based collaborations, they argue that psychologists have a responsibility to protect clients and research participants from human rights violations and to provide improved education and training about human rights statutes within the profession.

Together, the authors of this volume bring to the foreground the importance of practitioners, researchers, and educators engaging with the complexity of trauma and violence faced by racial minority immigrants and with the crisis of xenophobic and racist actions directed against racial minority immigrants both in the present and in the future. Bearing witness to trauma experienced by immigrants is especially critical in a historic state marked by turmoil and uncertainty. Furthermore, developing an in-depth understanding of the impact of the current sociopolitical climate on immigrant individuals and communities, and recognizing immigrants' resilience and resistance—both of which are ethical imperatives of psychologists—can guide future theory, research, practice, and training.

The book is intended for practitioners, researchers, and educators across different disciplines (e.g., psychology, social work, psychiatry) who are interested in traumatic stress and the experiences of racial minority immigrants and how these experiences are connected with broader American society. It will also be of benefit to graduate students in psychology, social work, and psychiatry training programs, where education concerning culturally informed and trauma-informed research and practice with immigrants is sorely needed.

REFERENCES

American Psychological Association Presidential Task Force on Immigration. (2012). *Crossroads: The psychology of immigration in the new century.* American Psychological Association. https://www.apa.org/topics/immigration/executive-summary.pdf

Bronfenbrenner, U., & Ceci, S. J. (1994). Nature–nurture reconceptualized in developmental perspective: A bioecological model. *Psychological Review, 101*(4), 568–586. https://doi.org/10.1037/0033-295X.101.4.568

Centers for Disease Control and Prevention. (2020). *COVID-19 in racial and ethnic minority groups.* https://www.cdc.gov/coronavirus/2019-ncov/need-extra-precautions/racial-ethnic-minorities.html

Clauss-Ehlers, C. S., Chiriboga, D. A., Hunter, S. J., Roysircar, G., & Tummala-Narra, P. (2019). APA Multicultural Guidelines executive summary: Ecological approach to context, identity, and intersectionality. *American Psychologist, 74*(2), 232–244. https://doi.org/10.1037/amp0000382

García Coll, C., & Marks, A. K. (Eds.). (2012). *The immigrant paradox in children and adolescents: Is becoming American a developmental risk?* American Psychological Association. https://doi.org/10.1037/13094-000

Pew Research Center. (2019). *Facts on U.S. immigrants, 2017.* https://www.pewresearch.org/hispanic/2019/06/03/facts-on-u-s-immigrants/

Zimbardo, P., & Sword, R. (2017). Unbridled and extreme present hedonism. In B. X. Lee (Ed.), *The dangerous case of Donald Trump* (pp. 25–50). St. Martin's Press.

CONTEXT OF XENOPHOBIA AND RACISM IN THE UNITED STATES

1

Wounds That Never Heal

The Proliferation of Prejudice Toward Immigrants in the United States

Angel D. Armenta, Miriam J. Alvarez, and Michael A. Zárate

For decades, the United States has been a leader in immigration by opening its doors to immigrants from across the globe (Radford, 2019). For many nations, the United States has become a model for immigration policies and legislation. For immigrants, the United States sells a dream of equality, opportunity, and fairness. Perceptions of outsiders differ from the reality of the sociopolitical context in the United States, where tensions between anti-immigration and pro-immigration proponents have created a nation divided. Although the United States is home to one of the largest populations of immigrants in the world, the sociopolitical climate since 2007 makes immigration one of the most divisive issues (Budiman, 2020). Immigration has become a flash point in the new political landscape of increasing political polarization. At the center of the political divisiveness is a debate over the changing American landscape. Does our country move forward in a more progressive way, or is change happening too rapidly and should our country revert to old times to "make America great again"?

This chapter provides an overview of how perceived threat felt by cultural change from the current immigration surge has facilitated the growth of individual and systemic bias, which has led to a hostile environment for racial minority immigrants. Through a cultural inertia perspective (i.e., the model asserts that cultural change leads to hostility; Zárate et al., 2019), we discuss the explanations for why individuals react to change and the perceived enactors of the change. Utilizing the biopsychosocial model and minority stress model

https://doi.org/10.1037/0000214-002
Trauma and Racial Minority Immigrants: Turmoil, Uncertainty, and Resistance,
P. Tummala-Narra (Editor)

(Clark et al., 1999), we further discuss the ways in which discrimination can have direct negative psychological and physiological outcomes. We end the chapter by shifting the discourse to address psychological theory (e.g., cultural inertia) and its implications concerning the growing anti-immigrant atmosphere.

THE CURRENT POLITICAL CLIMATE

One potential cause for the heightened negative immigrant attitudes is the rhetoric produced by the now-President Trump. As a candidate, Mr. Trump entered the race for the presidency by saying,

> When Mexico sends its people, they're not sending their best. They're not sending you. They're not sending you. . . . They're sending people that have lots of problems, and they're bringing those problems with us. They're bringing drugs. They're bringing crime. They're rapists. And some, I assume, are good people. (Kopan, 2016)

This now-controversial quote was followed by continued anti-immigrant rhetoric, protracted political battles over President Trump's desire to build a wall along the entire U.S.–Mexico border, family separation policies at the border (resulting in migrant kids dying in U.S. custody; Acevedo, 2019), and a "Muslim ban" to keep Americans "safe." Some policies were implemented (e.g., immigration restrictions), and those that needed congressional approval were not implemented (American Bar Association, 2018; Lind & Zarracina, 2019).

President Trump's political agenda and continuous targeting of immigration reform have created a platform that promotes negative immigration rhetoric and behavior, which have had damaging societal consequences. For example, in 2017, citizens of Charlottesville, Virginia, took to rallying and rioting to promote White nationalism. At the Charlottesville rally, a large crowd of far-right-wing individuals and White supremacists gathered with tiki torches and hateful chants to protest and share their disdain for immigrants and other groups. Common chants included "Blacks will not replace us!"; "Jews will not replace us!"; and "Immigrants will not replace us!" Those crowds were eventually met with antifascist protestors. Ultimately, the rally became violent, several people were injured, and one person was killed by a White supremacist. As a response, President Trump proclaimed that there were "very fine people on both sides" (McEldowney, 2018), further cementing his anti-immigrant reputation.

One should always be careful when drawing inferences from single actions such as the killing in Charlottesville. In line with the increasing anti-immigrant rhetoric and behavior, hate crimes toward racial minorities, including immigrants, have skyrocketed in the United States since President Trump was elected into office (Campbell et al., 2018). Two weeks after the presidential election, anti-Latinx hate crimes reported in major U.S. cities increased 176%, compared with the daily average (Campbell et al., 2018). Furthermore, 57% of Latinx immigrants reported feeling uneasy and unsure about their place in the United States, and 71% reported that policies under the Trump administration have harmed Latinxs as a group (Lopez et al., 2018). As a result of anti-Latinx immigrant discourse and policy, 66% of Latinx immigrants in the United States reported worrying tremendously about deportation (Lopez et al., 2018). Like Latinx immigrants, 62% of Muslim immigrants stated that they believe it has become more difficult to be Muslim in America, 74% reported that media coverage of Muslims is unfair, only 38% reported that they are satisfied with how things are going in the United States, and 85% reported that President Trump is unfriendly to Muslims (Pew Research Center, 2018).

The rise in feelings of worsening marginalization and prejudice among immigrants of color is partially due to increased contact with law enforcement officials. Historically, racial profiling markers have been used by law enforcement to aid in their search for immigrants. Some of these markers include but are not limited to accents, styles of clothing, generation status, English-language fluency, socioeconomic status, and ability to follow U.S. social norms. Profiling individuals through the use of the aforementioned markers has been labeled "citizenship profiling"—and the consequences of citizenship profiling are drastic. It is so widespread that in El Paso, Texas, first- and second-generation citizens are 93% and 89% more likely than third-generation (or later) residents, respectively, to be questioned about their citizenship. Additionally, El Paso residents who reside in low socioeconomic areas report more citizenship profiling and increased levels of surveillance than those in high socioeconomic areas. Furthermore, citizenship profiling through the use of external markers has facilitated the incarceration and deportation of immigrant groups of color (Morales et al., 2018).

MYTHS ABOUT IMMIGRATION

Another possible reason for the political divisiveness is the lack of knowledge regarding immigration and immigrants. Immigrants are often treated as a monolithic whole, the proverbial "them" to the "us" of American citizens. U.S. society often acts on myths that are not supported by fact. There are, in fact, multiple distinct immigrant groups, and the myths are often distinct from the stereotypes. Latinxs, for example, are viewed as foreigners, criminals, and low-skilled laborers. However, little or no empirical data support these myths, and the opposite tends to be true (Harris et al., 2020). Many people associate immigrants as Mexican (or Latinxs in the United States in general), but Latinx immigrants represent only a third of the Latinxs in the United States (Flores et al., 2017). Another commonly held belief is that most immigrants coming into the United States are from Mexico. In 2017, Asian immigrants outnumbered Latinx immigrants among new arrivals in the

United States (Budiman, 2020). Specifically, roughly 37% of new immigrant arrivals were Asian, whereas approximately 27% of new arrivals were Hispanic. Mexican immigration into the United States has been plummeting for years, although it is true that in 2019 the country saw a new surge of Latinx immigrants, primarily family units (Bialik, 2019).

The political rhetoric and myth is that Latinx immigration produces more crime. Data show, however, that as Latinx immigrants move into an area, crime is reduced (Martinez et al., 2010). In particular, as unauthorized and authorized immigration increases in the United States, violent crime decreases (Adelman et al., 2017), suggesting that communities become safer as immigrants, including those immigrating from Latin countries, move into U.S. neighborhoods. These findings were more fully described by Harris and colleagues (2020), who discussed how the Latinx crime myth is largely due to the unfair coverage of Latinx crime in the media, the disproportionate incarceration rates of Latinxs driven by stereotypes and myths, and the historical complexities (e.g., the war on drugs) that have shaped modern policy and institutional bias against Latinxs.

Latinx immigrants facilitate economic stability and improvement in the United States (Harris et al., 2020). Immigrants make up one of the largest groups in the United States who contribute to the economy through their leadership and the creation of jobs. Reports show that 19% of all self-employed U.S. workers are immigrants (Pew Research Center, 2015). Some racial minority groups are even outpacing U.S.-born residents in terms of ownership of new businesses. Rates for new business startups among Latinxs, for example, now outpace startup rates across all other race categories (Orozco et al., 2018). There is no evidence that job prospects for native-born Americans are negatively affected by the workforce participation of immigrants. If anything, immigrants have a positive effect on American job prospects (Zavodny, 2018). For example, studies show that for every 100 immigrants who have advanced degrees and are working in science, technology, engineering, and mathematics, an additional 262 jobs were created for U.S.-born Americans (American Enterprise Institute for Public Policy Research & the Partnership for a New American Economy, 2011).

Although we focus on Latinx immigration, it is important to stress that seemingly all immigrant groups, particularly immigrants of color, are negatively stereotyped. The prevailing stereotype of Asian immigrants is that they are clannish (B. E. Armenta et al., 2013; Zou & Cheryan, 2017); Muslims are perceived as vicious and coarse (Shaheen, 2003), and Arab immigrants are viewed as vindictive and hostile (Reyna et al., 2013). As with the myths and stereotypes concerning Latinx immigrants, no empirical data support these generalizations (Bellovary et al., 2020).

Although unsubstantiated, immigrant myths and stereotypes are theorized to drive perceived threat concerning so-called tangible resources and outcomes (e.g., jobs, salaries, politics, national security). This type of threat is known as *realistic threat* (LeVine & Campbell, 1972; Sherif, 1966) or *perceived realistic threat* (Esses et al., 1998). Examples of realistic threat are commonly found within anti-immigrant discourse. Latinx immigrants are viewed as "stealing" jobs from U.S. natives (Hoban, 2017). Asian immigrants are perceived to be industrious and diligent; thus, they are viewed as "unfair" competition for high-skilled occupations (Lee, 1996). Arab and Muslim immigrants are viewed as aggressive and revengeful; as a result, they are viewed as threats to U.S. national security (Hetherington & Suhay, 2011; Norris, 2017). Although no empirical data support or justify these beliefs (Bellovary et al., 2020), many people continue to propagate these dogmas.

Attitudes toward immigrants are occasionally nuanced. Attitudes toward involuntary immigrants tend to be more positive than attitudes toward voluntary immigrants. Specifically, those who involuntarily migrate (i.e., had no other choice but to migrate) for various reasons, such as threat of political assassination in their country of origin or war, are viewed more positively and garner more sympathy than those who voluntarily choose to do so (i.e., made the choice to migrate but did not absolutely need to; Verkuyten et al., 2018). However, there are some caveats. Authorized immigrants (i.e., those who are residing within the United States legally) are less likely than unauthorized immigrants to provoke realistic threat and intergroup anxiety and are less likely to be used as scapegoats for financial instability (Murray & Marx, 2013), despite authorized immigration normally falling under voluntary migration.

CONSEQUENCES OF PREJUDICE

The literature has linked prejudice and discrimination to negative psychological and physical outcomes (Williams & Mohammed, 2009). The biopsychosocial model and the minority stress model posit that prejudice and discrimination function as excess stress to which individuals from stigmatized social categories are exposed as a result of their social and minority position (Clark et al., 1999). These models argue that minority stress is additive to general stressors that are experienced by all people. Therefore, it requires additional adaptation efforts, which require extra cognitive, psychological, and physical resources (Meyer et al., 2008). Theoretically, exposure to prejudice and discrimination produces both physiological and psychological stress that can lead to decreased mental health, physical health, and cognitive performance (Pascoe & Smart Richman, 2009).

Psychological Consequences

Research consistently supports the relationship between discrimination and negative outcomes (Williams & Mohammed, 2009). Perceptions of discrimination are associated with increased depression, anxiety, and negative mood (Schmitt et al., 2014). Results from multiple meta-analytic reviews support these patterns of association, suggesting that prejudice and discrimination may contribute to the growing number of mental health disparities noted among minority groups (Williams & Mohammed, 2009).

Self-control refers to the mental effort individuals use to regulate one's own behavior (Muraven & Baumeister, 2000) and is an emergent psychological factor that has been linked to controlling one's emotions and feelings, eating and drinking in moderation, and delaying gratification (Muraven et al., 1998). An increasing body of evidence suggests that prejudice triggers a sustained activation of stress responses that decrease an individual's cognitive resources (i.e., self-control; Inzlicht et al., 2006). When self-control resources are used to control thoughts, behaviors, or emotions, performance on subsequent tasks requiring self-control can be diminished. For example, Salvatore and Shelton (2007) found that ambiguous racism produced the highest level of cognitive depletion (i.e., maintaining cognitive resources to make good decisions) among Black participants. This study is consistent with additional evidence supporting the argument that stress induced by perceiving racial discrimination leads to decreased executive function, self-control, and working memory (Richeson & Shelton, 2003).

Physiological Consequences

Prejudice and discrimination have also been linked to decreased physical health and increased risk of many health problems, such as digestive problems, heart disease, sleep problems, weight gain, and memory and concentration impairment. When one experiences discrimination, a variety of involuntary stress responses are activated (Inzlicht & Kang, 2010). For example, research shows that being a target and victim of discrimination produces increased anxiety and heart rate (Alvarez, 2019). Specifically, high-stress interactions, such as interacting with an individual with prejudiced beliefs regarding minorities, activate fight-or-flight responses and are characterized by changes to stress levels that transform from physiological to mental processes. Such changes may seem inconsequential when isolated but can have irreparable effects that can lead to chronic disease and allostatic load. To support this point, research has tested the psychophysiological mechanism associated with prejudice and discrimination. In one experiment, Latinas who anticipated interacting with a biased partner showed greater blood pressure increases and sympathetic nervous system activation during speech anticipation and reported more threat than did those who were led to believe that their partner was not biased (Sawyer et al., 2012).

Protective Factors

The involuntary responses activated by negative experiences such as discrimination should invoke coping strategies, including resilience (Luthar & Cicchetti, 2000). Resilience is defined as the ability to achieve positive developmental outcomes in the context of adversity and stress (Masten, 2001).

Resilience derives from the psychological, social, and material resources that protect individuals against the negative experiences that confront them (Min, 1995). This protective process provides a variety of ways for individuals to adjust positively and to flourish even in the worst of conditions (McCreary et al., 2006).

Alvarez (2019) showed that individuals high on resilience exhibited minor upsurges in heart rate and anxiety responses to discrimination. This finding suggests that individuals might find meaning in their adversity and emerge from negative racial interactions with increased resilience and intact well-being. Alvarez also showed that those high in trait levels of resilience reacted less negatively to the racist interaction than did those low in trait levels of resilience. In fact, some participants were rather dismissive of the racist confederate. Future work will further investigate the factors that lead to resilient reactions to hostile racism.

THREAT IN THE FACE OF CHANGE

America's racial tapestry is changing. By 2055, Whites are expected to be less than 50% of the population (Cohn & Caumont, 2016). And while most Americans agree that all citizens deserve equality regardless of background (Citrin et al., 1994), the changing environment is introducing both improvements and challenges (Amadeo, 2019). Change, in and of itself, can produce stress and resentment toward those who are perceived to be enacting the change (Zárate et al., 2019). The changing demographics provoke questions of national identity, realistic threat, and a host of other issues.

Who Is American?

Typically, when U.S. residents think of "Americans," they are thinking of White individuals (Devos & Banaji, 2005). When racial minorities such as Blacks, Asians, and Latinxs are asked "who is American," they also generally state that Whites are the most American (Devos et al., 2010). Even immigrant groups tend to associate American with White, wealth, and privilege (Bloemraad, 2013). These findings support the narrative that European Americans believe that they represent the prototypical American and that other groups are less American than they are and therefore less deserving of the rights that all Americans deserve.

Perceived otherness is a good indicator of prejudice toward minorities of various backgrounds, including immigrant groups (Esses et al., 1993). Specifically, those who do not "look" American are assumed to be foreigners who possess different moral and value systems in comparison to the prototypical American (Devos & Banaji, 2005; Devos et al., 2010). And because oftentimes immigrants who are also racial or religious minorities actually do look different than the prototypical White American, they are perceived to be less American.

These beliefs have major implications for the ways in which majority groups interact with minority groups, particularly once groups perceive that group dynamics are changing.

Cultural Inertia

As more immigrants come into the United States (and along with them, their cultures), the more that cultural nuances and stereotypes become perceived threats to the existing culture in the United States. The theory of cultural inertia posits that individuals avoid cultural change to maintain their existing culture systems (Zárate et al., 2019). The model asserts that the change, in and of itself, leads to negative interactions between majority and minority groups. When cultural change is perceived to be occurring, opponents of the change retaliate.

The model borrows heavily from Newton's three laws of motion and asserts that changing environments produce three basic principles (Zárate et al., 2019). First, static cultures desire to stay static. Second, cultures in motion desire to stay in motion. And third, for every action, there is an equal and opposite reaction. This last tenet applies to both static and dynamic cultures, such that static cultures push back against cultural change whereas dynamic cultures push back against cultural stability. By virtue of their size and perceived prototypicality in the United States, White populations are generally described as static cultures, while minority groups are described as the enactors of cultural change. As a result, White populations from static cultures often favor assimilation policies (i.e., legislation perceived to enact the least amount of change), whereas minority populations favor multicultural policies (i.e., legislation that allows them to integrate into mainstream U.S. culture and simultaneously preserve their own culture). White populations are also not monolithic. White liberals, for instance, are significantly more likely to endorse multicultural policies and perspectives, whereas White conservatives/Republicans are more likely to oppose them. Young, educated Whites are also more likely to believe that their race has been advantageous (Pew Research Center, 2016). Finally, the cultural inertia model posits that psychological anchors (e.g., group identity) and propellers (e.g., need for novelty) are theorized to facilitate cultural stagnancy and cultural motion, respectively.

In experimental tests of the cultural inertia model, perceived cultural change drives prejudice. When participants are made to believe that U.S. culture is changing as a result of immigration, they show significantly higher negative attitudes toward immigrants than those who believe that U.S. culture will remain stable despite immigration (Quezada et al., 2012). These findings mirror the social malady occurring in the real world. Across the country, counties that have been historically White have begun to experience shifts to their culture and racial makeup; along with the changing tapestry, feelings of bitterness toward those perceived to be causing the inertia (i.e., immigrants and racial minorities) begin to arise.

Changing Tapestry—A Case Study

Our own research is experimental in nature and uses typical experimental psychology samples. Reactions to societal shifts are seen anecdotally in small cities all over the United States (Norris, 2018). Hazleton, Pennsylvania, in particular, has gone from 7% Hispanic in 2000 to 46% Hispanic in 2014 (Norris, 2018). While immigration and diversity often introduce economic improvement (New American Economy, 2017), many residents of Hazleton have expressed their concerns regarding this sweeping demographic change. Feelings of being outnumbered and discontent with the changing tapestry and economy are common themes expressed by the White residents of Hazleton. Norris described a majority White town that went from an industrial coal mining town to a nearly deserted town, with a large Latinx population who work in distribution centers or run small businesses in the town. Despite the economic benefits of their new businesses and trade, the Latinx population are seen as the drivers of change and therefore bad.

On a larger scale, the cultural inertia model predicts political gains and losses. Several studies now show that many Whites who voted for Mr. Obama in 2012 voted for Mr. Trump in 2016. An estimated 6.7 million to 9.2 million voters are estimated to have made the jump from Obama to Trump (Skelley, 2017). The reason? Whites' racial resentment drove the outcome of the 2016 presidential election—more so than perceived economic instability (Schaffner et al., 2018). When Whites were asked whether they believe that being poor, Muslim, Black, or Hispanic helps or hurts these groups in society, 59% reported that they believe it helps these minority groups a little or helps a lot (Horowitz et al., 2019). In the same study, 62% of Whites reported that they believe that the United States has been about right or has gone too far in terms of giving Blacks equal rights with Whites. In experimental studies (Luttig et al., 2017), researchers have manipulated marketing materials regarding social policies such as housing, sometimes disseminated by a White person and sometimes disseminated by a racial minority. When the policy information is disseminated by a person from a racial minority group, White Trump supporters are less likely to support it than they are when the same policy is presented by a White person.

It is possible that in the eyes of many White Obama-to-Trump voters, Obama and his administration were changing the country too quickly, in particular, changing America to favor racial minorities and threatening the existing societal structures that traditional White Americans have grown to appreciate. Thus, as the cultural inertia model predicts, the political pendulum swung too far to the left for some, and, as a result of the perceived extreme cultural change, Whites voted in 2016 in a way that swung the political pendulum back toward the right—in the direction Whites perceived to be in their favor.

Given that the Trump administration's policies have been further to the right than past presidential administrations, it is possible that the political pendulum may swing further to the left during the next election. The United

States may even be currently witnessing sparks of cultural retaliation across the nation toward the rise in far-right political candidates. For example, many of the politicians that Trump endorsed lost their midterm elections in places that have been red for decades (Kamarck, 2018). Even Texas almost turned blue in 2018 (Milligan, 2018).

HOT TOPICS IN RESEARCH AND FUTURE DIRECTIONS

The changing tapestry in the United States (as well as around the world) has facilitated increasing interest in the ways in which cultural change affects intergroup relations. In this section, we discuss how focusing on the past (i.e., national nostalgia) hinders intergroup relations, while focusing on the future (i.e., national prostalgia) may facilitate positive intergroup relations. Recommendations for reducing intergroup hostility via community-based interventions are also discussed.

The Past

For many U.S. residents, desperately longing for the "good old days" when it was "just us" (Duyvendak, 2011) has become commonplace. These feelings are akin to what has been called "national nostalgia," formally defined as a sentimental longing for one's nation as it used to be in the past (Smeekes et al., 2015). In the modern context, the slogan "Make America Great Again" coupled with the anti-immigrant rhetoric strategically capitalizes on national nostalgia. By targeting Americans' discomfort with the changing tapestry and facilitating their longing for the past, anti-immigrant proponents are being spoon-fed their cravings: the possibility of reverting to a nation in which it was just "them."

While other forms of nostalgia (e.g., personal nostalgia) lead to positive consequences concerning one's well-being (e.g., social connectedness; Wildschut et al., 2010), national nostalgia leads to negative consequences, especially for intergroup relations. For instance, Smeekes et al. (2015) conducted four studies in which they primed participants with national nostalgia and then measured their attitudes toward Muslim immigrant rights (e.g., freedom of speech). The results consistently indicated that participants who were primed to feel nationally nostalgic expressed more opposition toward Muslim immigrant rights than those who did not feel nationally nostalgic. National nostalgia has also been found to be negatively correlated with attitudes toward Latinx immigrants and positively correlated with in-group protection and out-group derogation (A. D. Armenta et al., 2018).

The Future

Recent research has focused on reactions to the past and national nostalgia. From a cultural inertia perspective, national nostalgia becomes a personal anchor, bonding people to a past and making them resistant to change. Cultural inertia also suggests that attention to the future should be a propeller for more change. One potential future research direction, then, may be to focus on the future. Research suggests that future-thinking is positively linked to optimism and motivation (Vasquez & Buehler, 2007). Future-thinking is also pragmatic (Baumeister et al., 2018), allowing individuals to make "better decisions" in the present (Daniel et al., 2013).

If longing for the good old days predicts prejudice, it may also be the case that attention to the future reduces prejudice. "National prostalgia," a variable that we formally define as longing for the way in which Americans and American society will be in the future, may be advantageous for intergroup relations (A. D. Armenta et al., 2018). Although national nostalgia leads to more prejudice toward immigrants (A. D. Armenta et al., 2018; Smeekes et al., 2015), our preliminary data suggest that national prostalgia may serve as a prejudice reduction tool. In one study, for example, national prostalgia positively predicted attitudes toward Latinx immigrants and negatively predicted in-group protection and out-group derogation (A. D. Armenta et al., 2018). Future studies could address, through an experimental paradigm, whether national prostalgia causally leads to prejudice reduction toward immigrants and whether certain groups of individuals (e.g., those with a particular political affiliation) are more likely to reap the benefits of national prostalgia. On a larger scale, national prostalgia may be the catalyst through which political campaigns (i.e., those that are not run on disdain toward groups of people) are won.

Prejudice reduction programs may also benefit from national prostalgia. Practitioners, for example, could integrate national prostalgia in community-based interventions to reduce racial tension in U.S. neighborhoods. At the least, practitioners could develop interventions that increase the likelihood of focusing on possible futures rather than focusing on impossible pasts. National prostalgia could be a part of the solution for the social malady currently occurring in the modern world.

CONCLUSION

Prejudice and discrimination toward immigrants of color have been common themes across history. Modern examples such as the "Muslim ban" at the federal level are clear examples of disdain and perceived threat toward immigrants of color. The injustices faced by immigrants lead to negative psychological (e.g., decreased mental health) and physiological outcomes (e.g., stress). In more extreme examples, being an immigrant in America has led to death (e.g., migrant children and adolescents dying in U.S. custody; Acevedo, 2019). Perceived threat and cultural change have exacerbated these prejudices and acts of discrimination. Nevertheless, in the midst of the psychological and physiological toll facing immigrants, many immigrants find ways to cope (i.e., resiliency). In spite of the myths and stereotypes concerning immigrants,

Americans thrive on immigration. Immigrants serve as one of the strongest economic backbones of the United States—they are one of the largest groups who start new businesses, they create new jobs, and they hire Americans. Ultimately, the benefits of immigration enable the United States to progress as one of the leading countries in the world.

REFERENCES

Acevedo, N. (2019, May 29). *Why are migrant children dying in U.S. custody?* NBC News. https://www.nbcnews.com/news/latino/why-are-migrant-children-dying-u-s-custody-n1010316

Adelman, R., Reid, L. W., Markle, G., Weiss, S., & Jaret, C. (2017). Urban crime rates and the changing face of immigration: Evidence across four decades. *Journal of Ethnicity in Criminal Justice, 15*(1), 52–77. https://doi.org/10.1080/15377938.2016.1261057

Alvarez, M. (2019). *Under the skin: Psychophysiological consequences of racial discrimination* [Unpublished doctoral dissertation]. University of Texas at El Paso.

Amadeo, K. (2019, May 16). *Immigration's effect on the economy and you.* The Balance. https://www.thebalance.com/how-immigration-impacts-the-economy-4125413

American Bar Association. (2018). *The Trump immigration agenda.* https://www.americanbar.org/content/dam/aba/administrative/immigration/trump_immigration_agenda_timeline.pdf

American Enterprise Institute for Public Policy Research, & the Partnership for a New American Economy. (2011, December). *Immigration and American jobs.* https://www.newamericaneconomy.org/sites/all/themes/pnae/img/NAE_Im-AmerJobs.pdf

Armenta, A. D., Evans, N., & Zárate, M. A. (2018). [Unpublished raw data on national prostalgia and prejudice]. University of Texas, El Paso.

Armenta, B. E., Lee, R. M., Pituc, S. T., Jung, K. R., Park, I. J. K., Soto, J. A., Kim, S. Y., & Schwartz, S. J. (2013). Where are you from? A validation of the Foreigner Objectification Scale and the psychological correlates of foreigner objectification among Asian Americans and Latinos. *Cultural Diversity & Ethnic Minority Psychology, 19*(2), 131–142. https://doi.org/10.1037/a0031547

Baumeister, R. F., Maranges, H. M., & Sjastad, H. (2018). Consciousness of the future as a matric of maybe: Pragmatic prospection and the simulation of alternative possibilities. *American Psychological Association, 5*, 223–238.

Bellovary, A., Armenta, A., & Reyna, C. (2020). Stereotypes of immigrants and immigration in the United States. To appear in J. T. Nadler & E. Voyles (Eds.), *Stereotypes: The thinking person's guide to today's reality in the U.S.* (pp. 146–164). Praeger Publishing.

Bialik, K. (2019, January 16). *Border apprehensions increased in 2018—especially for migrant families.* Pew Research Center. https://www.pewresearch.org/facttank/2019/01/16/border-apprehensions-of-migrant-families-have-risen-substantially-sofar-in-2018/

Bloemraad, I. (2013). Being American/Becoming American: Birthright citizenship and immigrants' membership in the United States. *Law, Politics, & Society, 60*, 55–84.

Budiman, A. (2020). *Key findings about U.S. immigrants.* Pew Research Center. http://www.pewresearch.org/fact-tank/2018/09/14/key-findings-about-u-s-immigrants/

Campbell, B., Mendoza, A. Diestel, T., & News21 Staff. (2018, August 22). *Rising hate drives Latinos and immigrants into silence.* The Center for Public Integrity. https://publicintegrity.org/federal-politics/rising-hate-drives-latinos-and-immigrants-into-silence/

Citrin, J., Haas, E. B., Muste, C., & Reingold, B. (1994). Is American nationalism changing? Implications for foreign policy. *International Studies Quarterly, 38*(1), 1–31. https://doi.org/10.2307/2600870

Clark, R., Anderson, N. B., Clark, V. R., & Williams, D. R. (1999). Racism as a stressor for African Americans: A biopsychosocial model. *American Psychologist, 54*(10), 805–816. https://doi.org/10.1037/0003-066X.54.10.805

Cohn, D., & Caumont, A. (2016, March 31). *10 demographic trends that are shaping the U.S. and the world.* Pew Research Center. http://www.pewresearch.org/fact-tank/2016/03/31/10-demographic-trends-that-are-shaping-the-u-s-and-the-world/

Daniel, T. O., Stanton, C. M., & Epstein, L. H. (2013). The future is now: Reducing impulsivity and energy intake using episodic future thinking. *Psychological Science, 24*(11), 2339–2342. https://doi.org/10.1177/0956797613488780

Devos, T., & Banaji, M. R. (2005). American = White? *Journal of Personality and Social Psychology, 88*(3), 447–466. https://doi.org/10.1037/0022-3514.88.3.447

Devos, T., Gavin, K., & Quintana, F. J. (2010). Say "adios" to the American dream? The interplay between ethnic and national identity among Latino and Caucasian Americans. *Cultural Diversity & Ethnic Minority Psychology, 16*(1), 37–49. https://doi.org/10.1037/a0015868

Duyvendak, J. W. (2011). *The politics of home: Nostalgia and belonging in Western Europe and the United States.* Palgrave Macmillan.

Esses, V. M., Haddock, G., & Zanna, M. P. (1993). Values, stereotypes, and emotions as determinants of intergroup attitudes. In D. M. Mackie & D. L. Hamilton (Eds.), *Affect, cognition, and stereotyping: Interactive processes in group perception* (pp. 137–166). Academic Press.

Esses, V. M., Jackson, L. M., & Armstrong, T. L. (1998). Intergroup competition and attitudes toward immigrants and immigration: An instrumental model of group conflict. *Journal of Social Issues, 54*(4), 699–724. https://doi.org/10.1111/j.1540-4560.1998.tb01244.x

Flores, A., Lopez, G., & Radford, J. (2017, September 18). *Facts on U.S. Latinos, 2015.* Pew Research Center. https://www.pewhispanic.org/2017/09/18/facts-on-u-s-latinos-trend-data/

Harris, K., Armenta, A. D., Reyna, C., & Zárate, M. A. (2020). Latinx stereotypes: Myths and realities in the twenty-first century. In J. T. Nadler & E. C. Voyles (Eds.), *Stereotypes: The incidence and impacts of bias* (pp. 128–145). Praeger Publishing.

Hetherington, M. J., & Suhay, E. (2011). Authoritarianism, threat, and Americans' support for the war on terror. *American Journal of Political Science, 55*(3), 546–560. https://doi.org/10.1111/j.1540-5907.2011.00514.x

Hoban, B. (2017, August 24). *Do immigrants "steal" jobs from American workers?* Brookings. https://www.brookings.edu/blog/brookings-now/2017/08/24/do-immigrants-steal-jobs-from-american-workers/

Horowitz, J. M., Brown, A., & Cox, K. (2019, April 9). *Race in America 2019.* Pew Research Center. https://www.pewsocialtrends.org/wp-content/uploads/sites/3/2019/04/PewResearchCenter_RaceStudy_FINAL-1.pdf

Inzlicht, M., & Kang, S. K. (2010). Stereotype threat spillover: How coping with threats to social identity affects aggression, eating, decision making, and attention. *Journal of Personality and Social Psychology, 99*(3), 467–481. https://doi.org/10.1037/a0018951

Inzlicht, M., McKay, L., & Aronson, J. (2006). Stigma as ego depletion: How being the target of prejudice affects self-control. *Psychological Science, 17*(3), 262–269. https://doi.org/10.1111/j.1467-9280.2006.01695.x

Kamarck, E. (2018, November 7). *Trump endorsed 75 candidates in the midterms. How did they fare on Election Day?* Brookings. https://www.brookings.edu/blog/fixgov/2018/11/07/trump-endorsed-75-candidates-in-the-midterms-how-did-they-fare-on-election-day/

Kopan, T. (2016, August 31). *What Donald Trump has said about Mexico and vice versa.* CNN Politics. https://www.cnn.com/2016/08/31/politics/donald-trump-mexico-statements/index.html

Lee, S. J. (1996). *Unraveling the "model minority" stereotype: Listening to Asian American youth.* Teachers College Press.

LeVine, R. A., & Campbell, D. T. (1972). *Ethnocentrism: Theories of conflict, ethnic attitudes, and group behavior.* John Wiley & Sons.

Lind, D., & Zarracina, J. (2019, February 5). *By the numbers: How 2 years of Trump's policies have affected immigrants.* Vox. https://www.vox.com/policy-and-politics/2019/1/19/18123891/state-of-the-union-2019-immigration-facts

Lopez, M. H., Gonzalez-Barrera, A., & Krogstad, J. M. (2018, October 25). *More Latinos have serious concerns about their place in America under Trump.* Pew Research Center. https://www.pewhispanic.org/2018/10/25/more-latinos-have-serious-concerns-about-their-place-in-america-under-trump/

Luthar, S. S., & Cicchetti, D. (2000). The construct of resilience: Implications for interventions and social policies. *Development and Psychopathology, 12*(4), 857–885. https://doi.org/10.1017/S0954579400004156

Luttig, M. D., Federico, C. M., & Lavine, H. (2017). Supporters and opponents of Donald Trump respond differently to racial cues: An experimental analysis. *Research & Politics, 4*(4), 1–8. https://doi.org/10.1177/2053168017737411

Martinez, R., Jr., Stowell, J. I., & Lee, M. L. (2010). Immigration and crime in an era of transformation: A longitudinal analysis of homicides in San Diego neighborhoods, 1980–2000. *Criminology, 48*(3), 797–829. https://doi.org/10.1111/j.1745-9125.2010.00202.x

Masten, A. S. (2001). Ordinary magic. Resilience processes in development. *American Psychologist, 56*(3), 227–238. https://doi.org/10.1037/0003-066X.56.3.227

McCreary, M. L., Cunningham, J. N., Ingram, K. M., & Fife, J. E. (2006). Stress, culture, and racial socialization: Making an impact. In P. T. P. Wong & L. C. J. Wong (Eds.), *Handbook of multicultural perspectives on stress and coping* (pp. 487–513). Springer. https://doi.org/10.1007/0-387-26238-5_21

McEldowney, M. (2018, August 12). What Charlottesville changed: We asked 16 of the most thoughtful people we know to describe the impact of the violence—and how we should think about it a year later. *Politico Magazine.* https://www.politico.com/magazine/story/2018/08/12/charlottesville-anniversary-supremacists-protests-dc-virginia-219353

Meyer, I. H., Schwartz, S., & Frost, D. M. (2008). Social patterning of stress and coping: Does disadvantaged social statuses confer more stress and fewer coping resources? *Social Science & Medicine, 67*(3), 368–379. https://doi.org/10.1016/j.socscimed.2008.03.012

Milligan, S. (2018, November 7). Democrats make gains in formerly ruby red Texas. *U.S. News.* https://www.usnews.com/news/politics/articles/2018-11-07/democrats-make-gains-in-formerly-ruby-red-texas

Min, P. G. (1995). Korean Americans. In P. G. Min (Ed.), *Asian Americans: Contemporary trends and issues* (pp. 199–231). Sage.

Morales, M. C., Delgado, D., & Curry, T. (2018). Variations in citizenship profiling by generational status: Individual and neighborhood characteristics of Latina/os questioned by law enforcement about their legal status. *Race and Social Problems, 10*(4), 293–305. https://doi.org/10.1007/s12552-018-9235-3

Muraven, M., & Baumeister, R. F. (2000). Self-regulation and depletion of limited resources: Does self-control resemble a muscle? *Psychological Bulletin, 126*(2), 247–259. https://doi.org/10.1037/0033-2909.126.2.247

Muraven, M., Tice, D. M., & Baumeister, R. F. (1998). Self-control as limited resource: Regulatory depletion patterns. *Journal of Personality and Social Psychology, 74*(3), 774–789. https://doi.org/10.1037/0022-3514.74.3.774

Murray, K. E., & Marx, D. M. (2013). Attitudes toward unauthorized immigrants, authorized immigrants, and refugees. *Cultural Diversity & Ethnic Minority Psychology, 19*(3), 332–341. https://doi.org/10.1037/a0030812

New American Economy. (2017, December). *How Hispanics contribute to the U.S. economy.* http://research.newamericaneconomy.org/wp-content/uploads/sites/2/2017/12/Hispanic_V5.pdf

Norris, G. (2017). Authoritarianism and privacy: The moderating role of terrorist threat. *Surveillance & Society, 15*(3/4), 573–581. https://doi.org/10.24908/ss.v15i3/4.6607

Norris, M. (2018). As America changes, some anxious Whites feel left behind. *National Geographic.* https://www.nationalgeographic.com/magazine/2018/04/race-rising-anxiety-white-america/

Orozco, M., Oyer, P., & Porras, J. I. (2018, February). *2017 State of Latino entrepreneurship.* Stanford Graduate School of Business in collaboration with the Latino Business Action Network. https://www.gsb.stanford.edu/faculty-research/publications/state-latino-entrepreneurship-2017

Pascoe, E. A., & Smart Richman, L. (2009). Perceived discrimination and health: A meta-analytic review. *Psychological Bulletin, 135*(4), 531–554. https://doi.org/10.1037/a0016059

Pew Research Center. (2015, October 22). *Immigrants' contributions to job creation.* https://www.pewsocialtrends.org/2015/10/22/immigrants-contributions-to-job-creation/

Pew Research Center. (2016, June 27). *On views of race and inequality, Blacks and Whites are worlds apart.* https://www.pewsocialtrends.org/2016/06/27/on-views-of-race-and-inequality-blacks-and-whites-are-worlds-apart/

Pew Research Center. (2018, April 17). *Muslims in America: Immigrants and those born in U.S. see life differently in many ways.* https://www.pewforum.org/essay/muslims-in-america-immigrants-and-those-born-in-u-s-see-life-differently-in-many-ways/

Quezada, S. A., Shaw, M. P., & Zárate, M. A. (2012). Cultural inertia: The relationship between ethnic identity and reactions to cultural change. *Social Psychology, 43*(4), 243–251. https://doi.org/10.1027/1864-9335/a000125

Radford, J. (2019, June 17). *Key findings about U.S. immigrants.* Pew Research Center. https://www.pewresearch.org/fact-tank/2019/06/17/key-findings-about-u-s-immigrants/

Reyna, C., Dobria, O., & Wetherell, G. (2013). The complexity and ambivalence of immigration attitudes: Ambivalent stereotypes predict conflicting attitudes toward immigration policies. *Cultural Diversity & Ethnic Minority Psychology, 19*(3), 342–356. https://doi.org/10.1037/a0032942

Richeson, J. A., & Shelton, J. N. (2003). When prejudice does not pay: Effects of interracial contact on executive function. *Psychological Science, 14*(3), 287–290. https://doi.org/10.1111/1467-9280.03437

Salvatore, J., & Shelton, J. N. (2007). Cognitive costs of exposure to racial prejudice. *Psychological Science, 18*(9), 810–815. https://doi.org/10.1111/j.1467-9280.2007.01984.x

Sawyer, P. J., Major, B., Casad, B. J., Townsend, S. S., & Mendes, W. B. (2012). Discrimination and the stress response: Psychological and physiological consequences of anticipating prejudice in interethnic interactions. *American Journal of Public Health, 102*(5), 1020–1026. https://doi.org/10.2105/AJPH.2011.300620

Schaffner, B. F., Macwilliams, M., & Nteta, T. (2018). Understanding White polarization in the 2016 vote for president: The sobering role of racism and sexism. *Political Science Quarterly, 133*(1), 9–34. https://doi.org/10.1002/polq.12737

Schmitt, M. T., Branscombe, N. R., Postmes, T., & Garcia, A. (2014). The consequences of perceived discrimination for psychological well-being: A meta-analytic review. *Psychological Bulletin, 140*(4), 921–948. https://doi.org/10.1037/a0035754

Shaheen, J. G. (2003). Reel bad Arabs: How Hollywood vilifies a people. *The Annals of the American Academy of Political and Social Science, 588*(1), 171–193. https://doi.org/10.1177/0002716203588001011

Sherif, M. (1966). *Group conflict and cooperation.* Routledge & Kegan Paul.

Skelley, G. (2017, June 1). *Just how many Obama 2012–Trump 2016 voters were there?* Center for Politics. http://www.centerforpolitics.org/crystalball/articles/just-how-many-obama-2012-trump-2016-voters-were-there/

Smeekes, A., Verkuyten, M., & Martinovic, B. (2015). Longing for the country's good old days: National nostalgia, autochthony beliefs, and opposition to Muslim expressive rights. *British Journal of Social Psychology, 54*(3), 561–580. https://doi.org/10.1111/bjso.12097

Vasquez, N. A., & Buehler, R. (2007). Seeing future success: Does imagery perspective influence achievement motivation? *Personality and Social Psychology Bulletin, 33*(10), 1392–1405. https://doi.org/10.1177/0146167207304541

Verkuyten, M., Mepham, K., & Kros, M. (2018). Public attitudes toward support for migrants: The importance of perceived voluntary and involuntary migration. *Ethnic and Racial Studies, 41*(5), 901–918. https://doi.org/10.1080/01419870.2017.1367021

Wildschut, T., Sedikides, C., Routledge, C., Arndt, J., & Cordaro, F. (2010). Nostalgia as a repository of social connectedness: The role of attachment-related avoidance. *Journal of Personality and Social Psychology, 98*(4), 573–586. https://doi.org/10.1037/a0017597

Williams, D. R., & Mohammed, S. A. (2009). Discrimination and racial disparities in health: Evidence and needed research. *Journal of Behavioral Medicine, 32*(1), 20–47. https://doi.org/10.1007/s10865-008-9185-0

Zárate, M., Reyna, C., & Alvarez, M. (2019). Cultural inertia, identity, and intergroup dynamics in a changing context. *Advances in Experimental Social Psychology, 59*, 175–233. https://doi.org/10.1016/bs.aesp.2018.11.001

Zavodny, M. (2018, May). *Immigration, unemployment and labor force participation in the United States.* National Foundation for American Policy. https://nfap.com/wp-content/uploads/2018/05/IMMIGRANTS-AND-JOBS.NFAP-Policy-Brief.May-2018-1.pdf

Zou, L. X., & Cheryan, S. (2017). Two axes of subordination: A new model of racial position. *Journal of Personality and Social Psychology, 112*(5), 696–717. https://doi.org/10.1037/pspa0000080

2

Multifaceted Profiling and Violence

Experiences of Mexican and Central American Migrants to the United States

Hannah W. McDermott and Ricardo C. Ainslie

The violence that Mexican and Central American migrants to the United States experience is a defining feature of contemporary American immigration.[1] In this chapter, we examine four sources of violence faced by migrants: (a) the violence in their communities of origin, (b) the violence experienced during the migration journey, (c) the violence that forms the context of reception in the United States, and (d) the violence inherent in the American immigration system itself. Together, these elements create a complex web of violence that shapes the experience of many Mexican and Central American migrants to this country.

Exploring this web of violence, we draw from three theoretical frameworks: multicultural theory in counseling, trauma theory, and the theory of the social imaginary. Multicultural theory in counseling holds that psychology and mental health have been developed around White, Eurocentric experiences and perspectives, seeing these as healthy and "normal," and therefore the experiences of marginalized peoples are defined as abnormal as they deviate from this narrow standard (Sue & Sue, 2015). Intervening appropriately with

---

[1]In this chapter, we use the term "migrant" to reflect the reality that many people arriving at the U.S.–Mexico border fit neither into the category of immigrant (i.e., implying economic need) nor into the category of refugee (i.e., referring to a status that confers protections based on harms experienced in the country of origin). Refugee status reflects state acknowledgment of experiences of harm or persecution, rather than the reality of these experiences themselves. However, we use the term "immigration" in referring to U.S. policies and laws.

https://doi.org/10.1037/0000214-003
Trauma and Racial Minority Immigrants: Turmoil, Uncertainty, and Resistance,
P. Tummala-Narra (Editor)

nondominant culture populations, then, requires taking highly contextualized perspectives, including acknowledgment of the ways in which discrimination and marginalization affect health, histories of oppression, and collectivistic approaches (Arredondo et al., 2015). The concept of the social imaginary will help to frame our understanding of how larger social and cultural messaging impact and are incorporated into the psyches of migrants, producing an internalized dialogue between the individual's feelings and experiences and society's expectations (Ainslie & Ainslie, 2013; Castoriadis, 1987). Finally, we also use the lens of trauma theory, as outlined by Herman (1997), to understand the ways in which migrants are impacted by exposure to and experiences of violence and to understand society's difficulty holding these in consciousness. In highlighting these dimensions of the migration experience, we hope to sensitize providers and researchers working with this population to the complex intersection of past and present experiences of violence faced by migrants.

CLINICAL VIGNETTE: PAST AND PRESENT VIOLENCE

To introduce the multiple, complex dimensions of the violence experienced by contemporary migrants from Mexico and Central America and how these issues present in the context of therapy, we begin with a case example.[2]

Marta was a woman in her mid-30s who had migrated from Mexico to the United States a decade before. She was seen in therapy by the first author for symptoms of posttraumatic stress following an armed home invasion. Happily married and the mother of three daughters, at intake, she identified the home invasion as the only traumatic event she had experienced. However, after several sessions Marta reported having witnessed a gang-related double homicide while she was getting a haircut in her community of origin shortly before her immigration to the United States. Marta described a profound shift in her sense reality: She saw the shooting through the hair salon window; she and the other people in the salon dove to the floor; time froze, and they waited; they realized the danger had passed, and the two men lay dead in the street. She described a long wait for police, uncertainty about what to do, and an anticlimactic resolution when police arrived, covered the bodies, and did not speak to anyone in the hair salon as witnesses. Marta then went home, resuming her daily life as though nothing had happened.

However, something had happened to her sense of safety in the world; the shooting ended a long debate about migration between Marta, who wanted to stay, and her husband, who wanted to go. It was the tipping point. Within a year of witnessing this shooting, Marta agreed to move their small family to the United States. First, her husband crossed the river and found a

---

[2]All case material has been altered to protect confidentiality.

well-paying job in construction. Shortly thereafter, Marta and their then-only daughter joined him, overstaying a tourist visa.

Marta's previous experience of violence and her precarious legal position in the United States provided important context for her subsequent presentation in therapy. Her hypervigilance following the home invasion was fundamentally connected to this earlier traumatic event—this was not her first experience of the abrupt shift from a safe environment to a dangerous one. Marta also reported disturbed sleep due to both nightmares and frequent gunshots in her neighborhood; her economic marginalization rendered her at risk of violence because she could not afford to move her family to a safer community.

Furthermore, she lived with a profound distrust in the system's ability to protect her, despite a relatively positive interaction with police and the successful apprehension of the suspect following the home invasion. Her distrust was rooted in the lived experience of justice systems failing to prevent violence and produce justice. Her engagement with police was further complicated by her undocumented status. As a result of the crime committed against her, she became eligible for a U-Visa, a type of visa set aside for victims of a crime on U.S. soil. Yet this development also made her, and her status, visible to authorities and therefore put her at risk of deportation and separation from her U.S.-citizen children. In the Trump era, with heightened Immigration and Customs Enforcement presence and immigration raids in her neighborhood, Marta had reason to fear: U-Visa court proceedings were no guarantee of safety.

FOUR SOURCES OF VIOLENCE SHAPING IMMIGRANT EXPERIENCE

Migrants from Mexico and Central America have often experienced multiple forms of violence from multiple sources. As in Marta's case, these experiences intersect, compounding each other, and affect psychological presentation. We review four important sources of violence impacting these clients: violence in the community of origin, along the journey, in the context-of-reception, and inherent to the U.S. immigration system.

Violence in Community of Origin

Many migrants from Mexico and the Northern Triangle emigrate from communities experiencing unprecedented levels of violence. Four of the five most dangerous cities in the world, based on a 2019 report ranking cities by number of violent deaths per 100,000 inhabitants, are in Mexico—15 Mexican cities made the list altogether. Latin America has an additional 27 cities on the list, including four each in Honduras, El Salvador, and Guatemala. (Consejo Ciudadano Para la Seguridad Pública y la Justicia Penal, 2019). Honduras and El Salvador were identified as among the five most violent countries in the world in 2016, with some of the highest rates of armed violence. Homicide rates have decreased from highs seen in 2016 but remain extremely high (The World Bank, n.d.).

However, the number of murders is only one way of indexing the experience of violence in a community. The second author spent 2 years researching the impact of Mexico's drug war on Ciudad Juárez, at the time the most violent city in both Mexico and Latin America (in 2010 alone there were over 3,000 murders). In Ciudad Juárez, the murder rate was accompanied by high levels of other violent crime. Kidnappings, assaults, rapes, extortions, and disappearances were epidemic. Local gangs were in control of most neighborhoods, extorting, assaulting, and murdering residents with impunity. As a source of protection or a resource for justice, state authority (e.g., municipal, state, and federal law enforcement agencies) had no meaningful presence in these communities (Ainslie, 2013).

Residents were victimized by gangs to the extent that even using public transportation to get to work was dangerous. Contact with state authorities similarly carried the risk of extortion and violence and, occasionally, of being "disappeared." Most Ciudad Juárez residents, especially in poor neighborhoods, had nowhere to turn for protection. The murder rate was the tip of the iceberg in terms of the violence that these residents faced on a daily basis. This kind of chronic, multifaceted violence becomes traumatizing to many who endure it—affecting them, their families, their friends, and their neighbors (Ainslie, 2013).

Likewise, the countries of the Northern Triangle face critical security concerns beyond the murder rate. Extortion is rampant; estimates suggest Salvadorans pay $390 million, Hondurans pay $200 million, and Guatemalans pay $61 million per year in extortion to gangs, enormous sums considering the limited means of these communities (Isacson et al., 2017). Residents report forced gang conscription, in which adolescents and even children are pressured, under threat of violence, to join gangs. Young women and girls are threatened with violence to become gang members' "girlfriends" (Valdez et al., 2015). As in Mexico, enmeshment between police and gangs produces fear that reporting crimes will increase the likelihood of further victimization. Estimates vary but suggest widespread corruption of government officials, including police (Kennedy, 2013). As a result, law enforcement is ineffective at providing protection or achieving justice following victimization, with some estimates stating that 95% of crimes go unpunished and only 3% of murders are solved (Eguizábal et al., 2015). Reporting crimes is seen as ineffective at best and, at worst, potentially dangerous; few people report experiences of victimization (Parish, 2017).

Herman (1997) conveyed that traumatic events are "overwhelming systems of care that give people a sense of control, connection, and meaning" (p. 33); the violence and failure of justice systems endemic to communities in Mexico and Central America that drive migrants to leave their countries of origin do precisely that. Accordingly, people fleeing violence experience significant mental health problems, including trauma-related disorders, depression, anxiety, substance abuse, and comorbidities between these diagnoses (Goodman et al., 2017; Kaltman et al., 2010; Torres & Wallace, 2013).

Violence on the Immigration Journey

Migrants fleeing these communities undertake a long, difficult, and often violent journey. Increased enforcement of the U.S.–Mexico border, as well as pressure from the United States on Mexico to curb migration, has created increasingly dangerous conditions for migrants. Migrants from Central America must rely on *coyotes* to cross Mexico, and crossing the U.S.–Mexico border has become increasingly deadly as migrants must take remote routes to avoid detection (De León, 2015; Massey & Riosmena, 2010; Valdez et al., 2015). The challenges facing Mexican migrants and Central American migrants are different, however, because Central American migrants must cross Mexico clandestinely while Mexican migrants do not.

In the following two sections, participant quotes from the first author's research on Central American women's migration journeys (McDermott, 2019) illustrate the challenges of the clandestine migration journey through Mexico and the difficulty of crossing the U.S. border. This research examined the psychological impact of the migration journeys of women from Honduras, El Salvador, and Guatemala to help providers meet these individuals' needs. Using a hermeneutic phenomenological method and snowball sampling, the first author conducted semistructured interviews with 19 women from Honduras, El Salvador, and Guatemala who had migrated to the United States since 2000.

Crossing Mexico

The migration journey from the countries of the Northern Triangle to the United States is long and difficult. Migrants often seek the services of a *coyote*, a guide who arranges travel and lodging for a fee and who helps migrants avoid detection by authorities (Brigden, 2016). Travel occurs via multiple modes of transit, including bus, walking, car, taxi, semi-trailer, and riding on top of the trains (Kaltman et al., 2010). Evidence suggests that people with the fewest resources walk and ride the trains, the modes of transit with highest likelihood of victimization, while people who are better off take buses or private cars (Dominguez Villegas, 2014; Valdez et al., 2015).

Victimization is rampant, in no small part due to migrants' marginalization and need to stay hidden. Robbery, kidnapping, and assault are reportedly widespread (Vogt, 2013). Female migrants face significant risk of sexual assault, and sexual violence is understood to be an inherent danger of the migration journey (Parish, 2017; Simmons et al., 2015). One woman described her experience of being at risk while crossing Mexico:

> I was afraid because I saw that they raped women, and kidnapped people, and this and that. I felt, well, it was the first time I had left [Honduras] and I feared Mexico because you're migrating there. . . . And how the people looked at me . . . and they'd send a woman to whatever man liked her and he'd rape her. I was afraid in Mexico. I'm afraid of it. (McDermott, 2019)

She described an atmosphere of almost casual violence, in which she felt visible and endangered as a migrant and as a woman. Sexual violence, specifically, looms as a threat in which women's bodies are subject to men's whims.

Crossing the U.S.–Mexico Border

Increased U.S. border enforcement has relied on a policy known as "prevention through deterrence," which funnels migrants through increasingly remote and difficult-to-traverse desert terrain (D. Martínez et al., 2013; Slack et al., 2016). As a result of this policy, crossing the desert has become increasingly dangerous and deadly. Migrants picked up by border patrol often have serious physical ailments due to extreme temperatures, inadequate protective gear (e.g., clothes, shoes), and insufficient food and water (De León, 2012, 2015). For others, the desert is deadly. Numbers are imprecise, but in 2012 the bodies of 463 people were found in the desert (Slack et al., 2016). Extreme desert conditions cause extremely rapid decomposition, and it is likely that many are never found, leaving families without closure (De León, 2015).

Alejandra, whose asylum experience we discuss in detail later, described a multiplicity of threats inherent in crossing the U.S.–Mexico border with her 12-year-old son, Mateo:

> When I got there to cross the river I did have to pay a person to take me across. Well, you say "to take me across," but he didn't take me across. He just took my money and left me there [by the side of the river], and he said, "don't look back." And he didn't say anything else. I didn't know where to go. He left me in the middle of the river and let me tell you: I don't know how I crossed that river . . . It was like 11:00 at night and the man took me to the river . . . first he told me to go across and everything and he told me that he would carry my son, but I told him no, I will carry my son. And from there, he said, "take off your clothes," and I said to him, "No, I'm going to get in like this" and he said, "you can't get in with clothes on." "No," I said to him, "I'm going in like this." (McDermott, 2019)

Alejandra described having her money stolen and losing a guide to help them cross the desert, her fear that the coyote might take her son, and the looming threat of sexual violence. She described walking through the desert after crossing the river:

> We walked across all the whole *monte* . . . with the sounds of the animals . . . the night in the wilderness . . . the night . . . it's horrible, horrible. At that point I was afraid . . . any person could appear, and we wouldn't know if they were good or bad . . . In that moment, I didn't know where I was [whether in Mexico or in the United States]. (McDermott, 2019)

Crossing the U.S.–Mexico border, the unknown desert wilderness is terrifying and disorienting, with the looming threat that *bajadores* (i.e., bandits) could victimize them at any time. Border crossing involves facing multitude of threats yet going forward into the unknown regardless. Alejandra noted that her son won't talk about the experience; he denies remembering any of it.

Violence in the Context of Reception

Migrants to the United States from Mexico and Latin America arrive to a society that has a long history of anti-Latinx violence. This violence has been physical, rhetorical, and political, utilizing a discourse of fear to exert social control over Latinx people. The theory of the social imaginary is helpful for understanding how this history forms the context migrants enter on arriving in the United States. Castoriadis (1987) viewed the social imaginary as a system of meanings that defines the social structure that is created out of the interplay of individuals and society. These meanings become referenced and perceived as societal norms and prevailing attitudes, and they are internalized to become part of an internal dialogue that each individual has as they move through the social contexts in which they live. This internal dialogue shapes experience in a way not unlike the Freudian superego; however, it is social rather than familial in its derivation (Ainslie & Ainslie, 2013). In the present context we argue that part of the immigrant's social imaginary is shaped by the internalization of a view of a surrounding social word that is infused with anti-immigrant rhetoric that is intensely hostile to Latinx peoples and to migrants more generally.

History of Anti-Latinx Violence

Anti-Latinx violence in the United States stretches back to the 19th century and the turbulent conflicts around Texas independence, the Mexican–American War, and the Plan de San Diego uprising. The state-driven character of these conflicts often masks the racialized nature of the violence against people of Mexican ancestry during this period. Between 1910 and 1920, at the height of the Jim Crow era, many Latinx communities in Texas and elsewhere in the Southwest were subjected to state-sponsored and vigilante-driven violence (Montejano, 1987).

The January 28, 1918, massacre in the village of El Porvenir in West Texas is emblematic; Texas Rangers, supplemented by the U.S. Cavalry and Anglo ranchers, arrived at El Porvenir around 3:00 a.m. Going house-to-house, they turned men out of their homes and marched them a short distance before all 13 adults and two adolescents were summarily executed (Montejano, 1987). The pretext was a recent raid on a nearby Anglo ranch. However, a search of the El Porvenir homes found none of the stolen objects. In fact, no evidence was ever presented to support the accusations that anyone in the village had participated in the raid of the Anglo ranch. The victims of the El Porvenir massacre were racialized stand-ins against whom the Anglo settlers took revenge. Five of the Texas Rangers who participated in the massacre were eventually suspended, and their unit was disbanded. With this event having been swept under the rug (M. M. Martínez, 2018), only recently have journalists and historians begun to bring details to light.

While the El Porvenir massacre stands out for its brutality and vigilante character, the years between 1910 and 1920 were marked by widespread violence against Mexicans in the Southwest. This violence included lynchings as well as the imposition of Jim Crow–style laws in many communities, forbidding Latinx people from eating in restaurants or speaking in Spanish, forcing them into segregated residential areas, and requiring their children to attend segregated schools. During this same era, people were driven from their homes, lands were confiscated, and people were sometimes driven across the border into Mexico (Montejano, 1987). Thousands were murdered by mobs between 1848 and 1928, although surviving records document only 547 cases. These lynchings occurred primarily in the Southwest but were not limited to it, with documented instances as far north as Wyoming and Nebraska (Carrigan & Webb, 2013). Lynching of Mexicans often included direct participation by state and local authorities, as in the El Porvenir massacre (Carrigan & Webb, 2013).[3] Anyone who "looked Mexican" could readily be accused of being a "bandit" and become a target of violence (Carrigan & Webb, 2013). This kind of violence was especially prominent in states along the U.S.–Mexico border from California to Texas. In California alone, between 1848 and 1928, lynchings of Mexicans far outnumbered lynchings of Chinese immigrants, Native Americans, or African Americans (Pérez, 2019). Contemporary racial profiling and racist discourse eerily reflect this rhetoric (e.g., President Trump's invocation of the same stereotype, infamously calling Mexicans "bad hombres").

As today, anti-Latinx violence was often explained away as economic insecurity. There was tremendous ambivalence among the Anglo population regarding immigration and the use of Mexican labor. Nativist rhetoric was the framework for targeting Mexicans (Montejano, 1987). Between 1929 and 1940, in the aftermath of the Great Depression, estimates suggest that a million Mexicans were driven out of the United States, including American citizens who had been in the United States for generations, losing everything they owned (Balderrama & Rodríguez, 2006). Employers "encouraged" many to return to Mexico and paid train fares to the border amid the rhetoric that Mexicans and people of Mexican descent were taking "American" jobs (Balderrama & Rodríguez, 2006).

Current Anti-Immigrant Rhetorical Violence

Public discourse about immigration justifies and perpetuates harmful policies and causes harm to the individuals disparaged by this discourse. For example, President Trump has frequently used accounts of sexual violence against migrant women to fuel his anti-immigrant rhetoric and policy, stating that their experiences of sexual violence on the journey through Mexico is evidence that the United States must increase border security (Trump, 2019a, 2019b). Co-opting violence against migrant women to stoke anti-immigration fear doubly victimizes them, first by highlighting their sexual assault and then by excluding them from protections, justified on the grounds of their own victimization.

As immigration is debated on the national stage, migrants are subject to debasing, dehumanizing discourse of which they are acutely aware. For example, recently while working in a small, rural, and economically marginalized community in Mexico, the second author was struck by the extent to

---

[3]See also Bishop and Shu (2016); Villanueva (2017).

which people in the village were aware of the anti-immigrant rhetoric pervasive in contemporary America. As in many communities in Mexico, many households had family members who had migrated to work in the United States. One woman referred directly to the president of the United States, Donald Trump, as "el señor quien no nos quiere" (i.e., "the man who doesn't want us"). For a community with very limited access to the outside world, with no internet, limited cellular service, no newspapers, and radio or television limited to a handful of regional stations, the universality of this awareness was a testament to what loved ones in the United States were communicating to their families back home. The complexity of immigration policy was distilled down to a core, essential component: a sense of being hated.

There is an intimate connection between the rhetoric of hate and violence itself. Indeed, hateful rhetoric is a form of violence (Graumann, 2001). In his classic chapter "Aggression as Discourse," Gergen (1984) examined how speaking is a form of world construction in part because language is a collection of referents. In speech, the speakers invoke those referents and invite the listener to accept an ontological system. Language is also performative and therefore has social effects; words have a real impact on social processes. Studies examining this proposition directly have looked at the relationship between language used by leaders of ideologically motivated groups when talking about despised opponent out-groups and the acts of aggression committed by their groups. Results show linguistic differences between the speeches made by leaders of groups that go on to commit aggression and the leaders of groups that do not (Matsumoto & Hwang, 2013). Leaders whose groups go on to engage in violence expressed significantly more anger, contempt, and disgust when talking about the groups toward whom they felt hostility (Matsumoto et al., 2013; Matsumoto et al., 2014). Another series of experiments demonstrated that even mild violent metaphors increase support for political violence among individuals prone to aggression, especially younger people (Kalmoe, 2014).

Some evidence suggests a positive correlation between anti-immigrant political discourse and anti-immigrant sentiment in addition to a negative relationship between anti-immigrant political discourse and migrants' sense of belonging (Simonsen, 2019). Hjerm and Schnabel (2010) found that the threat of loss of territory was specifically linked to increases in anti-immigrant and nativist sentiment in Europe. Reconquest and lack of assimilation into the dominant culture in the United States have been prominent themes in right-wing discourse, evident in the use of words such as "invasion" and "invaders" by right-wing media and even the concept of building a wall along the southern border (Finley & Esposito, 2020). The 2018 FBI hate-crimes statistics report indicated that hate crimes rose 17% between 2016 and 2017, with a 24% increase in anti-Latinx hate crimes (U.S. Federal Bureau of Investigation, 2018). Although these statistics cannot definitively be tied to the anti-Latinx rhetorical violence apparent in the 2016 presidential election and the Trump administration, they suggest a troubling trend. History and social context not only represent external threats but become part of the internalized social imaginary, subjecting Latinx migrants to invalidating and threatening internal criticism.

The Violence of U.S. Immigration Policy

The U.S. immigration system itself is violent. People living in the United States with undocumented status or who are subject to detention, Alternative To Detention (ATD), or the ambiguity of the asylum process experience these circumstances as powerfully stressful. The U.S. immigration policy environment enacts violence on migrants from Mexico and Latin America, as it persecutes, dehumanizes, and punishes them.

Criminalizing Is Traumatizing

Immigration policy[4] since the 1980s has increasingly blurred the distinction between criminal law and immigration law through rhetoric, the expansion of policing (both inside the country and at the border), expansion of so-called "criminal" offenses for immigrants, and the use of the technology of crime and punishment (e.g., prison detention environments, ankle monitors, use of law enforcement; Menjívar et al., 2018). These policies have used race-neutral language in the creation of laws targeting Latinx people, conflating race and ethnicity with legal status (Asad & Clair, 2018). As immigration has been criminalized, the infrastructure supporting criminalization has grown. Budgets for Immigration and Customs Enforcement and Border Patrol have climbed exponentially (Kerwin, 2018). This growth has different but equally devastating impacts on undocumented people living in U.S. communities and on unauthorized migrants crossing the U.S.–Mexico border.

Migrants apprehended crossing the U.S.–Mexico border are impacted by the criminalization of immigration through their encounters with a punitive immigration and asylum system. This system uses the technology of crime and punishment via detention, postrelease monitoring, and legal battles. After apprehension, migrants are frequently held in short-term detention facilities, or *hieleras* (i.e., "ice boxes"), for up to 72 hours. These facilities are reported to be extremely cold with inadequate blankets or clothing, inadequate food, limited privacy, and insufficient medical care; they are sites of dehumanizing and abusive treatment (Cantor, 2015; Valdez et al., 2015). For many, the experiences are hard to understand. As one woman said to the first author, "I don't understand that . . . there has to be some reason they would treat us like that, treat us like animals . . . because that's the way you treat animals, no one should be treated like that."

---

[4]For detailed information about the history of U.S. immigration law, see Kerwin (2018), Menjívar et al. (2018), and Abrego et al. (2017), among many others.

Immigration detention itself, typically in former prisons or prison-like environments, has negative psychological consequences that worsen with length of detention, even when controlling for predetention experiences (Filges et al., 2016; Robjant et al., 2009). For many, it triggers feelings of powerlessness, helplessness, uncertainty about the future, isolation, and fear about the safety of loved ones (Coffey et al., 2010; Keller et al., 2003). Private prison companies also run ATD programs, which consist of combinations of electronic monitoring using GPS ankle monitors, other monitoring systems, home visits, and case management (Gómez Cervantes et al., 2017). Although more cost-effective and less restrictive than detention, ATD programs represent significant government control over migrant lives. Ankle monitors track all movements, and unauthorized travel can violate an immigration order. Monitors are reported to be very uncomfortable (producing rashes and lesions), stigmatizing, and cumbersome, needing to be charged frequently. Furthermore, migrants are sometimes required to pay the cost of these monitors, which can be extremely expensive (Gómez Cervantes et al., 2017).

For migrants from violent communities in Mexico and Central America, the act of being criminalized can be triggering of the traumatic events that caused them to flee their countries of origin. Criminalizing immigration for these migrants effectively tells them that they are what they flee. Considering the concept of the social imaginary, the impact of criminalization can clearly be understood as violent. The message that migrants receive about their so-called criminality becomes an internalized, invalidating judgment of their lived experiences by their host society. In the first author's research with women from Honduras, El Salvador, and Guatemala, almost every interviewee stressed the message "I am not a criminal." Most who were ordered to use a GPS monitor, called a *grillete* in Spanish—directly translated to "shackle"—reported that it was humiliating and isolating. One woman, who fled domestic and gang violence with her three young children, described that after being released from detention with a grillete she felt

> even more stressed . . . more than a year I had that . . . and how it felt to have el grillete . . . I felt like . . . I felt shame that people were looking at me thinking "that's a criminal" or "she did something to have go around like that [with the grillete]." It pained me to use it . . . and I had to use it for over a year. (McDermott, 2019)

The grillete was a scarlet letter of sorts: identifying her to the world as a criminal, isolating her from others—a constant shameful, painful reminder that she did not belong.

Asylum Seeking: A State of Limbo

The hostile U.S. immigration policy climate has implications for access to the asylum process as well. Officials may not solicit information about fear of removal appropriately and may disregard migrants' asylum claims (Kerwin, 2018). Individuals appropriately referred to the asylum process receive a credible fear interview (CFI) conducted by immigration officials to determine whether they will face persecution if returned to their community of origin.[5] This process is very difficult, and success often depends on access to legal counsel, which is difficult to come by and often prohibitively expensive (Kerwin, 2018).

Backlogs of these cases mean that individuals may wait years for their cases to be adjudicated (Haas, 2017; Kerwin, 2018). Seeking safety in the United States via asylum is, itself, prolonging a state of trauma. Migrants' asylum claims are based on the credibility of their fear; they must surrender the reality of perhaps the most traumatic experiences of their lives to a hostile state actor. For many, it is a struggle to understand a world in which their experiences are essentially rendered fraudulent by a system from which they sought protection and, as a result, experience feelings of helplessness, hopelessness, despair, and even suicidal ideation (Haas, 2017). The lack of congruence between migrants' lived experiences and the social imaginary can produce these extremely difficult feelings.

The excruciating waiting game of asylum seeking was evident in an interview the first author conducted with Alejandra, the woman described previously who fled Honduras with her youngest son, Mateo. Alejandra's older son had been murdered for refusing to join a gang. After his murder, she began to receive death threats, and gang members attempted to recruit Mateo, then 12 years old. Alejandra and Mateo fled through Mexico, traveling without a coyote to the U.S. border. Although initially her CFI was found credible, at the time of our interview she reported that her asylum case had been denied and that she was in the appeals process. Alejandra described the way in which the history of violence in her past intersects with the violence of the immigration system and the consequences:

ALEJANDRA: So, basically you are saved from the persecution in your country, but you become persecuted by immigration . . . so you're in the same situation. . . . It's the same, the same. I'm here, I feel good because I'm protected . . . because I know that here nothing is going to happen to us, nothing is going to happen to my son. But at the same time, I'm like "what's going to happen?" When are they going to say "No" definitively [that my asylum was denied] . . . right now I have to submit another statement for the first of August. I'm thinking: "I'll submit it, will they accept me or will they not accept me? Will they give me another chance or will they not give me another chance?"

---

[5]Under the Trump administration, Attorney General Jeff Sessions issued a decision that "private violence," such as domestic violence or gang violence, is not grounds for asylum because these acts are not perpetuated by a government (Benner & Dickerson, 2018). The decision was widely understood to target the large number of Central American migrants seeking asylum on these grounds (O'Toole, 2018). The decision is under appeal and continues to complicate the cases of individuals seeking asylum on these grounds (Human Rights Watch, 2019).

HANNAH: And the time they don't give you another chance you're at risk . . .?

ALEJANDRA: At risk of deportation, so yeah . . . I put in the statement, the appeal, now I can't even appeal . . . the lawyer put my request for permission [to stay in the United States] in for a year and they only give me 6 months. Every legal process is like this. I have to pay. I have to be paying to live . . . every 6 months I am paying. There isn't a future; I am stuck. I don't know if tomorrow I suddenly will have to make that phone call and I'll have to say "*Ay hijo,* we won't see each other again." I have no future. I can't have dreams. I can't . . . I don't know. I am stuck, basically my life has become like when they trap a wild beast in a cage. That's how I am.

The life-or-death persecution that Alejandra faced in Honduras, the persecution that drove her to flee, was being relived in the United States. She felt pursued by immigration, seeing them around every corner and, as she mentioned elsewhere in the interview, in every policeman. She was living with the constant fear that her next court appointment would be her last, separating her permanently from her son and perhaps condemning her to death. For every appeal, every legal filing, she had to pay enormous sums, which were even more burdensome because she had not been granted a work permit. She was paying to live, much like paying *renta* or *cuota* to gangs in Honduras. This system had caged her, depriving her of a future and of her dreams in much the same way her past experiences of gang violence did.

DISCUSSION AND CONCLUDING THOUGHTS

Herman (1997) described the way in which the dialectic between avoidance and reliving traumatic events is also reproduced at the societal level. We cannot hold or understand such unspeakable violence, and therefore we deny it. The multidimensional landscape of violence faced by contemporary Mexican and Central American migrants is often underrecognized, perhaps because it is too much to bear. We may fail to appreciate the scope of this violence because of attention to specific elements (e.g., violence in communities of origin, violence crossing the border) or because migrants may not find it easy to convey these experiences because of their trauma, a focus on survival, or stigma, or because, as in Marta's case, it did not seem extraordinary amid a multiplicity of experiences of violence. Herman's understanding of the dialectic of avoidance and reliving trauma is pertinent to both survivors of traumatic experience and those who might find themselves working with these individuals in a clinical context. The latter may be unconsciously motivated to avoid (and therefore not be receptive to) narratives in which the content would be too disquieting to hear. It is imperative that clinicians be alert to and adept at appreciating the myriad ways in which traumatic experience is presented (and sometimes not presented) when immigrants seek therapy as well as how the clinicians themselves might defensively avoid this painful and difficult material, to the detriment of their therapeutic efforts.

Our aim in this chapter has been to illustrate four facets of violence that many migrants from these countries may carry with them, namely, the violence that defines the communities from which they've emigrated, the violence of the journey itself, the violence of the context-of-reception's history of anti-Latinx racism, and, finally, the violence of the immigration system. Any one of these sources of violence constitutes a significant psychological stressor. Together, however, they represent an enormously complex challenge for migrants in an unfamiliar, unwelcoming culture far from support systems in their communities of origin. Multiple exposures to adverse or traumatic events (including witnessing community violence) are linked to poor mental health outcomes, including depression, anxiety, substance abuse, and post-traumatic stress disorder (Eisenman et al., 2003; Fortuna et al., 2008; Torres & Wallace, 2013).

The case of Marta, described at the beginning of the chapter, illustrates this complexity. Marta witnessed a double homicide in Mexico, living in a community in which the authorities could not provide protection or justice. She endured the dangers of migration and arrived in the United States amidst an anti-immigrant climate, then an armed intruder threatened her in her own home. She lived with the daily fear that she would be deported and separated from her American-born children. Presenting to treatment following the home invasion, she did not mention her prior exposure to violence; it emerged only later, providing important context to her current presentation. Appreciating the intersection of multiple vectors of violence, past and present, is critical to understanding our migrant clients, and creating a space in which these experiences can be spoken is essential to meeting clients' needs (Ainslie et al., 2018).

We wrote this chapter at a historical moment of unprecedented institutional violence against migrants by the U.S. state as well as unprecedented visibility of some of the many forms of violence that migrants face. However, it is not enough to appreciate the scope of this violence. We must also appreciate the strength and resilience of our clients as they navigate a hostile host country, carrying the weight of this past, and continue to persist. For example, Marta, in addition to being a victim of violence, was an active agent against it in her own life: examining her parents' abusive relationship and working to establish a healthy marriage; speaking often with her daughters about healthy relationships, sexuality, and consent. Participants in the first author's study reported spiritual faith and family connection as critical sources of resilience; they specifically identified the role of motherhood and their faith as allowing them to persist despite the odds. Some other participants also identified therapy and contact with Americans who listened to them and believed them as helpful resources.

We believe that clinicians' awareness of the nature and character of the immigrant experience is a vital tool in their efforts to be helpful when working with immigrant populations. Several of the women who shared their stories were quite explicit about the importance of feeling understood and believed when speaking to helping resources. Clinicians sometimes overlook this very basic aspect of a successful intervention process (i.e., listening and understanding). It is our hope that a more complex and nuanced understanding of the immigration experience will lead clinicians to be more sensitive to these experiences and will alert them to potential areas of importance to be explored therapeutically.

Limited research has addressed the population and issues we discuss in this chapter, in part because of the tendency in psychological research to divorce the social and contextual from the individual and in part because of the vast scope of the problem. However, attention to the complexity of this problem is essential. Studies examining mental health among migrants must recognize the potentially impactful events in the participants' countries of origin or during their migration process and must recognize that migrants may still be experiencing the trauma of undocumented status or asylum proceedings as well as trauma inflicted by a hostile sociopolitical climate. Mental health providers working with this population must recognize the complex interplay between past and present events as they may appear in the client's life. Recognizing the violence of the immigration system may mean reconceptualizing diagnosis and treatment for a population whose lives may have been threatened by multiple actors across years or may remain threatened throughout the course of treatment. Furthermore, providers must develop new forms of screening and assessment to bring these experiences to light and must recognize that the pervasive nature of this violence may make it invisible. The violence that migrants face is not extraordinary, and nor is their resilience as they continue to fight for safe, healthy, and prosperous lives in the United States.

REFERENCES

Abrego, L., Coleman, M., Martinez, D. E., Menjívar, C., & Slack, J. (2017). Making immigrants into criminals: Legal processes of criminalization in the post-IIRIRA era. *Journal on Migration and Human Security, 5*(3), 694–715. https://doi.org/10.1177/233150241700500308

Ainslie, R., & Ainslie, D. (2013). Looking north: Mexican immigration and the social imaginary. In D. Leal & J. Limón (Eds.), *Latinos in the 21st century* (pp. 86–104). University of Notre Dame Press.

Ainslie, R. C. (2013). *The fight to save Juarez: Life in the heart of Mexico's drug war.* University of Texas Press.

Ainslie, R. C., McDermott, H. W., & Guevara, C. (2018). Dying to get out: Challenges in the treatment of Latin American migrants fleeing violent communities. In

P. Gherovici & C. Christian (Eds.), *Psychoanalysis en el barrio: Race, class and the unconscious* (pp. 54–68). Routledge. https://doi.org/10.4324/9780429437298-4

Arredondo, P., Gallardo-Cooper, M., Delgado-Romero, E. A., & Zapata, A. L. (2015). *Latinas/os in counseling, in culturally responsive counseling with Latinas/os.* American Counseling Association. https://doi.org/10.1002/9781119221609

Asad, A. L., & Clair, M. (2018). Racialized legal status as a social determinant of health. *Social Science & Medicine, 199,* 19–28. https://doi.org/10.1016/j.socscimed.2017.03.010

Balderrama, F. E., & Rodríguez, R. (2006). *Decade of betrayal: Mexican repatriation in the 1930s.* University of New Mexico Press.

Benner, K., & Dickerson, C. (2018, June 11). Sessions says domestic and gang violence are not grounds for asylum. *The New York Times.* https://www.nytimes.com/2018/06/11/us/politics/sessions-domestic-violence-asylum.html

Bishop, M., & Shu, J. (2016, March 11). *The history of anti-Mexican violence and lynching.* Latino USA. https://www.latinousa.org/2016/03/11/the-history-of-anti-mexican-violence-and-lynching/

Brigden, N. K. (2016). Improvised transnationalism: Clandestine migration at the border of anthropology and international relations. *International Studies Quarterly, 60*(2), 343–354. https://doi.org/10.1093/isq/sqw010

Cantor, G. (2015). Hieleras *(iceboxes) in the Rio Grande Valley sector: Lengthy detention, deplorable conditions, and abuse in CBP holding cells.* American Immigration Council. https://www.americanimmigrationcouncil.org/sites/default/files/research/hieleras_iceboxes_in_the_rio_grande_valley_sector.pdf

Carrigan, W. D., & Webb, C. (2013). *Forgotten dead: Mob violence against Mexicans in the United States, 1848–1928.* Oxford University Press.

Castoriadis, C. (1987). *The imaginary institution of society.* MIT Press.

Coffey, G. J., Kaplan, I., Sampson, R. C., & Tucci, M. M. (2010). The meaning and mental health consequences of long-term immigration detention for people seeking asylum. *Social Science & Medicine, 70*(12), 2070–2079. https://doi.org/10.1016/j.socscimed.2010.02.042

Consejo Ciudadano Para la Seguridad Pública y la Justicia Penal, A. C. (2019). Metodología del ranking (2018) de las 50 Ciudades mas Violentas del Mund. *Seguridad, Justicia, y Paz. Ciudad de Mexico.*

De León, J. (2012). "Better to be hot than caught": Excavating the conflicting roles of migrant material culture. *American Anthropologist, 114*(3), 477–495. https://doi.org/10.1111/j.1548-1433.2012.01447.x

De León, J. (2015). *The land of open graves.* University of California Press.

Dominguez Villegas, R. (2014). *Central American migrants and "La Bestia": The route, dangers, and government responses.* Migration Policy Institute. https://www.migrationpolicy.org/article/central-american-migrants-and-%E2%80%9Cla-bestia%E2%80%9D-route-dangers-and-government-responses

Eguizábal, C., Ingram, M. C., Curtis, K. M., Korthuis, A., Olson, E. L., & Phillips, N. (2015). *Crime and violence in Central America's northern triangle.* Woodrow Wilson International Center for Scholars.

Eisenman, D. P., Gelberg, L., Honghu, L., & Shaprio, M. F. (2003). Mental health and health-related quality of life among adult Latino primary care patients living in the United States with previous exposure to political violence. *JAMA, 290*(5), 627–634.

Filges, T., Montgomery, E., & Kastrup, M. (2016). The impact of detention on the health of asylum seekers: A systematic review. *Research on Social Work Practice, 28*(4), 1–16.

Finley, L., & Esposito, L. (2020). The immigrant as bogeyman: Examining Donald Trump and the right's anti-immigrant, anti-PC rhetoric. *Humanity & Society, 44*(2), 178–197. https://doi.org/10.1177/0160597619832627

Fortuna, L. R., Porche, M. V., & Alegria, M. (2008). Political violence, psychosocial trauma, and the context of mental health services use among immigrant Latinos in the United States. *Ethnicity & Health, 13*(5), 435–463. https://doi.org/10.1080/13557850701837286

Gergen, K. (1984). Aggression as discourse. In A. Mummendey (Ed.), *Social psychology of aggression* (pp. 51–68). Springer-Verlag Heidelberg. https://doi.org/10.1007/978-3-642-48919-8_5

Gómez Cervantes, A., Menjívar, C., & Staples, W. G. (2017). "Humane" immigration enforcement and Latina immigrants in the detention complex. *Feminist Criminology, 12*(3), 269–292. https://doi.org/10.1177/1557085117699069

Goodman, R. D., Vesely, C. K., Letiecq, B., & Cleaveland, C. L. (2017). Trauma and resilience among refugee and undocumented immigrant women. *Journal of Counseling and Development, 95*(3), 309–321. https://doi.org/10.1002/jcad.12145

Graumann, C. (2001). Verbal discrimination: A neglected chapter in the social psychology of aggression. *Journal for the Theory of Social Behaviour, 28*(1), 41–61. https://doi.org/10.1111/1468-5914.00062

Haas, B. M. (2017). Citizens-in-waiting, deportees-in-waiting: Power, temporality, and suffering in the U.S. asylum system. *Ethos (Berkeley, Calif.), 45*(1), 75–97. https://doi.org/10.1111/etho.12150

Herman, J. L. (1997). *Trauma and recovery*. BasicBooks.

Hjerm, M., & Schnabel, A. (2010). Mobilizing nationalist sentiments: Which factors affect nationalist sentiments in Europe? *Social Science Research, 39*(4), 527–539. https://doi.org/10.1016/j.ssresearch.2010.03.006

Human Rights Watch. (2019, January 23). *US: Protect right to asylum for domestic violence*. https://www.hrw.org/news/2019/01/23/us-protect-right-asylum-domestic-violence

Isacson, A., Meyer, M., & Smith, H. (2017). *Mexico's southern border: Security, Central American migration, and U.S. policy*. https://www.wola.org/analysis/wola-report-mexicos-southern-border-security-central-american-migration-u-s-policy/

Kalmoe, N. P. (2014). Fueling the fire: Violent metaphors, trait aggression, and support for political violence. *Political Communication, 31*(4), 545–563. https://doi.org/10.1080/10584609.2013.852642

Kaltman, S., Green, B. L., Mete, M., Shara, N., & Miranda, J. (2010). Trauma, depression, and comorbid PTSD/depression in a community sample of Latina immigrants. *Psychological Trauma: Theory, Research, Practice, and Policy, 2*(1), 31–39. https://doi.org/10.1037/a0018952

Keller, A. S., Ford, D., Sachs, E., Rosenfeld, B., Trinh-Shevrin, C., Meserve, C., Leviss, J. A., Singer, E., Smith, H., Wilkinson, J., Kim, G., Allden, K., & Rockline, P. (2003). The impact of detention on the health of asylum seekers. *The Journal of Ambulatory Care Management, 26*(4), 383–385. https://doi.org/10.1097/00004479-200310000-00016

Kennedy, E. G. (2013). Refugees from Central American gangs. *Forced Migration Review, 43*, 50–52.

Kerwin, D. (2018). From IIRIRA to Trump: Connecting the dots to the current U.S. immigration policy crisis. *Journal on Migration and Human Security, 6*(3), 192–204. https://doi.org/10.1177/2331502418786718

Martínez, D., Reineke, C., Rubio-Goldsmith, R., Anderson, B., Hess, G., & Parks, B. (2013). A continued humanitarian crisis at the border: Undocumented border crosser deaths recorded by the Pima County Office of the Medical Examiner, 1990–2012. *SSRN*. https://doi.org/10.2139/ssrn.2633209

Martínez, M. M. (2018). *The injustice never leaves you: Anti-Mexican violence in Texas*. Harvard University Press.

Massey, D. S., & Riosmena, F. (2010). Undocumented migration from Latin America in an era of rising U.S. enforcement. *The Annals of the American Academy of Political and Social Science, 630*(1), 294–321. https://doi.org/10.1177/0002716210368114

Matsumoto, D., & Hwang, H. C. (2013). The language of political aggression. *Journal of Language and Social Psychology, 32*(3), 335–348. https://doi.org/10.1177/0261927X12460666

Matsumoto, D., Hwang, H. C., & Frank, M. G. (2013). Emotional language and political aggression. *Journal of Language and Social Psychology, 32*(4), 452–468. https://doi.org/10.1177/0261927X12474654

Matsumoto, D., Hwang, H. C., & Frank, M. G. (2014). Emotions expressed in speeches by leaders of ideologically motivated groups predict aggression. *Behavioral Sciences of Terrorism and Political Aggression, 6*(1), 1–18. https://doi.org/10.1080/19434472.2012.716449

McDermott, H. W. (2019). *En el camino: Central American women's migration experiences* [Unpublished manuscript]. Department of Education, University of Texas, Austin.

Menjívar, C., Gómez Cervantes, A., & Alvord, D. (2018). The expansion of "crimmigration," mass detention, and deportation. *Sociology Compass, 12*(4), e12573. https://doi.org/10.1111/soc4.12573

Montejano, D. (1987). *Anglos and Mexicans in the making of Texas 1836–1986.* University of Texas Press.

O'Toole, M. (2018, December 20). The nation: Asylum blocking policy ruled illegal; Judge overturns a Trump revision that limited claims by victims of gangs and domestic violence. *Los Angeles Times.* https://enewspaper.latimes.com/infinity/article_share.aspx?guid=1b059e01-2253-40a6-a7ac-11fb24e29615

Parish, A. (2017). *Gender-based violence against women: Both cause for migration and risk along the journey.* The Migration Policy Institute.

Pérez, M. (2019). A history of anti-Latino state-sanctioned violence: Executions, lynchings, and hate crimes. In A. Miranda (Ed.), *Gringo injustice: Insider perspectives on police, gangs, and law* (pp. 25–44). Routledge. https://doi.org/10.4324/9780429296857-2

Robjant, K., Hassan, R., & Katona, C. (2009). Mental health implications of detaining asylum seekers: Systematic review. *The British Journal of Psychiatry, 194*(4), 306–312. https://doi.org/10.1192/bjp.bp.108.053223

Simmons, W. P., Menjívar, C., & Téllez, M. (2015). Violence and vulnerability of female migrants in drop houses in Arizona: The predictable outcome of a chain reaction of violence. *Violence Against Women, 21*(5), 551–570. https://doi.org/10.1177/1077801215573331

Simonsen, K. B. (2019). The democratic consequences of anti-immigrant political rhetoric: A mixed methods study of immigrants' political belonging. *Political Behavior.* https://doi.org/10.1007/s11109-019-09549-6

Slack, J., Martínez, D. E., Lee, A. E., & Whiteford, S. (2016). Geography of border militarization: Violence, death and health in Mexico and the United States. *Journal of Latin American Geography, 15*(1), 7–32. https://doi.org/10.1353/lag.2016.0009

Sue, D. W., & Sue, D. (2015). *Counseling the culturally diverse: Theory and practice.* John Wiley & Sons.

Torres, J. M., & Wallace, S. P. (2013). Migration circumstances, psychological distress, and self-rated physical health for Latino immigrants in the United States. *American Journal of Public Health, 103*(9), 1619–1627. https://doi.org/10.2105/AJPH.2012.301195

Trump, D. J. (2019a, January 19). *Remarks by President Trump on the humanitarian crisis on our southern border and the shutdown.* https://www.whitehouse.gov/briefings-statements/remarks-president-trump-humanitarian-crisis-southern-border-shutdown/

Trump, D. J. (2019b, February 6). *Remarks by President Trump in State of the Union address.* https://www.whitehouse.gov/briefings-statements/remarks-president-trump-state-union-address-3/

U.S. Federal Bureau of Investigation. (2018). *2017 Hate crime statistics.* https://ucr.fbi.gov/hate-crime/2017

Valdez, E. S., Valdez, L. A., & Sabo, S. (2015). Structural vulnerability among migrating women and children fleeing Central America and Mexico: The public health impact of "humanitarian parole." *Frontiers in Public Health, 3,* 163. https://doi.org/10.3389/fpubh.2015.00163

Villanueva, N. (2017). *The lynching of Mexicans in the Texas borderlands.* University of New Mexico Press.

Vogt, W. A. (2013). Crossing Mexico: Structural violence and the commodification of undocumented Central American migrants. *American Ethnologist, 40*(4), 764–780. https://doi.org/10.1111/amet.12053

The World Bank. (n.d.). *Intentional homicides (per 100,000 people).* Retrieved July 10, 2019, from https://data.worldbank.org/indicator/VC.IHR.PSRC.P5

3

Xenophobia and Racism

Immigrant Youth Experiences, Stress, and Resilience

Amy K. Marks, G. Alice Woolverton, and Marit D. Murry

The number of overall hate crimes in the United States is increasing, with most recent national data showing an approximate 15% increase from 6,121 incidents in 2016 to 7,175 in 2017 (U.S. Federal Bureau of Investigation, 2017). According to the American Bar Association (2019), this recent increase is primarily driven by rising numbers of hate crimes based on ethnicity, ancestry, or race, which together made up the majority (59.6%) of hate crimes in 2017. The American Bar Association identified hate crimes directed at immigrant communities as fueled by increasing anti-immigrant rhetoric in the United States following the 2016 presidential election and noted that bias incidents are largely underreported. In addition, during the COVID-19 pandemic in April 2020, more than 1,000 hate crimes were reported in a 2-week period alone, primarily targeting members of Asian-origin immigrant communities (Nawaz, 2020). Both domestic and international anti-immigrant attitudes are easily read and viewed by youth and families on social media and in daily news articles online, including many instances of anti-Chinese and anti-immigrant hate speech during the COVID-19 pandemic (Roberg et al., 2020). Such public attitudes are fueling a crisis of discrimination in the United States aimed at children and adolescents from immigrant and refugee families, with deleterious consequences for youth health and well-being (Marks et al., 2018).

On an individual level, racism occurs when individuals hold prejudice against (i.e., have inaccurate and harmful thoughts or beliefs) and discriminate

https://doi.org/10.1037/0000214-004
Trauma and Racial Minority Immigrants: Turmoil, Uncertainty, and Resistance,
P. Tummala-Narra (Editor)

(i.e., act on those thoughts or beliefs) toward others based on their assumed or identified membership in a racial group (Hoyt, 2012). Racial groups themselves are socially defined based on observable and arbitrary differences in phenotypic features (Omi & Winant, 2014). Xenophobia includes the fear and negatively held beliefs about immigrants and perceived outsiders and often accompanies ethnocentrism, the belief that individuals from one's national group are superior to individuals from other nations (Yakushko, 2009). Whereas individuals enact racism and xenophobia person to person, oppressive social systems (including some schools, government organizations, corporations, and other large social groups) can both enable and bolster xenophobia and racism, thereby creating and perpetuating the negative health and behavioral consequences associated with them.

In the United States, a history of racism and systemic oppression against people of color means that anti-immigrant xenophobia and discrimination are often aimed in their strongest forms against racial minority youth and families. As such, immigrant youth and families of color may experience doubly marginalized statuses of both immigrant (i.e., xenophobia) and person of color (i.e., racism) social groups. A large majority of immigrants in the United States—89%—migrate from Latin America, Asia, Africa, or the Caribbean and are typically ascribed racial identities as people of color in the United States during their acculturation (Child Trends, 2013). Even for immigrant-origin youth born in the United States, skin color and other aspects of physical appearances that are not phenotypically Caucasian may lead to experiences of discriminatory *foreigner objectification*, in which U.S.-born children and youth are treated, based on physical appearance, as though they had been born abroad (Huynh et al., 2011; Kiang et al., 2019). While this marginalization can take the form of explicit xenophobia, the harmful microaggressions of foreigner objectification that U.S.-born immigrant youth face can also manifest through seemingly positive comments such as "you speak English so well," highlighting stereotypes and assumptions associated with presumed immigrant status (Kiang et al., 2019). Underlying foreigner objectification is the tendency shown in experimental studies for White Americans to define "American" as synonymous with "White" and to view anyone who appears racially not White as "less American" (Devos & Banaji, 2005). This finding supports the notion that many racial-minority immigrant children and families are treated as perpetual foreigners, based on their presumed immigrant status and presumed race, and thereby face repeated discrimination and xenophobia regardless of where they were born.

In addition, immigrant-origin children and youth (IOCY) experience exclusion, discrimination, and harassment based on other aspects of their identities and acculturation experiences. Being an individual who speaks English as a second language, for example, can serve as an identifying basis for microaggressions or harassment. In a sample of youth from Latinx backgrounds, lower English proficiency was associated with more foreigner objectification, which was linked to negative outcomes such as lower self-esteem (Kiang et al., 2019). Other aspects of acculturation that may lead to perceived discrimination against immigrant youth include assumptions or biases about legal status and religious or cultural practices. For example, youth living in families of mixed legal statuses in the United States experience marginalization and subsequent increased risk for anxiety, depression, and lower educational achievement outcomes (Landale et al., 2015). In terms of religious discrimination, post-9/11 Islamophobia in the United States has created environments in which Muslim American youth face bullying at school based on their religious identities (Britto, 2011).

As hate crimes targeting immigrant communities and individuals are on the rise in the United States (U.S. Federal Bureau of Investigation, 2017), it is a critical time to document and illuminate the many challenging experiences and stressors that IOCY experience because of xenophobia and discrimination. In this chapter, we first present a brief description of a recent integrative theoretical framework for understanding how xenophobia and discrimination impact the development of IOCY. Next, we present recent research demonstrating the negative effects of both xenophobia and discrimination on the development of IOCY, incorporating case studies from our original research with immigrant families of color. Finally, we present ideas for intervention efforts to help promote recovery and resilience among IOCY.

THEORETICAL FRAMEWORK: PROMOTING AND INHIBITING ENVIRONMENTS

To understand the many environmental facets that shape IOCY development, a recent theoretical framework was created to emphasize both risk and resilience factors unique to the immigration experience (Suárez-Orozco et al., 2018). In this theoretical framework (see Figure 3.1), the authors emphasize that ecological contexts of IOCY development can be sources of both risk and resilience—in other words, for example, schools can be sources of upward social mobility or sources of discrimination and barriers to economic advancement, depending on many factors, such as the cultural competence of school staff, federal and state policies, and other aspects of classroom and school environments. Although IOCY attend schools with widely varying characteristics, on average they are overrepresented in schools that lack economic and educational resources to ensure their success (Suárez-Orozco et al., 2015). Research has also shown that schools can play a unique role in fostering resilience among IOCY communities, promoting positive social relationships and community engagement (Motti-Stefanidi & Masten, 2017).

At the individual level of the model, coping with xenophobia and racism is a core task for IOCY as they then, in turn, build developmental, acculturative, and psychological competencies. These coping skills become paramount, as developmental milestones and outcomes will be influenced by how children learn to cope with the stigma, marginalization, discrimination, and social exclusion that exist in many of their ecological settings. Latinx students tend to perceive more discrimination in the school setting than their nonimmigrant

FIGURE 3.1. Integrative Risk and Resilience Model for the Adaptation of Immigrant-Origin Children and Youth to the Host Country

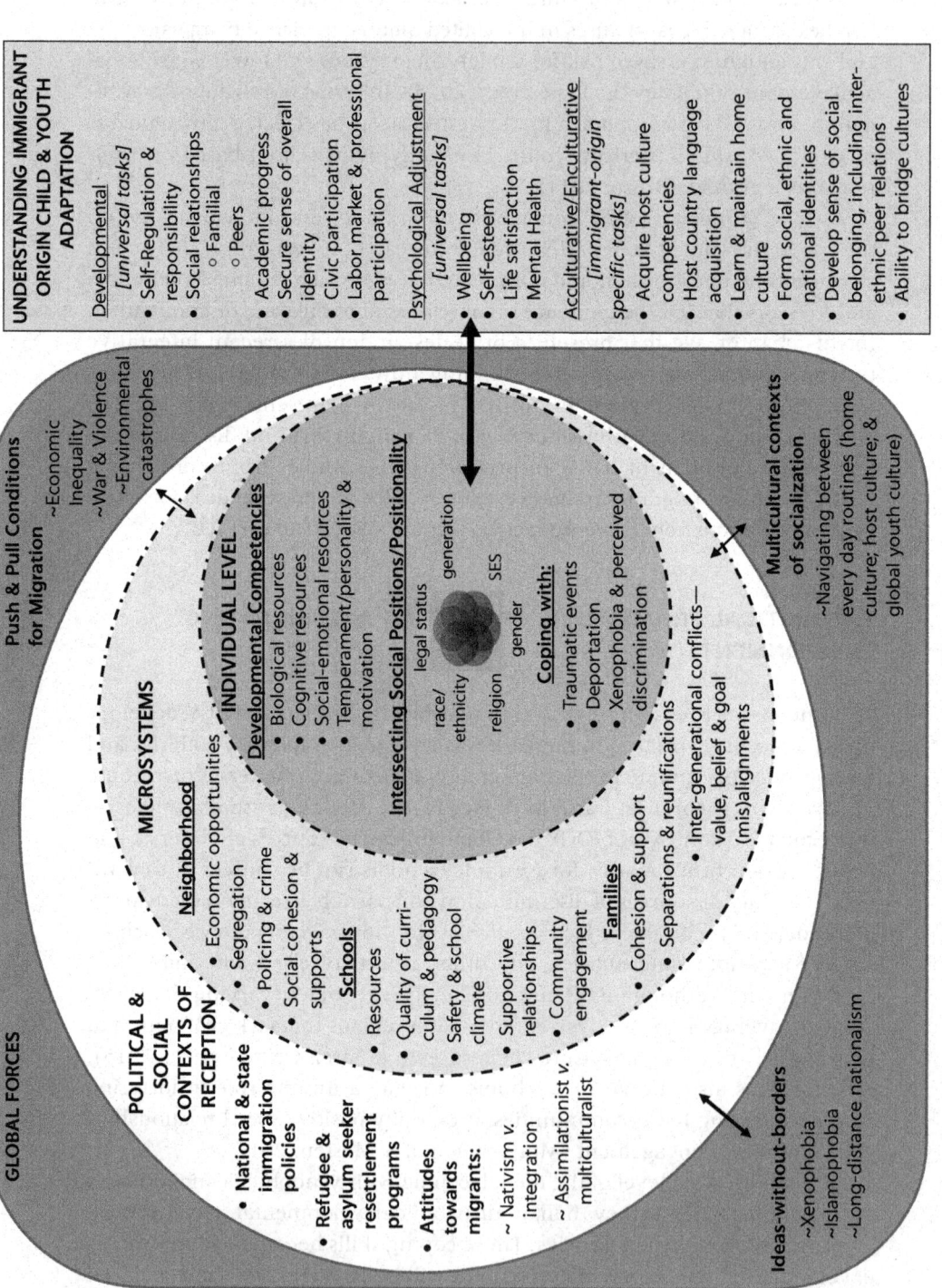

Note. SES = socioeconomic status. Reprinted from "An Integrative Risk and Resilience Model for Understanding the Development and Adaptation of Immigrant Origin Children and Youth," by C. Suárez-Orozco, F. Motti-Stefanidi, A. K. Marks, and D. Katsiaficas, 2018, *American Psychologist, 73*(6), p. 786. https://doi.org/10.1037/amp0000265. Copyright 2018 by the American Psychological Association.

peers (Brown & Chu, 2012). Importantly, multiculturalism—or the practice of valuing multiple cultural orientations in the school setting—is an important moderator of the school-based discrimination effects. When children attend schools that promote multiculturalism, perceived discrimination decreases and pride about students' ethnic/racial identities increases. For example, in a sample of Mexican American high school students, experiences at school that dispelled negative ethnic/racial stereotypes and instead valued skills like bilingualism as an asset (e.g., multicultural events and clubs, anti-bias curricula) were associated with increased feelings of ethnic/racial pride and decreased perceptions of discrimination (Gonzalez, 2009). Cultural competency of school staff, as well as systematic programming and curricula that support cultural inclusivity are necessary ingredients for promoting multicultural practices in school settings. Increasing staff or student diversity alone—without clear emphases on multicultural competency and inclusivity—is insufficient for addressing the many problems of xenophobia and discrimination so important to immigrant youth functioning in schools (Marks & Pieloch, 2015).

XENOPHOBIA: RESEARCH ON RISK AND RESILIENCE

Because IOCY are navigating both universal and acculturative developmental competencies (see Figure 3.1), and because immigration is often not voluntary for children in migrating families (Falicov, 2013), the impacts of xenophobia on immigrant youth are of unique importance. Current empirical studies specifically focusing on xenophobia are relatively scarce in the U.S.-based literature; however, mounting research suggests that experiences of xenophobia among immigrant youth affects their—and their family members'—mental and behavioral health and social experiences at school.

Taking a family-systems approach, in which stress experienced by immigrant families affects families as a whole and each family member individually, two studies to date examined parent and adolescent dyads with an emphasis on how xenophobia affects both parents and children. In a sample of 302 Latinx parent–adolescent dyads living in the United States, Lorenzo-Blanco and colleagues (2019) explored how experiences of cultural stress affected family functioning over time. In this research, cultural stress included factors such as discrimination, acculturative stress, and a xenophobic postmigration receiving context that together contribute to stress for Latinx immigrant families. Family functioning was defined by positive relational processes including family cohesion, positive parenting, and parental involvement. Baseline adolescent cultural stress, but not parental cultural stress, predicted lower adolescent and parent family functioning over time. Although cultural stress as measured by these researchers included more than xenophobia, this finding is particularly meaningful: The authors suggested that youth may be more sensitive to cultural stressors than their parents because of developmental challenges associated with adolescence or increased exposure to diverse settings (e.g., school) compared to their parents.

How cultural stress is psychologically manifested within a family was also addressed by Kiang et al.'s (2019) investigation into how foreigner objectification, a form of xenophobia focused on presumed foreigner status directed toward immigrant individuals, affected mental health among 173 Latinx mother–adolescent-child dyads living in the United States. Among mothers and their adolescent children, foreigner objectification was linked to negative psychological outcomes, symptoms of depression among mothers, and low self-esteem and high instances of internalization and externalization among youth. The authors highlighted the importance of this finding: Despite few overall instances of foreigner objectification in their study, even a small dose of this form of xenophobia can create traumatic stress and psychological harm.

While further U.S.-based investigations into the mental and behavioral health consequences of experiencing xenophobia as an immigrant youth are limited, international research provides support for Kiang et al.'s (2019) findings. For example, among Ecuadorian immigrant youth living in Spain, experiences of xenophobia and discrimination based on country of origin were linked to significantly greater risk for mental health disorders (i.e., depression, anxiety, somatic symptoms, and social dysfunction) than was found for nonimmigrant Spanish peers (Llácer et al., 2009). In terms of behavioral health, Martínez García and Martín López (2015) found that among Latin American-origin immigrant youth living in Spain, experiences of discrimination were linked to increased risk for gang involvement, a behavior that the authors suggested may stem from a desire to seek social support after negative experiences of xenophobia.

As social support is highly important among all youth and is often provided in school settings, emerging qualitative research examines the social experiences of in-school xenophobia among immigrant youth. In a study of 60 Ghanaian immigrant youth attending school in the United States (Kumi-Yeboah & Smith, 2017), many reported xenophobia. For example, a respondent explained, "Some students in my school will make derogatory statement and negative comments because I'm from Africa. I will say that this affected my emotions and social interactions in school. I felt like I am not welcome in that class. No motivation to study in that class. . . . In the beginning of this class, nobody wanted me to be in a group with them just because I came from Africa . . . felt so rejected" (p. 445). Participants also noted that linguistic and cultural differences were significant challenges at school.

With linguistic differences among immigrant youth attending school in the United States in mind, many public schools in the United States separate immigrant students into English as a second language (ESL) classrooms. Speaking with 13 Taiwanese recent-immigrant youth attending school in the United States about their experiences of ESL programs revealed that ESL programs perpetuated youths' feelings of otherness and decreased their opportunities to form friendships with nonimmigrant peers (Tsai, 2006). One participant noted that she felt accepted by nonimmigrant peers because "they know that I am not ESL" (p. 293), a statement that highlights stigma and feelings of nonbelongingness associated with English language-learning segregation.

DISCRIMINATION: RESEARCH ON RISK AND RESILIENCE

Whereas little research has addressed xenophobia, the ill effects of discrimination have been studied for decades, with particular attention paid in post-9/11 research (Marks et al., 2015). An abundance of compelling evidence demonstrates that discrimination has widespread detrimental impacts on immigrant youth, spanning physical, psychological, academic, and social consequences (Brown, 2015). Recent research (Lo et al., 2017; Sirin et al., 2015) has supported previous findings that immigrant origin children and adolescents experience high levels of overt and covert discrimination across contexts and ethnic groups. Refugee and immigrant youth likely hold multiple disadvantaged statuses (e.g., religious beliefs, immigration status, ethnicity/ race, poverty) that may increase their risk of experiencing discrimination (Ellis et al., 2010). Some scholars have argued that prejudice and discrimination are normative experiences for immigrant youth (Ayón et al., 2017; Mirpuri et al., 2019). However, recent longitudinal, cross-sectional, and meta-analytic studies have elaborated on the associations among discrimination and a host of negative mental health and developmental outcomes (Davis et al., 2016), such as lower self-esteem, depression, anxiety, poor academic achievement, and risky behavior (Benner et al., 2018; Cano et al., 2015; Mirpuri et al., 2019).

Mixed-methods studies conducted by Pachter et al. (2018) and Patel et al. (2015) found discrimination to be particularly harmful to the psychological well-being and adjustment of recently arrived immigrant adolescents. Patel et al. identified cognitive appraisal to be a significant mediator of discriminatory events and suggested that the mediating effect of discrimination appraisal is strong for early adolescents, who may be more likely to view discriminatory experiences as serious threat. Furthermore, they identified strong, significant associations between negative attribution of ambiguous events and a decrease in self-esteem and between negative attribution of ambiguous events and an increase in depressive symptoms.

Relinquished control and peer discrimination have also been identified as important mediating factors between discrimination and depression and ethnic private regard (Chithambo et al., 2014; Huq et al., 2016). Multiple studies have shown that peer discrimination has a multiplicative negative effect on internalizing and externalizing symptoms among immigrant youth, including threats to youth ethnic private regard (i.e., sense of internal ethnic identity). Experiencing aggressive and negative feedback from peers, such as being harassed and disliked, exacerbates youth's feelings of marginalization and stigmatization, which can lead to greater internalizing symptoms, particularly given the uncontrollable nature of such negative environments (Benner et al., 2018; Cavanaugh et al., 2018).

Undocumented immigrant youth are also more likely to be victimized than their native-born youth peers, even after controlling for age, gender, race/ ethnicity, grade level, and familial affluence (Maynard et al., 2016). Findings indicate their victimization includes but is not limited to bullying, crimes, and exposure to pervasive violence (Rodriguez & Dawkins, 2017). Bullying victimization experienced among immigrant youth is linked to negative outcomes, including difficulty with interpersonal relationships, poor socioemotional health, academic-related distress, and substance use problems (Brown, 2015; Maynard et al., 2016; Stein et al., 2015).

When considering peer discrimination as a dynamic process involving perpetrators and victims, researchers often overlook the identity of the perpetrator relative to the victim. However, Stein et al. (2019) documented the adverse effects of peer discrimination perpetuated by in-group peers (i.e., Latinx) and outgroup peers (i.e., not Latinx) on Latinx adolescents. Findings showed that adolescents at highest risk of discrimination perpetuated by both in- and outgroup members reported significantly more internalizing and externalizing symptoms and more maladjustment than adolescents who were at risk for only in- or outgroup discrimination and adolescents who were not at risk for either. This research highlights that immigrant youth experience discrimination from peers of multiple identities, including those with shared identities, and that discriminatory experiences from multiple perpetrators appear to have an accumulative effect on victims (Stein et al., 2019).

Moreover, discrimination acts as a social stressor that can manifest biologically, promoting biochemical changes that increase the risk for poor physical and mental health. Prolonged exposure to these stressors can negatively impact brain development and threaten short- and long-term health through the disruption of developing neural circuitry and regulatory systems that influence physiology and behavior (Linton & Gutierrez, 2020). Therefore, some researchers assert that ethnic/racial discrimination is not only stressful but potentially traumatizing in itself (Perreira & Ornelas, 2013).

Research has demonstrated that trauma occurs frequently in the lives of immigrant youth and their parents. Perreira and Ornelas (2013) found that among 29% of foreign-born adolescents experiencing trauma during migration, 9% were at risk of developing posttraumatic stress disorder (PTSD), which was further amplified by undocumented status and discrimination postmigration. Events such as exposure to war or other forms of violence that occur in one's country of origin prior to migration also increase immigrant youth's risk for later developing PTSD (Ngo & Schleifer, 2005). Keller and colleagues (2017) found that 83% of Central American immigrants leaving their home country cited violence as a reason for fleeing, with a majority of individuals not reporting events to the police because of fear of gang-related retaliation, pressure to join, and/or corruption. Together, these findings suggest that many Latinx migrants seeking security in the United States likely have significant mental health symptoms in response to violence and persecution experienced in their origin countries.

Once immigrants enter the United States, they are often immediately disadvantaged, simply because of the ethnic/racial group they belong to. As a result, they are precluded from accessing the institutional resources that could help ameliorate the stresses of migration. In an increasingly unequal society, immigrant youth and their families find themselves segregated into more impoverished and high-crime neighborhoods and schools, where additional exposure to violence and discrimination is more likely to occur. These traumatic experiences, compounded by premigration vulnerabilities, put immigrant youth and their parents at risk for development of PTSD, generalized anxiety, and a number of acute and chronic mental health problems (Perreira & Ornelas, 2013). Furthermore, transgenerational trauma expands the severity of traumatic migration experiences on mental health concerns of entire families and across multiple generations. Research has indicated that youth whose parents experienced trauma were more likely to exhibit unique vulnerability to PTSD, to have higher levels of mistrust, and to experience identity confusion and isolation (Diaz & Fenning, 2017).

Despite all this hardship, studies have shown that immigrant adolescents in general have unique developmental patterns of strength, resilience, and increasing mental health heading into adulthood (Sirin et al., 2015). Although Latinx adolescents' strong sense of *familismo* (i.e., strong loyalty to family, family communication, and family values) may provide a vulnerability to transgenerational trauma, it has also been identified as a significant protective factor in the face of discrimination (Cavanaugh et al., 2018; Diaz & Fenning, 2017; Perreira et al., 2013). In a longitudinal study, Cavanaugh and colleagues (2018) found that despite high levels discrimination and foreigner objectification, Latinx youth reporting a high number of cultural assets reported protection against externalizing and internalizing symptoms. Reflecting prior research (cf. Umaña-Taylor et al., 2015), Cavanaugh et al. found that academic motivation and prosocial behavior are promoted by an embodiment of a strong enculturation orientation guided by cultural values, a strong racial/ethnic identity, and strong connection to family. Davis et al. (2016) analogously identified prosocial altruistic behaviors as a powerful protective factor against depressive symptoms linked to experiences of discrimination. Additionally, social support can be an essential protective factor, particularly peer support that attenuates the negative consequences associated with peer discrimination (Gonzalez et al., 2014). Religious identity may also serve as a protective factor in communities in which religion plays a central role. Studies with Mexican and Muslim immigrant adolescents have identified positive religious coping as a strategy to combat sociocultural stressors (e.g., stigma, social marginalization; Ahmed et al., 2011; Sirin & Katsiaficas, 2011). These promotive factors are directly associated with positive psychological outcomes and increased life satisfaction and serve as a buffer against acculturative stress (Ahmed et al., 2011).

Finally, considering the social characteristics of immigrant-origin children's and youths' national receiving contexts is imperative for understanding the effects of discrimination on their development (Marks et al., 2018). Negative social discourse and restrictive immigration laws have significant impacts on immigrant youth and families (Ayón et al., 2017). Institutions that work with immigrant youth have unique opportunities and obligations to harness resilient qualities and institute programs and policies that foster positive development for immigrant youth. Migration provides an opportunity for institutions to offer prosocial development, self-growth, self-efficacy, and self-affirmation gained through experiences that force individuals to use various skills in new experiences (Adair, 2015; Brown, 2015). Schools are positioned to provide a context that cultivates equity and inclusion, principles that have been shown to reduce prejudice and discrimination. Education and learning-based initiatives (e.g., culturally responsive teaching, multicultural education) in addition to identity-affirming programs amongst immigrant and ethnic/racial minority students have shown positive effects for immigrant and nonimmigrant students and for overall school climate (Schachner, 2019). Among immigrant adolescents, a sense of purpose in life (e.g., obligation to help family) and support-seeking behaviors are adaptive coping strategies that buffer against the stressful effects of undocumented status, discrimination, stereotypes, and family obligation (Ayón et al., 2017). Youth who respond to discrimination in a proactive way through discussion, community engagement, and self-affirmation tend to have higher self-esteem (Ayón, 2016; Sirin & Katsiaficas, 2011). Similarly, immigrant children who employ active coping such as reporting an incident or approaching the perpetrator are more empowered and display increased motivation and reduced stress (Ayón, 2016; Brown, 2015).

CASE STUDIES FROM COMMUNITY-BASED RESEARCH: PROFILES OF TRAUMA, STRESS, AND RESILIENCE

Aligned with the integrative risk and resilience model that emphasizes multisystem effects on risk and resilience associated with developmental adaptations for IOCY, our research is aimed at hearing directly from youth who have recently immigrated to the United States and their family members about their stories of challenges and resilience. Our qualitative research approaches allow for participants to discuss multiple dimensions and spaces in which postmigration adjustment and related experiences unfold. Taken directly from our research study of the psychological experiences of Latinx immigrant families living in the Northeast United States, the following descriptions of family experiences with migration, discrimination, and adjustment to the United States exemplify both the traumatic stress and the resilience of these parents and children during migration and acculturation.

The stories presented here were collected in 2018 and 2019 as part of a study designed to capture the lived experiences of families who currently fear deportation from the United States. The participants were parents and children living in an urban area of the Northeast United States. Most participants originally came from Latin American countries whose temporary protected status had recently been revoked or was threatened to be revoked, or they were Latinx community members residing in the United States without legal documentation. The families' reasons for relocating to the United States typically involve premigration trauma and include fleeing from domestic violence, gang violence, extreme poverty, and armed conflict.

Ana[1] was born in the United States in 2010. She currently lives with her mother, Maria, who crossed the U.S.–Mexico border twice. At the first border crossing, Maria was detained for 54 days at a U.S. jail and was then transported back across the U.S. border to Mexico in the trunk of an authority's truck. She sustained several burns to her neck and back in the trunk, which was hot and unventilated, and still bears a scar from that trip. Maria then moved to Portugal and received asylum due to domestic abuse. After living there for 2 years, she received a tourist visa to come to the United States, where she has been living for the past 13 years with Ana's father.

Ana is a sweet girl with a soft demeanor. She told us about being harassed by her peers at school: "There's three kids in my school that have been bothering me for a year. . . . One in particular . . . she really scares me. She makes me feel unprotected. She is really mean to me." Ana described ridicule and physical abuse, including name calling, hair pulling, and physical pushing, and she sensed that she was not accepted in general. She said that her classmates make fun of her for speaking Portuguese, and when she is not harassed, she is ignored. When we asked her whether she had any fears, she stated, "The only fear I have is that my parents are not going to come back home, or for some reason they might disappear." When asked what she does to help herself feel better, she said she likes to write: "Usually when I get really upset I like to write . . . and I am writing a story about my life."

In another family, we met with a mother of three children, originally from Guatemala. When we asked this mother to complete a PTSD checklist to assess her current psychological symptoms prior to her interview, she scored very high and well into the clinical range. Her parenting stress levels were also extremely high, and her anxiety and depression scores were elevated but subclinical. She had never received mental health services. Seño's[2] children were living in Mexico, where her husband is originally from, and though her children dreamed of coming to live with her, she said she couldn't imagine how that would happen "now that the way things are going here politically." Seño began her migration story stating that she crossed the border in Texas with the help of *coyotes*—mob-like individuals who smuggle people across the border through dangerous terrain. She initially minimized her telling of her migration as "a lot like other people . . . not that bad," stating that she also "does not remember" many details of the crossing and does not like to talk about it. After some time talking with us about her life, however, she recounted a story of being confined to an abandoned house with dozens of other migrants for 2 months, halfway through her journey, without communication to her family or anyone other than the coyotes. She then told of her elation when they were finally allowed to begin their journey again. Notably, she left us with a resounding message of resilience and hope when we asked her what she wanted others to know about what it is like to be an immigrant

---

[1] All case material has been altered to protect confidentiality.
[2] Her chosen pseudonym, *seño*, is Spanish for "ma'am."

in the United States today: "You just have to keep going as long as you can, you just have to push forward. . . . Help other people while you can. The way you help me, I help others. And we have to help everyone else too. Everyone needs some help."

In many ways, the stories of Ana and Maria and of Seño are typical narratives we hear from our community partners and research participants. They are stories that include hardship and trauma from their lives before migration and during the migration process, as well as stories of challenge and harassment living in the United States. We also hear countless examples of strength and resilience—of persistence through hardship and coping skills that help children and adults live meaningful lives and adjust to the challenges of being an immigrant in the United States As researchers, we work closely alongside community workers who help protect immigrant workers' rights, provide after-school care for immigrant youth, and promote physical and mental health care for mixed-legal-status and undocumented families. As researchers, we attend community events, engage in volunteerism, and listen closely to the stories shared with us. Our research team is multicultural and multilingual, and we take a community-based participatory action approach to our work, enabling us to identify and provide resources directly back to our community partners as we gain insight into the most pressing challenges they currently face.

INTERVENTION EFFORTS AND FUTURE DIRECTIONS

In this final section, we turn our attention to some recent efforts that are aimed at helping children, youth, and adults to cope with racism and discrimination. Because xenophobia and discrimination can occur at multiple ecological levels—and across all contexts of reception during migration—interventions must be designed in multiple settings on behalf of IOCY. Although we are currently unaware of interventions targeting discrimination and xenophobia specifically designed within immigrant communities, there are numerous empirically supported interventions for helping families of color to cope positively with racism. One prominent area of this intervention literature has sought to capture the positive, resilient aspects of forming a strong ethnic/racial identity (ERI) as a buffer against discrimination. ERI is a developmental construct that captures how an individual feels about themselves with respect to their membership in an ethnic or racial social group. ERI includes feelings such as pride and shame, cognitions such as self-labeling, and behaviors that develop throughout the lifespan such as ethnic/racial socialization in the family (Williams et al., 2020). Studies are increasingly documenting the benefits of having a strong, positive ERI for coping with discrimination (e.g., Motti-Stefanidi & Masten, 2017), as ERI has been shown to foster higher self-esteem and positive psychological adaptation skills within immigrant communities. Among a sample of immigrant adolescents, ERI had a protective effect, with stronger feelings of belonging associated with fewer reports of discrimination

1 year later. Adolescents with less well-developed ERIs reported more discrimination (Gonzales-Backen et al., 2018). Importantly, research suggests that schools can actively foster positive ERI development among students. Meaningful discussions at school about race and ethnicity and school-organized events that dispel negative stereotypes associated with immigrants contribute to positive ERI development among youth (Aldana & Byrd, 2015; Gonzalez, 2009).

Scholars have already begun synthesizing the research base on behalf of IOCY and students of color to be applied to new interventions and policies (see the review by Jones & Neblett, 2016). Although not specifically addressing immigrant youth, Anderson and Stevenson (2019) presented the racial encounter coping appraisal socialization theory (RECAST) to support African American youth and families facing racism and race-related trauma. The model combines aspects of behavioral and cognitive approaches to understanding and coping with racism, focusing on adaptive psychological skills such as reappraisal, decision making, and resolution of the discriminatory experience. This type of program also emphasizes positive family socialization practices and behaviors and cognitive understanding of self-efficacy to promote positive outcomes related to identity and psychological, academic, and social well-being. A key component of such approaches is taking a family-systems perspective, providing education and support to parents to help their children (and themselves) understand racism and talk openly about how to cope with instances of discrimination. Support programs designed within immigrant communities could be particularly helpful and useful today and should include components focused not only on discrimination and ERI but also on the psychological experiences of anxiety, fear, and PTSD that are brought about by harassment due to legal statuses and fear of deportation.

Another recent intervention, the Identity Project, combined a universal mental health promotion approach with a focus on helping youth to consolidate—or reconcile in a positive way—their ERIs (Umaña-Taylor, Kornienko, et al., 2018). Umaña-Taylor and colleagues (2018) took a multicultural approach to promote positive ERI development among adolescents from all ethnic/racial backgrounds, focusing on *identity consolidation*, the meaning making necessary to integrate a sense of self as one currently is with an identity one hopes to become (Erikson, 1968). Using a randomized controlled design, this program promoted ERI consolidation and positive psychosocial well-being outcomes, including increased self-esteem and improved academic grades. This type of programming could easily be adapted for use with immigrant communities, measuring outcomes related to coping with perceived discrimination or the psychological effects of xenophobia. For example, moving beyond ERI consolidation, the intervention might include elements specifically targeting effective behaviors for coping with xenophobia. Additionally, increasing the capacity for safe reporting of and systemic response to acts of discrimination and hate crimes in schools, neighborhoods, and other settings may help further promote the healthy adaptation of IOCY.

CONCLUSION

This chapter presents theory and research demonstrating the challenges faced by IOCY in a social receiving context of increasing xenophobia and discrimination in the United States. Using a new theoretical framework emphasizing that social settings can be both risk promoting and resilience promoting, we outlined the various ways children's ecological settings—particularly schools—can be both detrimental to and facilitating of the development of IOCY. Case studies from our research with immigrant families provide a rich picture of the lived experiences of children and parents, who shared their challenges of fear of deportation and xenophobia as well as their resilience during the acculturation process. Future studies should focus on community-based approaches to ameliorate the deleterious effects of discrimination on the development of IOCY.

REFERENCES

Adair, J. K. (2015). *The impact of discrimination on the early schooling experiences of children from immigrant families.* Migration Policy Institute.

Ahmed, S. R., Kia-Keating, M., & Tsai, K. H. (2011). A structural model of racial discrimination, acculturative stress, and cultural resources among Arab American adolescents. *American Journal of Community Psychology, 48*(3–4), 181–192. https://doi.org/10.1007/s10464-011-9424-3

Aldana, A., & Byrd, C. M. (2015). School ethnic–racial socialization: Learning about race and ethnicity among African American students. *The Urban Review, 47*(3), 563–576. https://doi.org/10.1007/s11256-014-0319-0

American Bar Association. (2019). *The rising tide of hate: How welcoming the stranger in a nation of immigrants has turned violent.* https://www.americanbar.org/groups/public_interest/immigration/events-and-cle/the-rising-tide-of-hate--how-welcoming-the-stranger-in-a-nation-/

Anderson, R. E., & Stevenson, H. C. (2019). RECASTing racial stress and trauma: Theorizing the healing potential of racial socialization in families. *American Psychologist, 74*(1), 63–75. https://doi.org/10.1037/amp0000392

Ayón, C. (2016). Talking to children about race, inequality, and discrimination: Raising families in an anti-immigrant political environment. *Journal of the Society for Social Work and Research, 7*(3), 449–477. https://doi.org/10.1086/686929

Ayón, C., Valencia-Garcia, D., & Kim, S. (2017). Latino immigrant families and restrictive immigration climate: Perceived experiences with discrimination, threat to family, social exclusion, children's vulnerability, and related factors. *Race and Social Problems, 9*(4), 300–312. https://doi.org/10.1007/s12552-017-9215-z

Benner, A. D., Wang, Y., Shen, Y., Boyle, A. E., Polk, R., & Cheng, Y.-P. (2018). Racial/ethnic discrimination and well-being during adolescence: A meta-analytic review. *American Psychologist, 73*(7), 855–883. https://doi.org/10.1037/amp0000204

Britto, P. R. (2011, September 23). *Global battleground or school playground: The bullying of America's Muslim children.* Institute for Social Policy and Understanding. https://www.ispu.org/global-battleground-or-school-playground-the-bullying-of-americas-muslim-children/

Brown, C. S. (2015). *The educational, psychological, and social impact of discrimination on the immigrant child.* Migration Policy Institute. https://www.migrationpolicy.org/research/educational-psychological-and-social-impact-discrimination-immigrant-child

Brown, C. S., & Chu, H. (2012). Discrimination, ethnic identity, and academic outcomes of Mexican immigrant children: The importance of school context. *Child Development, 83*(5), 1477–1485. https://doi.org/10.1111/j.1467-8624.2012.01786.x

Cano, M. Á., Schwartz, S. J., Castillo, L. G., Romero, A. J., Huang, S., Lorenzo-Blanco, E. I., Unger, J. B., Zamboanga, B. L., Des Rosiers, S. E., Baezconde-Garbanati, L., Lizzi, K. M., Soto, D. W., Oshri, A., Villamar, J. A., Pattarroyo, M., & Szapocznik, J. (2015). Depressive symptoms and externalizing behaviors among Hispanic immigrant adolescents: Examining longitudinal effects of cultural stress. *Journal of Adolescence, 42,* 31–39. https://doi.org/10.1016/j.adolescence.2015.03.017

Cavanaugh, A. M., Stein, G. L., Supple, A. J., Gonzalez, L. M., & Kiang, L. (2018). Protective and promotive effects of Latino early adolescents' cultural assets against multiple types of discrimination. *Journal of Research on Adolescence, 28*(2), 310–326. https://doi.org/10.1111/jora.12331

Child Trends. (2013). *Dual language learners and social-emotional development: The benefits for young children.* http://www.childtrends.org/dual-language-learners-and-social-emotional-development-understanding-the-benefits-for-young-children/

Chithambo, T. P., Huey Jr, S. J., & Cespedes-Knadle, Y. (2014). Perceived discrimination and Latino youth adjustment: Examining the role of relinquished control and sociocultural influences. *Journal of Latina/o Psychology, 2*(1), 54. https://doi.org/10.1037/lat0000012

Davis, A. N., Carlo, G., Schwartz, S. J., Unger, J. B., Zamboanga, B. L., Lorenzo-Blanco, E. I., Cano, M. Á., Baezconde-Garbanati, L., Oshri, A., Streit, C., Martinez, M. M., Piña-Watson, B., Lizzi, K., & Soto, D. (2016). The longitudinal associations between discrimination, depressive symptoms, and prosocial behaviors in U.S. Latino/a recent immigrant adolescents. *Journal of Youth and Adolescence, 45*(3), 457–470. https://doi.org/10.1007/s10964-015-0394-x

Devos, T., & Banaji, M. R. (2005). American = White? *Journal of Personality and Social Psychology, 88*(3), 447–466. https://doi.org/10.1037/0022-3514.88.3.447

Diaz, Y., & Fenning, P. (2017). Toward understanding mental health concerns for the Latinx immigrant student: A review of the literature. *Urban Education.* Advance online publication. https://doi.org/10.1177/0042085917721953

Ellis, B. H., MacDonald, H. Z., Klunk-Gillis, J., Lincoln, A., Strunin, L., & Cabral, H. J. (2010). Discrimination and mental health among Somali refugee adolescents: The role of acculturation and gender. *American Journal of Orthopsychiatry, 80*(4), 564–575. https://doi.org/10.1111/j.1939-0025.2010.01061.x

Erikson, E. H. (1968). *Identity, youth and crisis.* W. W. Norton & Company.

Falicov, C. J. (2013). *Latino families in therapy* (2nd ed.). Guilford Press.

Gonzales-Backen, M. A., Meca, A., Lorenzo-Blanco, E. I., Des Rosiers, S. E., Córdova, D., Soto, D. W., Cano, M. Á., Oshri, A., Zamboanga, B. L., Baezconde-Garbanati, L., Schwartz, S. J., Szapocznik, J., & Unger, J. B. (2018). Examining the temporal order of ethnic identity and perceived discrimination among Hispanic immigrant adolescents. *Developmental Psychology, 54*(5), 929–937. https://doi.org/10.1037/dev0000465

Gonzalez, L. M., Stein, G. L., Kiang, L., & Cupito, A. M. (2014). The impact of discrimination and support on developmental competencies in Latino adolescents. *Journal of Latina/o Psychology, 2*(2), 79–91. https://doi.org/10.1037/lat0000014

Gonzalez, R. (2009). Beyond affirmation: How the school context facilitates racial/ethnic identity among Mexican American adolescents. *Hispanic Journal of Behavioral Sciences, 31*(1), 5–31. https://doi.org/10.1177/0739986308328387

Hoyt, C., Jr. (2012). The pedagogy of the meaning of racism: Reconciling a discordant discourse. *Social Work, 57*(3), 225–234. https://doi.org/10.1093/sw/sws009

Huq, N., Stein, G. L., & Gonzalez, L. M. (2016). Acculturation conflict among Latino youth: Discrimination, ethnic identity, and depressive symptoms. *Cultural Diversity & Ethnic Minority Psychology, 22*(3), 377–385. https://doi.org/10.1037/cdp0000070

Huynh, Q. L., Devos, T., & Smalarz, L. (2011). Perpetual foreigner in one's own land: Potential implications for identity and psychological adjustment. *Journal of Social and Clinical Psychology, 30*(2), 133–162. https://doi.org/10.1521/jscp.2011.30.2.133

Jones, S. C., & Neblett, E. W. (2016). Racial-ethnic protective factors and mechanisms in psychosocial prevention and intervention programs for Black youth. *Clinical Child and Family Psychology Review, 19*(2), 134–161. https://doi.org/10.1007/s10567-016-0201-6

Keller, A., Joscelyne, A., Granski, M., & Rosenfeld, B. (2017). Pre-migration trauma exposure and mental health functioning among Central American migrants arriving at the US border. *PLOS ONE, 12*(1), e0168692. https://doi.org/10.1371/journal.pone.0168692

Kiang, L., Broome, M., Chan, M., Stein, G. L., Gonzalez, L. M., & Supple, A. J. (2019). Foreigner objectification, English proficiency, and adjustment among youth and mothers from Latinx American backgrounds. *Cultural Diversity & Ethnic Minority Psychology, 25*(4), 461–471. https://doi.org/10.1037/cdp0000216

Kumi-Yeboah, A., & Smith, P. (2017). Cross-cultural educational experiences and academic achievement of Ghanaian immigrant youth in urban public schools. *Education and Urban Society, 49*(4), 434–455. https://doi.org/10.1177/0013124516643764

Landale, N. S., Hardie, J. H., Oropesa, R. S., & Hillemeier, M. M. (2015). Behavioral functioning among Mexican-origin children: Does parental legal status matter? *Journal of Health and Social Behavior, 56*(1), 2–18. https://doi.org/10.1177/0022146514567896

Linton, J. M., & Gutierrez, J. R. (2020). Latinx child health: Challenges and opportunities to build a healthy future. In A. Martínez & S. Rhodes (Eds.), *New and emerging issues in Latinx health* (pp. 63–95). Springer Nature Switzerland. https://doi.org/10.1007/978-3-030-24043-1_4

Llácer, A., Amo, J. D., García-Fulgueiras, A., Ibáñez-Rojo, V., García-Pino, R., Jarrín, I., Díaz, D., Fernández-Liria, A., García-Ortuzar, V., Mazarrasa, L., Rodríguez-Arenas, M. A., & Zunzunegui, M. V. (2009). Discrimination and mental health in Ecuadorian immigrants in Spain. *Journal of Epidemiology and Community Health, 63*(9), 766–772. https://doi.org/10.1136/jech.2008.085530

Lo, C. C., Hopson, L. M., Simpson, G. M., & Cheng, T. C. (2017). Racial/ethnic differences in emotional health: A longitudinal study of immigrants' adolescent children. *Community Mental Health Journal, 53*(1), 92–101. https://doi.org/10.1007/s10597-016-0049-8

Lorenzo-Blanco, E. I., Meca, A., Piña-Watson, B., Zamboanga, B. L., Szapocznik, J., Cano, M. A., Cordova, D., Unger, J. B., Romero, A., Des Rosiers, S. E., Soto, D. W., Villamar, J. A., Pattarroyo, M., Lizzi, K. M., & Schwartz, S. J. (2019). Longitudinal trajectories of family functioning among recent immigrant adolescents and parents: Links with adolescent and parent cultural stress, emotional well-being, and behavioral health. *Child Development, 90*(2), 506–523. https://doi.org/10.1111/cdev.12914

Marks, A. K., Ejesi, K., McCullough, M., & Garcia Coll, C. (2015). The development and implications of racism and discrimination. In M. Lamb, C. Garcia Coll, & R. Lerner (Eds.), *Handbook of child psychology and developmental science* (7th ed., Vol. 3; pp. 324–365). John Wiley & Sons.

Marks, A. K., McKenna, J., & Garcia Coll, C. (2018). National receiving contexts: A critical aspect of native-born, immigrant, and refugee youth well-being. *European Psychologist, 23*(1), 6–20. https://doi.org/10.1027/1016-9040/a000311

Marks, A. K., & Pieloch, K. (2015). The school contexts of U.S. immigrant children and adolescents. In C. Suarez-Orozco, M. Abo-Zena, & A. K. Marks (Eds.), *Transitions: The development of children of immigrants* (pp. 47–60). NYU Press.

Martínez García, J. M., & Martín López, M. J. (2015). Group violence and migration experience among Latin American youths in justice enforcement centers (Madrid, Spain). *The Spanish Journal of Psychology, 18*, E85. https://doi.org/10.1017/sjp.2015.87

Maynard, B. R., Vaughn, M. G., Salas-Wright, C. P., & Vaughn, S. (2016). Bullying victimization among school-aged immigrant youth in the United States. *The Journal of Adolescent Health, 58*(3), 337–344. https://doi.org/10.1016/j.jadohealth.2015.11.013

Mirpuri, S., Ray, C., Hassan, A., Aladin, M., Wang, Y., & Yip, T. (2019). Ethnic/racial identity as a moderator of the relationship between discrimination and adolescent outcomes. In H. Fitzgerald, D. Johnson, D. Qin, F. Villarruel, & J. Norder (Eds.), *Handbook of children and prejudice* (pp. 477–499). Springer Nature Switzerland. https://doi.org/10.1007/978-3-030-12228-7_27

Motti-Stefanidi, F., & Masten, A. S. (2017). A resilience perspective on immigrant youth adaptation and development. In N. Cabrera & B. Leyendecker (Eds.), *Handbook on positive development of minority children and youth* (pp. 19–34). Springer Science & Business Media. https://doi.org/10.1007/978-3-319-43645-6_2

Nawaz, A. (2020, April 1). *Asian Americans report rise in racist attacks amid pandemic.* PBS NewsHour. https://www.pbs.org/newshour/show/what-anti-asian-attacks-say-about-american-culture-during-crisis

Ngo, H., & Schleifer, B. (2005). Immigrant children and youth in focus. *The Canadian,* (Spring), 29–33.

Omi, M., & Winant, H. (2014). *Racial formation in the United States.* Routledge. https://doi.org/10.4324/9780203076804

Pachter, L. M., Caldwell, C. H., Jackson, J. S., & Bernstein, B. A. (2018). Discrimination and mental health in a representative sample of African-American and Afro-Caribbean youth. *Journal of Racial and Ethnic Health Disparities, 5*(4), 831–837. https://doi.org/10.1007/s40615-017-0428-z

Patel, S. G., Tabb, K. M., Strambler, M. J., & Eltareb, F. (2015). Newcomer immigrant adolescents and ambiguous discrimination: The role of cognitive appraisal. *Journal of Adolescent Research, 30*(1), 7–30. https://doi.org/10.1177/0743558414546717

Perreira, K. M., Kiang, L., & Potochnick, S. (2013). Ethnic discrimination: Identifying and intervening in its effects on the education of immigrant children. In E. L. Grigorenko (Ed.), *U.S. immigration and education: Cultural and policy issues across the lifespan* (pp. 137–161). Springer.

Perreira, K. M., & Ornelas, I. (2013). Painful passages: Traumatic experiences and post-traumatic stress among immigrant Latino adolescents and their primary caregivers. *The International Migration Review, 47*(4). https://doi.org/10.1111/imre.12050

Roberg, R., Murry, M., Ramos, Z., Zhang, L., & Marks, A. K. (2020, May). *What we know about the social and emotional impacts of COVID-19 on immigrant families.* Research to Policy Collaboration.

Rodriguez, F. A., & Dawkins, M. (2017). Undocumented Latino youth: Migration experiences and the challenges of integrating into American society. *Journal of International Migration and Integration, 18*(2), 419–438. https://doi.org/10.1007/s12134-016-0484-y

Schachner, M. K. (2019). From equality and inclusion to cultural pluralism—Evolution and effects of cultural diversity perspectives in schools. *European Journal of Developmental Psychology, 16*(1), 1–17. https://doi.org/10.1080/17405629.2017.1326378

Sirin, S. R., & Katsiaficas, D. (2011). Religiosity, discrimination, and community engagement: Gendered pathways of Muslim American emerging adults. *Youth and Society, 43*(4), 1528–1546. https://doi.org/10.1177/0044118X10388218

Sirin, S. R., Rogers-Sirin, L., Cressen, J., Gupta, T., Ahmed, S. F., & Novoa, A. D. (2015). Discrimination-related stress effects on the development of internalizing symptoms among Latino adolescents. *Child Development, 86*(3), 709–725. https://doi.org/10.1111/cdev.12343

Stein, G. L., Cavanaugh, A. M., Supple, A. J., Kiang, L., & Gonzalez, L. M. (2019). Typologies of discrimination: Latinx youth's experiences in an emerging immigrant community. *Developmental Psychology, 55*(4), 846–854. https://doi.org/10.1037/dev0000638

Stein, G. L., Gonzalez, L. M., Cupito, A. M., Kiang, L., & Supple, A. J. (2015). The protective role of familism in the lives of Latino adolescents. *Journal of Family Issues, 36*(10), 1255–1273. https://doi.org/10.1177/0192513X13502480

Suárez-Orozco, C., Hernández, M. G., & Casanova, S. (2015). "It's sort of my calling": The civic engagement and social responsibility of Latino immigrant-origin young adults. *Research in Human Development, 12*(1–2), 84–99. https://doi.org/10.1080/15427609.2015.1010350

Suárez-Orozco, C., Motti-Stefanidi, F., Marks, A., & Katsiaficas, D. (2018). An integrative risk and resilience model for understanding the adaptation of immigrant-origin children and youth. *American Psychologist, 73*(6), 781–796. https://doi.org/10.1037/amp0000265

Tsai, J. H. (2006). Xenophobia, ethnic community, and immigrant youths' friendship network formation. *Adolescence, 41*(162), 285–298.

Umaña-Taylor, A. J., Kornienko, O., Douglass Bayless, S., & Updegraff, K. A. (2018). A universal intervention program increases ethnic-racial identity exploration and resolution to predict adolescent psychosocial functioning one year later. *Journal of Youth and Adolescence, 47*(1), 1–15. https://doi.org/10.1007/s10964-017-0766-5

Umaña-Taylor, A. J., Tynes, B. M., Toomey, R. B., Williams, D. R., & Mitchell, K. J. (2015). Latino adolescents' perceived discrimination in online and offline settings: An examination of cultural risk and protective factors. *Developmental Psychology, 51*(1), 87–100. https://doi.org/10.1037/a0038432

U.S. Federal Bureau of Investigation. (2017). *2017 hate crime statistics released.* https://www.fbi.gov/news/stories/2017-hate-crime-statistics-released-111318

Williams, C. D., Byrd, C. M., Quintana, S. M., Anicama, C., Kiang, L., Umaña-Taylor, A. J., Calzada, E. J., Dyer, J., Gautier, M. P., Ejesi, K., Tuitt, N. R., Martinez-Fuentes, S., White, L., Marks, A. K., Rogers, L. O., & Whitesell, N. (2020). *A lifespan model of ethnic-racial identity* [Unpublished manuscript]. University of Virginia.

Yakushko, O. (2009). Xenophobia: Understanding the roots and consequences of negative attitudes toward immigrants. *The Counseling Psychologist, 37*(1), 36–66. https://doi.org/10.1177/0011000008316034

4

Racism and Xenophobia on U.S. College Campuses

Anmol Satiani and Sindhu Singh

Given the current social and political climate in the United States, including current immigration policies, university students are being challenged with a range of forms of racism, xenophobia, sexism, heterosexism, classism, and other forms of oppression. Although these experiences have been an ongoing problem over the course of decades, the past 3 years have seen a rise in explicit displays of xenophobia and racism on college campuses across the United States (Kerr, 2018; Quinton, 2019). The COVID-19 crisis has further led to displacement of many college students from their campuses and has resulted in a rise of racial prejudice and attacks against Asian American students.

This chapter includes a discussion of trends in the broader sociopolitical climate in the United States and the impact on university campuses, such as the effects of White supremacy and threats of violence. We review scholarship focused on the experiences of college students of color, including racial minority children of immigrants and international students, with respect to racism and other forms of sociocultural oppression and prejudice. We then discuss, through clinical case vignettes, how these experiences shape students' psychological well-being and identity. These case examples from our clinical practice in a university counseling center illustrate some of the complexities of working with students in the contemporary climate. We address how college students work to resist social injustice on their campuses and elsewhere, and we provide recommendations for psychologists working with and supporting college students in coping with and resisting these challenges.

https://doi.org/10.1037/0000214-005
Trauma and Racial Minority Immigrants: Turmoil, Uncertainty, and Resistance,
P. Tummala-Narra (Editor)

We approach our work from ecological and systemic lenses in that we examine the impact of the current social and political context on college students' health (Bronfenbrenner, 1979). From this approach, we recognize that the student is influenced by several spheres or systems, including the immediate university environment and the larger sociopolitical climate, and that these spheres are interacting with and influencing each other and the experiences of the student. We consider the student to be an active participant in multiple contexts and acknowledge that we, as practitioners, are also influenced by our contexts.

IMPACT OF THE BROADER SOCIOPOLITICAL CLIMATE ON COLLEGE CAMPUSES: WHITE SUPREMACY AND THREATS OF VIOLENCE

The broader climate of xenophobia and racism in the United States has significantly impacted college campuses across the nation. The Anti-Defamation League issued a report in 2018 stating that "racist fliers, banners and stickers were found on college campuses 147 times in fall 2017, a more than threefold increase over the 41 cases reported one year before" (Kerr, 2018). They attributed this increase to White supremacist groups being more active on college campuses and recruiting more members as national politics shifted. "White supremacists are targeting college campuses like never before," the Anti-Defamation League's chief executive, Jonathan Greenblatt, stated in a news release (cited in Kerr, 2018). "They see campuses as a fertile recruiting ground, as evident by the unprecedented volume of propagandist activity designed to recruit young people to support their vile ideology." White supremacist groups such as Identity Evropa, Patriot Front, and Vanguard America are some of the most influential on college campuses. In fact, Identity Evropa is responsible for nearly half of the reported incidents of propaganda (Kerr, 2018). These efforts of White supremacist groups have had important consequences. One significant example was the August 2017 rally that attracted White supremacists to the University of Virginia; it ultimately resulted in a person driving a car into counterprotesters and causing the death of a 32-year-old woman (Binkley, 2018).

The Southern Poverty Law Center (SPLC; 2017) released a publication entitled *The Alt-Right on Campus: What Students Need to Know.* They explained that the reason that these groups are targeting university campuses is that universities "embrace diversity, tolerance, and social justice. They strive for equality and have created safe spaces for students of every gender and identity. College campuses are home to the highest ideals of human rights." One trend has been for alt-right or conservative student groups on campus to invite speakers who are provocateurs and who wish to incite violence. The SPLC made several suggestions for students who are trying to counteract this trend, as it may be difficult to stop. For instance, they suggested that students "deprive the speaker of the thing he or she wants most—a spectacle" and hold an alternative event that focuses on hope, inclusion, and democratic values. Within the context of these developments on campuses, students of color and other marginalized students have to navigate White supremacy in new forms. In particular, external groups are igniting violence by capitalizing on vulnerabilities, fears, and belief systems of some White students.

One of the "headliners" in this SPLC publication is Milo Yiannopolus, a British public speaker, writer, and former editor for Breitbart News who has routinely made racist, sexist, and heterosexist comments in his writing and speaking events. He was invited to our campus (DePaul University) to speak in May 2016 by the student Republican group on campus, an experience that was difficult for our campus because a riot resulted when student protesters shut down this event. The university later revised some policies and procedures and examined questions of free speech and hate speech. Students of color and LGBTQ-identified students were physically attacked at the event, with security standing by and witnessing the attacks. For days and months after this event, students who had protested the event were harassed, threatened, and intimidated, both in person and on social media. One student of color, a known activist on campus who was at this event, disclosed to Anmol (first author) that she was being followed by men in the Young Republican groups on campus. For example, she described an experience in which she was followed into an elevator by four or five White male students: "They were trying to intimidate me." Minoritized students described feeling fearful for their physical and emotional safety both during and after this event. This experience of fear has been shared by many students of color and students with marginalized identities, such as LGBTQ-identified students, across the United States on their respective campuses.

Furthermore, in recent years, many students recognize the possibility of being physically attacked or victimized by some other form of violence. Gun violence, in particular, poses a serious risk to safety on U.S. college campuses. The Gun Violence Archive Staff (2019) estimated that there were 418 mass shootings in the United States in 2019. One consequence is significant fear of gun violence on college campuses. For example, we have heard from students of color activists on campus that they worry about White supremacy taking the form of violence on their campus. These students are often being targeted on social media because of their activism, resulting in fears of being in public spaces on campus or anywhere and fears of being followed.

RACIST LANGUAGE ON COLLEGE CAMPUSES

Earlier in this chapter, we discussed the infiltration of White supremacist groups on campus, supported by college students who harbor and act on racist views. Bauer-Wolf (2017) reported a list of racist incidents in September 2017, which included the assault of a Black student and racist language and symbols, such as a note on a student's door that read "filthy [N-word]," a swastika carved into a campus elevator, the N-word written on a whiteboard, and the N-word written on door name tags of Black students. A number of campuses across the country have also reported racist graffiti in residential halls and classrooms. It is noteworthy that "N-word" seems to have expanded to apply to multiple groups of color, not just Black students. *The Chronicle of Higher Education* and other news outlets continue to publish logs of racist events occurring on college campuses, highlighting that they are continually occurring and that they are expected to continue (Dreid & Najmabadi, 2016).

Some have also observed, more anecdotally, that certain uses of language have now become more acceptable on college campuses, mirroring what is happening on the national scene. For example, the use of the N-word by White students seems more acceptable on college campuses. I (Anmol) have worked with several White cisgender heterosexual-identified men who come to counseling with unrelated presenting concerns but disclose in the course of counseling that they routinely use the N-word with their friends. One male student used this term and other derogatory terms toward women and people of color on a dating app; the woman with whom he was corresponding—a person of color—contacted the student's university and reported his offensive language. A staff person in the Student Affairs office, concerned about the student's level of distress after he was informed of the report, referred him to the counseling service. The student was concerned that there would be some consequence for his use of language; he seemed incredulous and very upset that someone would mistake his language as serious commentary about the woman with whom he was corresponding, because he had intended it as a joke. He had difficulty understanding why "this was such a big deal." This example speaks to the casual ways in which offensive, damaging language is used and the lack of understanding of the historical and the current implications of using such language. Another disturbing issue is that some of this language is used on social media. Individuals are not using this language in face-to-face interactions and perhaps not recognizing the impact that it can have on others: Students of color experience tremendous anxiety, fear, and anger on the other side of these interactions.

EXPERIENCES OF STUDENTS OF COLOR ON COLLEGE CAMPUSES

Research indicates that many students of color on college campuses experience significant racism-related stress. For example, Harwood and colleagues (2012) identified over 70 distinct racial microaggressions experienced by students of color on a predominately White campus. These microaggressions included racial jokes and verbal comments, racial slurs in shared spaces, segregated spaces, and unequal treatment. Student athletes of color can be racially targeted by opponents, fans, or even by their own team members (Zestcott & Brown, 2015).

Within classrooms, when race is discussed, students of color often find the discourse shifted to ease the discomfort of White students within the classroom, leaving little room for students of color to process and develop (Linder et al., 2015). Research also indicates that some White students have difficulty aligning with narratives on race relations within the United States, likely because the experience of examining these dynamics makes them aware of how they may be complicit in the system (Alemán & Gaytán, 2017). Some students of color face intersectional discrimination, such as that based in heterosexism, homophobia, transphobia, classism, xenophobia, ableism, and religious discrimination. Furthermore, many students of color experience certain forms of discrimination, such as classism, differently than White students who are coping with economic struggles do, as students of color do not benefit from race privilege (Cattaneo et al., 2019). Additionally, class differences are evident between many U.S. students of color and international students. Specifically, many U.S. students of color have fewer economic privileges than some international students. These experiences are further complicated for U.S. students of color with undocumented status, who face significant stress with regard to the uncertainty of changing immigration policies and fears of deportation.

EXPERIENCES OF INTERNATIONAL STUDENTS ON U.S. COLLEGE CAMPUSES

Some literature concerning international students describes experiences similar to those of students of color, while noting some important distinctions. International students, particularly those who are non-White, have reported negative experiences, including lack of cultural understanding, insults, direct confrontations, and social isolation (Lee & Rice, 2007). Experiences of stereotyping and racism can be related to various social identities, including gender (Green & Kim, 2005), race (Houshmand et al., 2014), and country of origin (Lee & Rice, 2007). For example, Liu et al. (2016) focused on the "triple threat" experienced by Asian women who are international students. That is, they are women, racial minorities, and foreigners, and these identities can be targeted in specific forms of discrimination and oppression. Liu et al. found that loneliness mediated the relationship between perceived discrimination and life satisfaction and that gender solidarity was a protective factor that mitigated loneliness when these women experienced gender-based discrimination.

There is also evidence that White students are more likely than students of color to have negative attitudes toward international students and that these attitudes are determined by multiple factors. In one study, Quinton (2019) found four factors that predicted negative views of international students: identifying as White, holding high levels of negative stereotypes of people of international origin, holding conservative views, and supporting Trump. Given the alt-right movements on campus and the research regarding conservative political views and support of Trump, international students are facing significant challenges related to discrimination and racism on college campuses today.

The Institute of International Education (2015; as cited by Volpone et al., 2018) reported that about 5% of students in higher education are foreign born. Amongst international students, Asian students are often largely represented, with Chinese students being the largest international group (Liao & Wei, 2014). As international students relocate and adjust to the host country, they wish for a sense of belonging. Cartmell and Bond (2015) conducted a qualitative study that looked at aspects of belonging for newly arrived international students. They discovered that sense of belonging correlated positively with intrinsic motivation and engagement with academic obligations: When belonging was absent or low, students were less motivated and engaged. They also found that some factors were related to their environment and other factors were related to their own personality styles. This sense of belonging can be fostered by attending to the relationships between faculty and students and those among students. It would be important to attend to the broader cultural attitudes towards international students on campuses. Furthermore, it is critical that counseling center staff be trained and familiar with systemic concerns related to international students and provide education to host students about interacting with international students. This intervention is, in fact, emphasized in studies with Indian international graduate students and Chinese international students, which found that social support, decreased financial concerns, and ability to build connections within and across cultural lines are associated with decreased depressive symptoms and increased life satisfaction (Du & Wei, 2015; Meghani & Harvey, 2016).

Negative Consequences of Racism and Xenophobia on Mental Health and Identity

Research demonstrates that racism and discrimination negatively impact the health of people of color (Alvarez et al., 2016). Prolonged exposure to racism can lead to significant psychological stress, physical stress, and traumatic stress (French et al., 2020). With regard to international students, studies such as that conducted by Wei et al. (2012) indicate that perceived racial discrimination is associated with posttraumatic stress symptoms among Chinese international students. At the same time, Asian and Asian American students and U.S. students of color more broadly are the least likely to seek services, despite experiencing high levels of distress (Lipson et al., 2018). It is important to note that the experiences of international students of color may be distinct from the experiences of 1.5- or second-generation U.S. students of color. International students arriving in the United States may face being racialized for the first time and may be less likely to identify with the term "student of color," whereas 1.5- and second-generation U.S. students of color may have been coping with racism, implicitly or explicitly, since childhood (Tummala-Narra, 2013; Tummala-Narra et al., 2011).

Acculturative processes and identity development also interact with xenophobic and discriminatory experiences. These processes are closely influenced by the constant evaluations of internal experiences, other members of their ingroups, other marginalized communities, and dominant groups (Sue & Sue, 2003). Internal experiences include but are not limited to emotional reactions, memories, value systems, and self-regard.

To demonstrate the impact of racism and xenophobia on students' mental health and identity, we present several case examples. These case vignettes provide a lens into how the psychological impact of racism and xenophobia manifests in the therapeutic relationship within a college counseling center.

Sam, a Second-Generation Immigrant-Origin Client

Sam, whose full name is Samir, is a 21-year-old heterosexual-identified, Indian American, single cisgender man who is a senior in the arts.[1] He initially presented with concerns about mood swings, erratic and impulsive behaviors, and a recent increase in substance use. He had been seen previously by another therapist in the university counseling service but had dropped out of treatment. In this new course of treatment, Sam began to consider the possibility that a bipolar II diagnosis reflected his experience and began to observe his moods and behaviors in this context.

Sam discussed identity and family concerns in the course of counseling. When I (Anmol) asked in the initial meeting about experiences of discrimination or oppression at the university or broadly in society, Sam responded, "Boilerplate stuff . . . you know with TSA . . . [Name of university] is so White. I have played the assimilation game well." During counseling, these themes were explored further. Sam noted that he goes by "Sam" at the university and "Samir" at home with his parents, who reside in another part of the country, "I am two different people at home and here." He discussed difficulties connecting with his Indian immigrant parents and their culture, and he described a complicated relationship between his parents. He felt that his parents lacked understanding of his experience growing up in the United State and that he had to "beat their success." He described experiences of being bullied because of his race while growing up and adults in his life not intervening. He also discussed feeling the need to distance himself from his family and Indian culture in order to progress. For example, Sam experienced pressure in his field to "fit in," and his friends and peers in his field were all White. Sam noted that he was unlikely to succeed in his field if he didn't "seem White" and feared that he would not be accepted as Samir and therefore would not be successful professionally. We connected some of his fears to incidents occurring more broadly in U.S. society, and he disclosed witnessing racism experienced by his parents. These experiences broadly led to him to minimize or deny parts of his Indian identity and his identity as a person of

---

[1]All case material has been altered to protect confidentiality.

color, causing significant internal conflict. We discussed our shared identity as South Asian Americans, and he seemed to appreciate my validation of his dilemmas.

Through counseling and medication management, Sam's symptoms began to improve. He reduced his substance use and was tracking his mood states; he expressed that he wished to engage in longer term treatment in the community following graduation. As graduation approached, he discussed more distress: "Two worlds will collide . . . my life here and my life at home," as his parents planned to attend graduation.

This case illustrates the interplay of racial trauma with mental health concerns. Sam's racial trauma and mental health concerns were exacerbated in the current political climate such that larger systemic forces cannot be ignored in understanding his concerns. Some of the mood concerns he described were directly related to his experiences of race and culture. The context of university and his field of study felt very "White" to Sam and, therefore, he felt he could not fully be himself in these contexts. He also did not feel that he could be whole in his family, as he felt his family members did not fully understand him. He often referenced the broader political climate when discussing his concerns, for example mentioning President Trump's treatment of immigrants.

Racial identity models, which examine how individuals take in racial stimuli and understand themselves and their relationships in the context of a racist society, can be helpful in understanding Sam. He seemed to be using a dissonance or encounter lens in understanding his racial identity in that he experienced some ambivalence and confusion around his own racial group (Helms, 1995). He also acknowledged the dominance of White people in his field and expressed a valid concern that he might not succeed as he did not fit into this "club." Although we could not work with each other long term because of his graduation, he seemed to benefit from discussing the complexity of his identity, his experiences growing up in the United States as a child of color, and his experiences of race and racism on campus with a South Asian American therapist. Inviting discussion concerning identity and oppression in the early stages of counseling was critical to this process.

Another salient context to consider with students of color is their legal status within the United States, as the anxiety related to detention and deportation has been heightened in the current sociopolitical context. The case of Paula highlights these dynamics.

Paula, an Undocumented Student of Color and Child of Undocumented Parents

Paula is a 21-year-old Latinx, heterosexual-identified, single cisgender junior. She presented with stress and anxiety related to political climate, family, finances, and academic concerns. She expressed that her main concerns were the national dialogue about the Deferred Action for Childhood Arrivals policy (DACA) and the impact of the larger political environment on her mental health. Paula reported that she had a panic attack when discussing immigration during a class, that she left class, and that she spent a great deal of time crying. She discussed some of the content and perspectives shared by other students in the class as "triggering" for her. Paula reported difficulty sleeping, persistent anxiety, and some concerns about her concentration and motivation, although was able to complete her academic work.

A significant theme we (Anmol and Paula) explored was her identity as an activist and advocate on campus for DACA students. She described being sought out by professors, staff, and students on campus to speak at events and attend rallies. She was also often outed as a DACA student in public spaces. I inquired further about this and reflected to her the conflict of wanting to advocate for herself and others and "get the right messages out there" and feeling fatigued about "being in the spotlight" when her legal status could disappear at any moment. Paula described her motivation to be active on campus given President Trump's rhetoric about undocumented people and DACA and the overall hostile tone of these messages. She expressed feeling fear and stress about her and her family members' documentation status. She also experienced microaggressions by well-intentioned faculty and staff about her race and immigration status. In our work, we were able to identify that the stress of both being a DACA student and being in the spotlight were directly related to her symptoms, including her sleep disturbance, fatigue, diminished motivation, and poor concentration. In addition, her grades had declined.

We met only twice; my interventions focused on helping Paula to make sense of her experiences, taking care of herself in a difficult political climate, and identifying supports. I reflected her ambivalence about continuing to speak up and also feeling fatigued by acknowledging the wish to help her community and also the costs for her. I wondered if she could encourage other students to "take up the torch" to allow herself some time to rest. Since the summer break was approaching, she felt that this would make things easier for her. We further discussed her connection with her allies on campus and ways she might be more genuine with them about her experiences of fatigue and anxiety, as she had not been open with them because she felt she had to be "perfect" and a model for others. She was responsive to these ideas.

The experience of working with Paula raised my awareness of the various ways that I can help students in similar situations, particularly DACA students and activists from minoritized groups. Since working with Paula, I have sought more training about undocumented students on campus and have invited trainers to my department. It has been clear to me the burden some students may carry in holding the torch and the impact of this burden on their health.

Students Resisting

In these case examples, students are grappling with concerns related to race, racial identity, racism, and cultural identity in the United States. Previous studies have highlighted that experiences of discrimination may be especially difficult for adolescents given that this is a time when they are exploring their identities and may be particularly sensitive to how they are viewed (Greene et al., 2006; Sirin & Fine, 2008). The social and political climate in which these students live makes this process more complex in that it is a particularly hostile and unwelcoming environment. There are constant messages in the mainstream media, particularly from the current administration, that people of color are not valued. Furthermore, the college environment does not always offer students the growth-promoting and supportive contexts and experiences they may need to address these concerns.

We underscore that students resist racist, sexist, classist, and heterosexist ideologies on college campuses. Every day, students are resisting on many levels. Some of the ways they resist are obvious, such as coordinating or attending a protest, while others are more subtle, such as gently challenging a classmate or a professor in class. Some students are collectively resisting, sometimes collaborating across several student organizations to promote social justice on their campuses. A powerful example that continues to be discussed on college campuses is the series of protests at University of Missouri in 2015. After weeks of student and faculty protests related to the mishandling of racist incidents on campus, the football players threatened to strike if the president of the university didn't resign. The president did resign in this case (New, 2015). One of the most salient aspects of this case is the collective force and solidarity across students and faculty in the university that led to systemic change.

When discussing resistance, we must also consider its relationship to power within the therapeutic relationship. Resistance can hinder the progress of therapy if the power dynamics in the room become rigid or go unnamed, but resistance can also be used to deepen therapeutic work. Although resistance can easily be labeled as uncooperativeness or nonresponsiveness to treat-ment, relationally it is always a form of communication. Similar to power dynamics within a relationship, the way resistance plays out can be obvious or subtle. From a psychodynamic perspective, resistance helps clients to avoid expression of unacceptable thoughts and feelings while allowing them to maintain their agency and sense of self. Resistance can extend beyond fight-ing against the expression of internal feelings and may include hiding how the client feels about the therapist (Messer, 2002). It is important to consider that these dynamics of power and resistance can reflect social inequities related to race, ethnicity, religion, gender, immigration status, social class, sexual orientation, gender identity, and dis/ability.

Relatedly, a student with whom I (Anmol) recently worked received some racist and sexist feedback from a professor and realized it would be difficult to challenge that professor directly. Instead, she sought other faculty in her department and described her experiences. They agreed with her and noted that they would consider how they might approach this faculty member, who has a history of providing discriminatory feedback. It is important that colleagues be able to challenge each other when we notice microaggressions or policies that are harmful.

Tsai and Wei (2018) noted different forms of resistance and coping. For example, internalization and resistance are two forms of coping used by many Chinese international students. Tsai and Wei found that women tended to use internalization more than men, looking inward and refocusing on their cultural views rather than focusing on racism. This finding highlights the complexities of students' responses to racism and ways of coping with racism. These complexities are important to recognize as we work with students of different social locations, cultural backgrounds, value systems, and access to varying levels of resources and power.

Adia, a First-Generation College Student and Child of Immigrants

Adia is a 24-year-old cisgender woman who is Black, West African, heterosexual, Christian, and single. Her primary presenting concerns were a long-term struggle with depressive symptoms and an inability to feel engaged with her environment. Being a first-generation college student, one of the only Black students in her courses, and a transfer student, she lacked a sense of belonging and trust within her campus.

Sitting in the room with Adia felt awkward in the beginning, as she used one-word responses and never made eye contact with me (Sindhu); however, she returned to therapy each week on time. Adia's nonverbals softened only slightly over the next few weeks, when she began looking at me briefly a few times a session and started to sit more leisurely in her chair. However, as I turned the conversation to visible identities and began to talk about the privileges awarded to me as a South Asian woman despite being a woman of color, Adia started to express her anger and vulnerability in session. I mirrored her emotions by verbally and nonverbally sharing my anger with the systemic oppression faced by people of color and specifically Black women. Adia started to share more details of her personal life, started to smile and laugh in session, but continued to be reserved about some interpersonal and family traumas. Weeks later, Adia shared with me that "this worked a whole lot better when you dropped your White girl act." I believe the awkwardness I experienced in the beginning of our work resulted in me treating her with more fragility, in the form of softened language and questions that required indirect processing. I believe that once I stopped softening my language, Adia saw me as an authentic subject in the room, a person with whom she could relate. By developing a more secure and trusted relationship, I was able to help her take an interpersonal risk to seek psychiatric consultation and pursue medical care for underlying health concerns. Previously, she had been reluctant to seek help because she had experienced various traumas and had historical mistrust of the medical system.

Another notable moment with Adia arose in the weeks before our scheduled termination. She fell back into a pattern of withdrawing during a session and then engaging again the next. I directly observed this pattern to Adia and explored what she was feeling internally when these shifts occurred. I also shared that I felt disconnected from her when she withdrew and wondered if she felt similarly. Part of our processing indicated that Adia was fearful of starting over with a new therapist and felt that she would not be understood elsewhere. While distancing herself in session, she avoided discussing her feelings about our relationship and the fear of the upcoming loss, in order to maintain a sense of self.

ROLE OF PSYCHOLOGISTS IN ADDRESSING RACISM AND XENOPHOBIA ON CAMPUSES

Universities can focus more on campus climate, making campuses more welcoming toward U.S. students of color and international students. Alt-right and nationalist movements and increased threats of violence across U.S. college campuses have heightened this need. Quinton (2019) argued that universities and colleges can play a critical role in reducing prejudicial attitudes. Quinton suggested, for example, that increasing socialization between domestic and international students and fostering a greater university identity can reduce prejudice. Quinton further argued that integrating international students into the campus would help other students' perceptions of them as fellow students rather than as "the Other" (p. 12). In this section, we use an ecological framework (Bronfenbrenner, 1979) to provide some suggestions that psychologists can use when considering how to address racism on campus.

As psychologists, we are accustomed to supporting individual students who are experiencing racial trauma. We can help to normalize and validate their reactions, providing support and suggestions for how to address and move through difficult periods. Psychologists can help them to learn about their strengths and resilience and help to inspire *critical consciousness*, defined as "an individual's capacity to critically reflect and act upon their sociopolitical environment" (Diemer et al., 2006, p. 445). In individual and group counseling, we can encourage students to challenge systemic oppression and support them as they take actions to address issues of equity and inclusion on the campus. Psychologists might also suggest that students connect with other allies on campus, such as faculty, staff, other students, or student groups who might have similar experiences or some knowledge to help them. We have connected students of color with staff and faculty on campus who share their backgrounds or who have a great deal of interest or experience working with students from particular backgrounds. Our own connections on campus are critical in assisting students who are experiencing racial trauma and who may benefit from additional support outside of counseling. Psychologists can also advocate for subgroups of students. For example, when we hear from multiple students in a specific department or area on campus that they are experiencing similar kinds of racism and/or sexism, we have worked toward making this known in a way that protects students' confidentiality.

Psychologists can, of course, help to support students individually, but we need to move beyond this and engage students, faculty, and staff who may not visit our offices. Outreach programming is critical to meeting the needs of students who are coping with racial trauma and/or with being marginalized and who might not engage with a university counseling center (Banks, 2020). This programming can also include students who, knowingly or unknowingly, perpetrate microaggressions or discriminatory behaviors. We can help students to find language to articulate their experiences and facilitate dialogues about race, racism, and intersectionality. We can collaborate with our colleagues in cultural centers or multicultural student offices on campus and offer our expertise and perspectives. We can also offer consultation to offices on campus that serve students struggling with racism and other -isms.

Psychologists have significant opportunities to reach broader audiences and provide some opportunities to have difficult dialogues to challenge oppression and to form connections with faculty, staff, and students with whom we would not ordinarily meet. I (Anmol) am reminded of an outreach program that I cofacilitated with a White female trainee. The purpose of the program was to provide a group of academic advisors with some suggestions for working with students in emotional or psychological distress. The trainee was surprised by the turn that the program took when the advisors, all White women, began describing a "difficult" Muslim student from the United Arab Emirates, noting that this student was difficult because "he refuses to shake our hands." I took the opportunity to discuss some cultural differences around gender role norms that may have been salient and to encourage them to reflect on their own biases and assumptions, such as those occurring during the training (e.g., assuming he is not cooperative because he chose not to shake hands, assuming he was "aggressive" because he was Muslim). After the training, the trainee asked me, "How did all of that come up? Does that usually happen to you?" She understood quickly that this shift in the program was related to their assumptions about my identities and that it was also an opportunity to challenge. Many opportunities like this will arise if we choose to venture out of our offices and engage with the larger university community. Furthermore, psychologists can help to inform colleagues who are not in the clinical field about ways in which institutional racism may be operating within universities and can provide education about the emotional and psychological impact on students of color, children of immigrants, and international students.

CONCLUSION

In this chapter, we have highlighted some key experiences of students of color and international students on U.S. college campuses and have discussed how their well-being and identity are impacted by systemic influences, including the current sociopolitical environment. As college students are often a convenient sample in psychological research, much of the literature reviewed in this chapter was conducted with undergraduates. However, this sample limits understanding of the experiences of others within higher education, such as graduate students at varying levels and departments. Furthermore, researchers often examine the experiences of racial minority and international students as homogenous groups, and these studies may fail to capture the nuances that exist within and between groups. Our work in counseling centers challenges us to think about our role on campus beyond what we do with individual students in our counseling offices. Future research within college contexts can explore how campus-wide community-based interventions that foster a culture of inclusion and equity can be created. We are in a sociopolitical climate that demands that clinicians, researchers, and educators engage in coalition building with others on campus, including students, faculty, and staff who are invested in addressing racism and xenophobia on campus.

REFERENCES

Alemán, S., & Gaytán, S. (2017). "It doesn't speak to me": Understanding student of color resistance to critical race pedagogy. *International Journal of Qualitative Studies in Education, 30*(2), 128–146. https://doi.org/10.1080/09518398.2016.1242801

Alvarez, A. N., Liang, C. T. H., & Neville, H. A. (Eds.). (2016). *The cost of racism for people of color: Contextualizing experiences of discrimination*. American Psychological Association. https://doi.org/10.1037/14852-000

Banks, B. M. (2020). Meet them where they are: An outreach model to address university counseling center disparities. *Journal of College Student Psychotherapy, 34*(3), 240–251. https://doi.org/10.1080/87568225.2019.1595805

Bauer-Wolf, J. (2017, September 22). *A September of racist incidents*. Inside Higher Ed. https://www.insidehighered.com/news/2017/09/22/racist-incidents-colleges-abound-academic-year-begins

Binkley, C. (2018, February 1). *Report says racist messages are appearing on college campuses in surging numbers*. Public Broadcasting System. https://www.pbs.org/newshour/politics/report-says-racist-messages-are-appearing-on-college-campuses-in-surging-numbers

Bronfenbrenner, U. (1979). *The ecology of human development: Experiments by nature and design*. Harvard University Press.

Cartmell, H., & Bond, C. (2015). What does belonging mean for young people who are international new arrivals? *Educational and Child Psychology, 32*(2), 89–101.

Cattaneo, L. B., Chan, W. Y., Shor, R., Gebhard, K. T., & Elshabassi, N. H. (2019). Elaborating the connection between social class and classism in college. *American Journal of Community Psychology, 63*(3–4), 476–486. https://doi.org/10.1002/ajcp.12322

Diemer, M. A., Kauffman, A., Koenig, N., Trahan, E., & Hsieh, C. A. (2006). Challenging racism, sexism, and social injustice: Support for urban adolescents' critical consciousness development. *Cultural Diversity & Ethnic Minority Psychology, 12*(3), 444–460. https://doi.org/10.1037/1099-9809.12.3.444

Dreid, N., & Najmabadi, S. (2016, December 13). Here's a rundown of the latest campus-climate incidents since Trump's election. *The Chronicle of Higher Education*. https://www.chronicle.com/blogs/ticker/heres-a-rundown-of-the-latest-campus-climate-incidents-since-trumps-election/115553

Du, Y., & Wei, M. (2015). Acculturation, enculturation, social connectedness, and subjective well-being among Chinese international students. *The Counseling Psychologist, 43*(2), 299–325. https://doi.org/10.1177/0011000014565712

French, B. H., Lewis, J. A., Mosely, D. V., Adames, H. Y., Chaves-Duenas, N. Y., Chen, G. A., & Neville, H. A. (2020). Toward a psychological framework of radical healing in communities of color. *The Counseling Psychologist, 48*(1), 14–46. https://doi.org/10.1177/0011000019843506

Green, D. O., & Kim, E. (2005). Experiences of Korean female doctoral students in academe: Raising voice against gender and racial stereotypes. *Journal of College Student Development, 46*(5), 487–500. https://doi.org/10.1353/csd.2005.0048

Greene, M. L., Way, N., & Pahl, K. (2006). Trajectories of perceived adult and peer discrimination among Black, Latino, and Asian American adolescents: Patterns and psychological correlates. *Developmental Psychology, 42*(2), 218–236. https://doi.org/10.1037/0012-1649.42.2.218

Gun Violence Archive Staff. (2019). *Gun violence archive.* Retrieved June 13, 2019, from https://www.gunviolencearchive.org/

Harwood, S. A., Huntt, M. B., Mendenhall, R., & Lewis, J. A. (2012). Racial microaggressions in the residence halls: Experiences of students of color at a predominantly White university. *Journal of Diversity in Higher Education, 5*(3), 159–173. https://doi.org/10.1037/a0028956

Helms, J. E. (1995). An update on Helms's White and People of Color (POC) racial identity models. In J. G. Ponterotto, J. M. Casas, L. A. Suzuki, & C. M. Alexander (Eds.), *Handbook of multicultural counseling* (pp. 181–198). Sage.

Houshmand, S., Spanierman, L. B., & Tafarodi, R. W. (2014). Excluded and avoided: Racial microaggressions targeting Asian international students in Canada. *Cultural Diversity and Ethnic Minority Psychology, 20*(3), 377–388. https://doi.org/10.1037/a0035404

Kerr, E. (2018, February 1). "White supremacists are targeting college campuses like never before." *The Chronicle of Higher Education.* https://www.chronicle.com/article/White-Supremacists-Are/242403

Lee, J. J., & Rice, C. (2007). Welcome to America? International student perceptions of discrimination. *Higher Education, 53*(3), 381–409. https://doi.org/10.1007/s10734-005-4508-3

Liao, K. Y., & Wei, M. (2014). Academic stress and positive affect: Asian value and self-worth contingency as moderators among Chinese international students. *Cultural Diversity & Ethnic Minority Psychology, 20*(1), 107–115. https://doi.org/10.1037/a0034071

Linder, C., Harris, J., Allen, E., & Hubain, B. (2015). Building inclusive pedagogy: Recommendations from a national study of students of color in higher education and student affairs graduate programs. *Equity & Excellence in Education, 48*(2), 178–194. https://doi.org/10.1080/10665684.2014.959270

Lipson, S., Kern, A., Eisenberg, D., & Breland-Noble, A. (2018). Mental health disparities among college students of color. *Journal of Adolescent Health, 63*(3), 348–356. https://doi.org/10.1016/j.jadohealth.2018.04.014

Liu, T., Wong, Y. J., & Tsai, P.-C. (2016). Conditional mediation models of intersecting identities among female Asian international students. *The Counseling Psychologist, 44*(3), 411–441. https://doi.org/10.1177/0011000016637200

Meghani, D., & Harvey, E. (2016). Asian Indian international students' trajectories of depression, acculturation, and enculturation. *Asian American Journal of Psychology, 7*(1), 1–14. https://doi.org/10.1037/aap0000034

Messer, S. B. (2002). A psychodynamic perspective on resistance in psychotherapy: Vive la résistance. *Journal of Clinical Psychology, 58*(2), 157–163. https://doi.org/10.1002/jclp.1139

New, J. (2015, November 11). *The power of a football boycott.* Inside Higher Ed. https://www.insidehighered.com/news/2015/11/11/u-missouri-football-boycott-demonstrates-economic-power-athletes

Quinton, W. J. (2019). Unwelcome on campus? Predictors of prejudice against international students. *Journal of Diversity in Higher Education, 12*(2), 156–169. https://doi.org/10.1037/dhe0000091

Sirin, S. R., & Fine, M. (2008). *Muslim American youth: Understanding hyphenated identities through multiple methods.* New York University Press.

Southern Poverty Law Center. (2017, August 10). *The alt-right on campus: What students need to know.* https://www.splcenter.org/20170810/alt-right-campus-what-students-need-know

Sue, D. W., & Sue, D. (2003). *Counseling the culturally diverse: Theory and practice* (4th ed.). John Wiley & Sons.

Tsai, P.-C., & Wei, M. (2018). Racial discrimination and experience of new possibilities among Chinese international students. *The Counseling Psychologist, 46*(3), 351–378. https://doi.org/10.1177/0011000018761892

Tummala-Narra, P. (2013). Psychotherapy with South Asian women: Dilemmas of immigrant and first generations. *Women & Therapy, 36,* 176–197. https://doi.org/10.1080/02703149.2013.797853

Tummala-Narra, P., Inman, A. G., & Ettigi, S. P. (2011). Asian Indians' responses to discrimination: A mixed-method examination of identity, coping, and self-esteem. *Asian American Journal of Psychology, 2*(3), 205–218. https://doi.org/10.1037/a0025555

Volpone, S. D., Marquardt, D. J., Casper, W. J., & Avery, D. R. (2018). Minimizing cross-cultural maladaptation: How minority status facilitates change in international acculturation. *Journal of Applied Psychology, 103*(3), 249–269. https://doi.org/10.1037/apl0000273

Wei, M., Wang, K. T., Heppner, P. P., & Du, Y. (2012). Ethnic and mainstream social connectedness, perceived racial discrimination, and posttraumatic stress symptoms. *Journal of Counseling Psychology, 59*(3), 486–493. https://doi.org/10.1037/a0028000

Zestcott, C., & Brown, K. (2015). From the crowd to the competition: White collegiate athletes' response to racism directed at a teammate of color. *Current Psychology, 34*(4), 634–643. https://doi.org/10.1007/s12144-014-9276-8

5

Microaggressions Toward Racial Minority Immigrants in the United States

D. R. Gina Sissoko and Kevin L. Nadal

The Center for Immigration Studies reported that there were 44.5 million foreign-born residents in the United States—comprising 13.7% of the population, or one in seven U.S. residents. The same report revealed 17.1 million U.S.-born minor children had a foreign-born parent (Camarota & Zeigler, 2018). In 2013, the Pew Research Center reported that the combined number of first-generation immigrants (i.e., foreign-born individuals who arrived in the United States as adults), 1.5-generation immigrants (i.e., foreign-born individuals who arrived in the United States as children), and second-generation immigrants (i.e., individuals who were born and raised in the United States and have at least one foreign-born parent) equates to 76 million people; it is projected that by 2050, first-, 1.5-, and second-generation immigrants will compose 37% of the total U.S. population (Pew Research Center, 2013).

With this growth in immigration has come anti-immigrant sentiment. After the controversial presidential election of 2016, the Southern Poverty Law Center reported a rapid increase in the number of hate groups (e.g., White supremacists, anti-Muslim groups, anti-immigrant groups) in the United States; between 2016 and 2017, the number of anti-immigrant hate groups rose from 14% to 22% (Beirich & Buchanan, 2018). Furthermore, in the month following the 2016 election, 315 hate crimes toward immigrants were reported—the largest number of hate crimes toward any targeted group at the time (Nadal, 2017).

https://doi.org/10.1037/0000214-006
Trauma and Racial Minority Immigrants: Turmoil, Uncertainty, and Resistance,
P. Tummala-Narra (Editor)

Although these numbers are alarming, anti-immigration bias is not new; decades of research have shown that immigrants have historically been stigmatized and oppressed on the basis of nationality, citizenship status, accent, and cultural values and customs (Sue et al., 2019). In recent years, authors have described how racial and ethnic discrimination has evolved over time—with a decrease in overt, blatant, and explicit prejudice and discriminatory behavior and an increase of subtle, less obvious forms of modern racism and covert discrimination (Kassin et al., 2018; Sue, 2010). Some authors have labeled these incidents as *racial microaggressions,* "brief and commonplace daily verbal, behavioral, and environmental indignities, whether intentional or unintentional, that communicate hostile, derogatory, or negative racial slights and insults to the target person or group" (Sue et al., 2007, p. 271). In this context, "micro" refers to the way in which these incidents can manifest (e.g., brief verbal exchanges, subtle behaviors) and not to their impact, which can be thought of as death by a thousand cuts. With a vast emergence of research on microaggressions since 2007, microaggression theory has been used to understand how multiple manifestations of oppression (e.g., systemic, interpersonal, overt, covert) may impact daily psychological experiences of people of historically marginalized groups (Nadal, 2018; Sue, 2010; Torino et al., 2019).

The purpose of this chapter is to explore how racial minority immigrants in the United States experience microaggressions. In particular, we contextualize the interpersonal and systemic microaggressions encountered by racial minority immigrants, highlighting common themes and lived experiences. We conclude with case vignettes illustrating how microaggressions manifest, along with recommendations for research, practice, and policy.

REVIEW OF RACIAL MICROAGGRESSIONS

Although the concept of racial microaggressions was first coined by Pierce et al. (1978), the term *microaggression* did not become well known until Sue and colleagues (2007) reintroduced the concept in *American Psychologist.* According to Sue et al., microaggressions are categorized into three classifications: microassaults, microinsults, and microinvalidations. *Microassaults* are overt behavioral or verbal insults mirroring traditional discrimination (e.g., calling Africans "savages" or "dirty"). *Microinsults* are behavioral or verbal interactions communicating stereotypes about a group of people (e.g., security guards following Black men in retail stores, someone suspiciously staring at a Muslim or Arab American person on an airplane or train). Finally, *microinvalidations* are communicated verbally and dismiss or undermine people's realities (e.g., telling a Black woman that she is oversensitive and that her perceptions of racism or sexism are irrational; complimenting a Latinx or Asian American student who was born and raised in the United States for speaking "good" English).

Sue et al. (2007) proposed a taxonomy of racial microaggressions experienced by people of color in the United States, and Nadal et al. (2010) proposed a taxonomy of religious microaggressions experienced by people of religious minority groups. Both taxonomies underscore several themes of micro-aggressions. Examples include

- *alien in own land:* experiences in which a U.S.-born individual may be assumed to be foreign-born, communicating that the person is not really American

- *ascriptions of intelligence:* experiences in which people are deemed less or more intelligent based on their race (e.g., surprise at an Asian American student's struggle or a Black student's success on a math test)

- *assumptions of criminality:* experiences in which a person is negatively stereotyped as dangerous or criminal on the basis of their race or religion

- *denial of individual racism:* experiences in which a White person denounces their own racial biases, resulting in the invalidation of people's lived experience

- *myth of meritocracy:* statements promoting the false notion that economic and scholastic advancement are based solely on merit and ignoring systemic barriers to achievement

- *pathologizing cultural values and communication styles:* experiences in which White American communication styles and cultural values are idealized, while others are viewed as abnormal or inferior

- *second-class citizen:* experiences in which a White American person is given preferential treatment over a person of color or a member of a religious minority group

Microaggressions can be particularly challenging for marginalized groups because they often occur briefly and seem unintentional. By the time the target has processed and identified the encounter as a microaggression, the moment to address the situation has often passed, leaving the target with feelings of anger, confusion, and guilt or shame for not having responded or called out the microaggressions (Sue, 2010). Meanwhile, people who enact microaggressions are likely to hold negative stereotypes toward other groups—a notion supported by social categorization theory, which posits that people categorize themselves and others into groups based on similar characteristics, such as physical features, nationality, or age (Kassin et al., 2018). Specific to race, researchers have found that cognitive racial classification is automatic, implicit, and spontaneous (Eberhardt, 2005); thus, people who commit micro-aggressions may not be aware of their biased behaviors or statements.

The experiences of racial and ethnic microaggressions have been measured both qualitatively and quantitatively, with some authors acknowledging that the number of studies of microaggressions has increased faster than that of studies of most other psychology phenomena (Torino et al., 2019). In general, studies have shown that cumulative encounters with microaggressions are predictive of various mental and physical health outcomes, including depressive symptoms (Nadal et al., 2014), suicidal ideation (O'Keefe et al., 2015), trauma symptoms (Moody & Lewis, 2019; Torres & Taknint, 2015), and lower psychological well-being (Nadal et al., 2015). While initially centered on experiences of race, microaggression theory and subsequent literature has expanded to include people of other historically marginalized groups, including queer and transgender people, women, people with disabilities, and people of religious minority groups (Nadal, 2018; Sue, 2010; Torino et al., 2019).

Despite this growth in academic scholarship, there is a dearth of literature exploring immigrants' experiences with microaggressions in the United States. Although many of the themes proposed by Sue and colleagues (2007) and Nadal and colleagues (2010) allude to immigrant experiences, only a few studies have examined how racial minority immigrants specifically navigate microaggressions as compared with their American-born counterparts. For example, one study with Latinx participants suggested that immigrants were more likely than U.S.-born participants to experience microaggressions in which they were treated as intellectually inferior (Nadal et al., 2014), whereas a study with Asian American participants showed no significant differences between immigrants and U.S.-born participants in the types of racial microaggressions they encountered (Nadal et al., 2015). Because these results are both limited and mixed in their findings, the need for research that addresses microaggressions toward racial minority immigrants is evident.

TAXONOMY OF MICROAGGRESSIONS TOWARD RACIAL MINORITY IMMIGRANTS

Given the lack of literature on microaggressions toward immigrants, we propose a taxonomy of the types of microaggressions that racial minority immigrants may encounter in their everyday lives. Expanding on the taxonomy of racial microaggressions proposed by Sue et al. (2007) as well as the taxonomy of religious microaggressions proposed by Nadal et al. (2010), we propose eight themes of microaggressions that target racial minority immigrants. Each theme reflects the ways in which racial minority immigrants may differentially experience systemic and interpersonal microaggressions based on nativity, immigration status, language barriers, and multicultural identity. Furthermore, the themes reflect the ways that immigrants may navigate complex family and community dynamics, including multigenerational members with different immigration statuses, language proficiency, and conflicting cultural values that potentially result in different types of acculturative stress. Table 5.1 highlights each of our proposed themes, along with the generational status of the target, the potential perpetrators, examples of the microaggression, and the conveyed message. The taxonomy highlights that immigrants face unique circumstances under which microaggressions might be perpetrated not only by members of mainstream U.S. culture but

TABLE 5.1. Examples of Microaggressions Experienced by Immigrants in the United States

Theme	Target	Perpetrator	Microaggression	Message
Alien in own land	1.5- and second-generation immigrants	Americans/nonmembers of immigrant culture	"Where are you from?"	You are not really American.
Questioning of cultural authenticity	1.5- and second-generation immigrants	Members of immigrant culture	"You are too American."	You are not really [part of your national and heritage culture].
Ascriptions of intelligence and language-related microaggressions	First-generation immigrants	Americans/nonmembers of immigrant culture	Questioning an immigrant's professional credentials based on their nativity or accent	You are incomprehensible and unintelligent.
Assumptions of homogeneity	First-, 1.5-, and second-generation immigrants	Americans/nonmembers of immigrant culture	Categorizing an African immigrant as African American	Your national and cultural background does not matter.
The myth of meritocracy/denial of individual and systemic racism	First-, 1.5-, and second-generation immigrants	Americans/nonmembers of immigrant culture	"You need only to work hard to achieve success in America."	You are a personal failure and lazy if you are not successful.
	1.5- and second-generation immigrants	Americans/nonmember of immigrant culture	"People raised in America have every opportunity to achieve success."	You are a personal failure and lazy if you are not successful.
Pathologizing cultural values and communication styles	First-, 1.5-, and second-generation immigrants	Americans/nonmember of immigrant culture	Telling a second-generation immigrant their family is too involved in their life	Your family system is pathological.
Criminalization	All generations, especially undocumented immigrants	Systemic/interpersonal	Immigration and Customs Enforcement targets and arrests immigrants	You are deviant.
Second-class citizenship	All generations, especially undocumented immigrants	Systemic/interpersonal	Barriers to obtaining educational funding, permanent legal residency, and access to basic human rights	You are worth less than "real" Americans.

potentially also by members of one's own cultural heritage group or by members of other racial minority groups. Although not exhaustive, the taxonomy sheds light on the unique microaggressions experienced by racial minority immigrants, above and beyond the microaggressions that they may experience based on race, ethnicity, or religion alone.

Theme 1: Alien in Own Land

Second- and 1.5-generation immigrants are vulnerable to experience unique microaggressions based on their multicultural identities. First-generation immigrants, who arrived in the United States as adults, may have developed primary social identities separate from other racial minorities (e.g., some African Americans, Native Americans). However, their offspring—1.5- and second-generation immigrants—are multicultural by nature and may identify with several cultural groups, including mainstream American culture, racial minority groups in the United States, and their heritage culture. In these cases, social identity formation can create a cultural conflict for multicultural individuals—especially when two or more cultures are perceived as having fundamentally different values. Stroink and Lalonde (2009) tested this assumption among Asian Canadian students and found that higher levels of perceived differences between cultures led to less identification with either group. In this context, experiencing microaggressions might reinforce this de-identification with either culture.

Studies of microaggressions have highlighted that racial minorities consistently report being treated as an alien in their own land. In a qualitative study by Sue et al. (2009), Asian American participants (i.e., Chinese Americans, Filipino Americans, Korean Americans, and multiracial Asian Americans) described experiences in which people frequently assumed that they were not American (e.g., asking about their birthplace, providing compliments about their English-language skills). Participants perceived these microaggressions as uncomfortable and distressing and as conveying the message that only White people are viewed as authentic Americans. In a qualitative study by Nadal, Escobar, et al. (2012), Filipino Americans shared similar experiences—from being called an alien to being aggressively told to "go back where [you] came from" (p. 163), despite being U.S.-born.

Theme 2: Questioning of Cultural Authenticity

Second- and 1.5-generation immigrants may face microaggressions from both people in mainstream American culture and people in their own ethnic communities, in which they are told that they are not culturally authentic (e.g., "not Mexican enough," "not Indian enough") because they were born or raised in the United States, do not hold stereotypes associated with that ethnic group, or are not intimately familiar with—or adhere to—specific cultural traditions and values. The questioning of authenticity as an example of a microaggression has been discussed previously in the context of the experiences of multiracial people, who are often told that they do not belong to any of their racial groups (Johnston & Nadal, 2010). However, the concept has been discussed in previous literature for different immigrant subgroups. For example, in Waters's (1994) study of second-generation Black immigrants in New York, one Haitian American participant shared the following:

> Some people just think I am American because I have no accent. So, I talk like American people. I don't talk Brooklynese. They think I am from down south or something. . . . A lot of people say you don't look Haitian. I think I look Haitian enough. I don't know, maybe they are expecting us to look fresh off the boat. I was born here and I grew up here, so I guess I look American and I have an American accent. (pp. 807–808)

For 1.5- and second-generation immigrants, cultural authenticity is based on whether or not they speak the language of their ancestral country or practice any of the traditions. For example, one Japanese American shared,

> You can't live your life feeling guilty. It doesn't make me any less of a person because I can't speak the language. It doesn't make me any less of a person because I don't make sushi. There are other things I teach my children. (Tuan, 2002, p. 227)

Theme 3: Ascriptions of Intelligence and Language-Related Microaggressions

Racial minority immigrants may experience intelligence- or language-related microaggressions in ways that are different from those of their U.S.-born and White immigrant counterparts. First-generation immigrants may be vulnerable to *accent bias*, prejudice and discrimination based on how they sound to others when speaking English. In a meta-analytic review of 20 studies, Fuertes et al. (2012) found that people who spoke English with a nonstandard accent were rated as significantly less educated, intelligent, and successful than people who spoke with a standard American English accent. Gluszek and Dovidio (2010) found that people with nonnative accents perceived stigmatization based on the strength of their accents—and perceived stigmatization, in turn, was associated with a lower sense of belonging in the United States. Similarly, Nadal, Mazzula, et al. (2014) found that foreign-born Latinx participants reported significantly more microaggressions involving intellectual inferiority as compared to their U.S.-born Latinx counterparts.

In the professional work-related context, Shenoy-Packer (2015) identified three types of microaggressions faced by first-generation immigrant workers: (a) verbal microaggressions disguised as sarcasm (e.g., coworkers making fun of an accent), (b) professional microinvalidations in the form of communicating skepticism about their credentials and qualifications and attributing these experiences to their accents, and (c) attitudinal microaggressions based on stereotypes (e.g., being told that one does not look Mexican). Furthermore, workers who were employed in the fields of education, agriculture, and information technology said they frequently questioned compliments they believed to be rooted in stereotypes (e.g., being called a "smart man" based on stereotypes linking Asians with intelligence). This finding is consistent with literature on international students' experiences of accent-related micro-aggressions in the university context, which may lead to feelings of incompe-tence and social isolation (Kim & Kim, 2010). Similarly, in a study with undocumented 1.5- and second-generation Chicana/Latina students, Huber and Cueva (2012) identified several microaggressions, including assumptions of intellectual inferiority based on learning English as a second language and the valuing of monolingual English speakers over bilingual speakers. Finally, in a study on colonial mentality, David and Okazaki (2006) described the ways that Filipino Americans may discriminate against Filipino immigrants who are less Americanized or whom they view as "fresh off the boat" ("FOBs"; p. 243) because they are inferior, backwards, or weird. This finding supports the claim that intelligence and language-related microaggressions occur within ethnic groups also.

Theme 4: Assumptions of Homogeneity

Immigrants may experience microaggressions related to the outgroup homo-geneity effect, which posits that members of the outgroup (e.g., a group of immigrants) are perceived as less variable than members of the in-group (Judd & Park, 1988). In practice, this means that U.S.-born Americans might perceive immigrants from a particular region of the world (i.e., out-group) as more similar than they perceive Americans (i.e., themselves) as a group. For example, people of color frequently experience microaggressions related to perceived physical homogeneity. In one study, Asian Americans reported being mistaken as Chinese or hearing statements indicating that all Asians look alike (Sue et al., 2009). Other studies reveal that many African immigrants report being mistaken as Black American, a mistake that inval-idates their cultural and ethnic backgrounds (Louis et al., 2017; Shenoy-Packer, 2015).

Furthermore, although first-generation immigrants might see themselves as separate from racial minority groups in the United States, 1.5- and second-generation immigrants often have a better understanding of racial dynamics in the United States, resulting in an identification with their respective racial minority groups regardless of immigration status and cultural differences (Hall & Carter, 2006). In fact, immigrants who have lived in the United States for a long time or were born and raised in the United States might develop a shared identity with a particular racial minority group (e.g., Africans or West Indians identifying as Black or Black Americans). As a result, some racial minority immigrants may experience the same microaggressions experienced by their U.S.-born counterparts in addition to microaggressions that specifi-cally target their immigration status or identity.

Theme 5: The Myth of Meritocracy and Denial of Systemic Racism

Many first-generation immigrants migrate to the United States in hopes of pursuing the American Dream, a colorblind utopia with endless educational and occupational opportunities and where all hard work inevitably leads to success (Hill & Torres, 2010). While many immigrants have been able to succeed (Pew Research Center, 2013), this idealized sentiment invalidates the systemic racial barriers to success faced by most people of color in the United States. Furthermore, research has consistently shown that foreign-born immigrants report lower levels of perceived racism than U.S.-born racial minorities (e.g., Dominguez et al., 2009). First-generation immigrants may believe that the United States is a meritocracy and deny the impact of systemic racism. This is consistent with system justification theory, which argues that people want to retain a sense of control and predictability in an unjust world (Jost et al., 2004).

Given these factors, meritocracy and the denial of systemic racism may affect different generations of immigrants in unique ways. For first-generation immigrants, encountering racism and other systemic barriers may be difficult to acknowledge, particularly if they had believed premigration that the United States was the land of opportunity and if they sacrificed significantly to migrate to the United States. Therefore, when they encounter microaggressions, they may struggle with labeling such experiences as biased, resulting in internalized oppression and psychological distress. For 1.5- and second-generation immigrants who were born or raised in the United States, it may be difficult to experience microaggressions from immigrant family members who uphold the American Dream and meritocracy. For example, some studies have shown that second- and third-generation Latinx immigrants show lower educational achievement than more recent immigrants (Hill & Torres, 2010). This achievement gap frustrates immigrant parents who migrated to the country with high expectations for the education system and upward mobility, resulting in conflicting worldviews, family tensions, and distress.

Theme 6: Pathologizing Cultural Values and Communication Styles

Immigrants often experience microaggressions in which their cultural values and communication styles are perceived or labeled as abnormal and/or inferior. In a study examining microaggressions toward Latinx Americans, participants described how their values, food, religion, dress, and language were viewed as inferior or deviant (Rivera et al., 2010). Specifically, participants reported being shamed for living with their parents, for speaking "too fast," and for exhibiting their "Latin temper" in conversations (p. 69). In a study exploring microaggressions toward Asian Americans, Chinese students reported they felt at a disadvantage compared with White American students because of their perceived passive or indirect communication styles (Sue et al., 2009).

These types of microaggressions convey the idea that immigrants should assimilate to mainstream culture, which further isolates them (Kim & Kim, 2010).

Theme 7: Criminalization

In recent years, immigrants of all statuses (e.g., undocumented, visa holders, citizens) have been subject to both systemic and interpersonal discrimination, resulting in microaggressions in which they are criminalized or made to feel like deviants. First, biased laws and policies have historically targeted immigrants, particularly those from non-White countries, for over a century. At the "founding" of the United States in the late 1770s, European immigrants were able to migrate to the United States without any documents or legal procedures; however, as Asian immigrants started to arrive, the Chinese Exclusion Act of 1882 was introduced as the first of many laws attempting to limit the number of Asian immigrants into the country (Dong, 2019). As more immigrants (particularly those from non-White countries) have entered the United States, more laws and policies have been created and enforced. For example, since 2008, federal immigration policies have resulted in the deportations of 3 million undocumented people in the United States, resulting in thousands of family separations and psychological trauma for both the deportees and the families and children left behind (Lovato et al., 2018). Furthermore, in 2017, an executive order that banned individuals from seven predominantly Muslim countries from entering the United States was signed into law (Collingwood et al., 2018).

While these policies have caused significant distress for immigrants (especially undocumented immigrants), anti-immigrant sentiment is fueled by racist rhetoric of elected officials who have painted immigrants as dangerous, violent, or criminal. For example, when Donald Trump first announced his campaign for president in 2015, he described Mexicans as "rapists and criminals." While many pundits presumed that his biased sentiment would be his demise, it only made him more popular and resulted in his election (Nadal, 2018).

After the 9/11 terrorist attacks, hate crimes and discrimination toward Muslim Americans and those perceived to be Muslim Americans (e.g., Sikh men) significantly increased (Ahluwalia & Pellettiere, 2010; Nadal, Griffin, et al., 2012). In addition to physical violence, Muslim Americans (and those assumed to be Muslim) experienced a variety of Islamophobic microaggressions, such as being called "terrorist," "Taliban," or "Osama." In addition, participants experienced microaggressions related to the theme of being seen as an alien in their own land; they were told to "go back to [their] country" and were perceived as anti-American (Ahluwalia & Pellettiere, 2010; Nadal, Griffin, et al., 2012). Research suggests that undocumented immigrants are afraid to engage in everyday activities because they fear that immigration officers will arrest and deport them or someone in their family (Lovato et al., 2018). As such, both undocumented and documented immigrants may experience microaggressions, including microassaults (e.g., people telling them to go back to their country) and microinvalidations (e.g., people telling them their fears are unwarranted).

Theme 8: Second-Class Citizen

In addition to being treated as criminals, racial minority immigrants may experience systemic and interpersonal microaggressions in which they feel like second-class citizens, particularly when they are also undocumented. Nienhusser et al. (2016) identified a variety of microaggressions experienced by undocumented college students, including interpersonal and environmental microassaults, such as discriminatory financial aid policies that rendered students ineligible for federal or state support for college tuition. Students also reported feelings of hopelessness, anger, and frustration during the college application process, due to overwhelming perceived and explicitly stated barriers structured to prevent life opportunities, such as internships, volunteer work, and job opportunities.

While international students usually migrate to the United States with valid yet restricted visas to pursue their studies, they may experience a variety of systemic and interpersonal microaggressions in university contexts, which may make them feel dehumanized, rejected, or like second-class citizens. Kim and Kim (2010) described an array of microaggressions faced by international students, including exclusion and social rejection by domestic peers or being ignored altogether. Other systemic barriers for international students include lack of resources, lack of inclusion in new student orientation, and limitations in financial aid or work study due to their international status.

A final example in which immigrants are treated as second-class citizens is the way in which migrant children have been managed after being detained and separated from their parents and families. In 2017, the American Association of Pediatrics released a policy report asserting that the conditions of detention centers in which migrant children were housed at the time were alarming and traumatizing (Linton et al., 2017). The report stated,

> The conditions in which children are detained and the support services that are available to them are of great concern to pediatricians and other advocates for children. . . . Immigrant and refugee children should be treated with dignity and respect and should not be exposed to conditions that may harm or traumatize them. The Department of Homeland Security facilities do not meet the basic standards for the care of children in residential settings. (Linton et al., 2017, p. 1)

Treating undocumented people in inhumane ways should be viewed as problematic, and the fact that innocent children are being treated without regard for their humanity is even more cruel and heinous.

The literature presented here suggests that microaggressions faced by racial minority immigrants might have implications for identity development across the lifespan. Experiencing microaggressions is associated with a variety of negative physical and negative health outcomes, including overall lower psychological well-being (Nadal, Griffin, et al., 2014), depressive symptoms and suicidal ideation (Nadal, Griffin, et al., 2014; O'Keefe et al., 2015), and posttraumatic stress symptoms (Moody & Lewis, 2019; Torres & Taknint, 2015). As a result, it is important to expand our understanding of how micro-aggressions may manifest toward racial minority immigrants.

CASE EXAMPLES

To highlight the potential manifestation and impact of microaggressions among racial minority immigrants, we present three fictional case studies that illustrate several themes from our taxonomy. These examples are drawn from the first author's personal and clinical experiences.

The Case of Amari

Amari is a 22-year-old second-generation Arab American college senior who presented at her college's counseling center with feelings of isolation, hopelessness, and suicidal ideation.[1] Amari's fiancé, Omar, had recently ended their engagement after she asked to postpone their wedding so that she could pursue a law degree after graduation. Although Amari wanted to get married, she was worried that having children would diminish her chances of getting accepted into law school—she was especially aware of stereotypes involving passive Arab wives. Amari's family and some close friends placed blame on Amari for the breakup, stating that she was "too American" and that she had "shamed her parents," who had always been supportive of her. Amari felt guilty that her parents were being questioned by their family and community, but she also felt betrayed and angry, as her parents had previously encouraged her to follow her dreams. In addition, Amari was unable to confide in her American friends, who lacked understanding of her culture and pressured her to disregard opinions from her "controlling" family. Her friends insisted she was American—and can and should, therefore, do what she wants to do. Amari felt hopeless, misunderstood, tense, and alone.

The Case of Aisha

Aisha is a 25-year-old 1.5-generation Senegalese immigrant who sought therapy to deal with her anxiety. Aisha moved to the United States when she was 8 years old, and she is the oldest of five siblings. Aisha grew up in a primarily Black American neighborhood, and although she did not necessarily struggle to make friends, she always felt somewhat different than her Black American peers because she was one of the only children of immigrants.

---

[1]All case material has been altered to protect confidentiality.

Aisha shared that her parents always spoke English with her and her siblings and never actively taught her to speak Wolof (their native language) or French (their secondary language). When Aisha was a child, some extended family members used to joke that Aisha and her siblings were not authentically Senegalese because they did not speak Wolof, but it did not bother her much. Two years ago, Aisha met her current boyfriend, Sekou, who is a second-generation Senegalese American. Having a shared ethnicity was one of the reasons that Aisha was attracted to Sekou and was why she decided she wanted to marry him. When the couple became engaged, they proceeded to introduce each other to their parents. Sekou's parents were appalled by the fact that Aisha did not learn to speak Wolof, which they equivocated with her being "too Americanized." Aisha's parents took offense at Sekou's parents' statements and forbade Aisha to marry Sekou because his family was poor, from a working-class background, and unable to assimilate to Western culture. Although Sekou was optimistic that their parents would reconcile in due time, Aisha was experiencing anxiety, depressed mood, shame, and guilt because she believed that if she were "Senegalese enough," none of these problems would have started in the first place.

The Case of Swapnil

Swapnil is a 30-year-old Bengali Muslim gay lawyer who immigrated to the United States with his family when he was 17 years old. He sought counseling to address work-related stress, difficulties in romantic relationships, and consequent social isolation. Swapnil lived at home with his parents and younger siblings and was having difficulties adjusting to his new job at a law firm. Swapnil's job involved frequent business meetings, involving alcohol consumption, with clients and coworkers. As a practicing Muslim, Swapnil did not consume alcohol but felt pressure to adhere to social-mainstream business practices. In addition, Swapnil had been fighting with his long-term boyfriend, Jonathan, a U.S.-born South Asian American, because Jonathan did not understand why Swapnil still lived with his family and why he did not officially come out to them. Over the previous few weeks, Swapnil had slowly entered a depressive state and was having difficulty eating, sleeping, and getting out of bed. He reported feeling isolated and miserable.

Case Discussion

In the first example, Amari experienced multiple microaggressions based on her identities as an Arab American, an Arab woman, and an Arab immigrant. While her extended family and community criticized her desire to pursue her individual career goals over marriage, her American friends stereotyped her family as controlling and dismissed the importance of her relationships with her family and culture.

The second example illustrates how 1.5- and second-generation immigrants might experience microaggressions related to (a) perceived identification with mainstream American culture and (b) perceived missing ties with their heritage culture. The meetings of Aisha's and Sekou's families reflect complex family dynamics and the multiple types of microaggressions that can manifest (e.g., classist microaggressions toward Sekou's family, questioning of cultural authenticity toward Aisha for not speaking Wolof). The case illustrates how language- and culture-related microaggressions may present unique circumstances for second-generation immigrants as they navigate their identities in both mainstream American culture and their respective heritage cultures.

The third example shows how microaggressions may function simultaneously on an interpersonal and on a systemic level. At work, Swapnil experienced microaggressions related to his religious beliefs and cultural practices, which affected his day-to-day functioning (e.g., inability to get out of bed), relationships, and work performance. In addition, the case reflects the ways in which intersectional identities complicate experiences with microaggressions—while Jonathan's boyfriend likely wanted Swapnil to come out because he perceived that doing so would make Swapnil feel happier, it is also important that he respect Swapnil's process and the cultural factors that may prevent him from coming out by Western standards. Finally, because Swapnil felt microaggressions from different parts of his life, he felt unable to talk about his experiences with anyone, resulting in his total isolation.

Taken together, it is clear that microaggressions may negatively affect the mental health of racial minority immigrants. As shown by previous research addressing people of color and other historically marginalized groups (see Torino et al., 2019, for a review), racial minority immigrants may experience an array of negative psychological outcomes, including depression, anxiety, and low self-esteem. Furthermore, these cases demonstrate how microaggressions may have a negative impact on identity development, career development, and even physical health; they reveal a critical need for microaggressions among racial minority immigrants to be addressed. These case examples show that racial minority immigrants face microaggressions from multiple sources, including mainstream American culture and heritage cultures, based on their intersecting identities. In the context of the proposed taxonomy, the cases illustrate how microaggressions toward racial minority immigrants threaten the target person's mental health and have the power to fundamentally influence immigrant's self-concept. For immigrants, microaggressions are not only perpetrated by outgroups; they often occur in close familial and intimate relationships and lead to isolation—the perhaps greatest known risk factor for mental health problems.

RECOMMENDATIONS FOR RESEARCH, CLINICAL WORK, AND POLICY

Because racial minority immigrants face unique circumstances that place them in vulnerable positions that can encourage stigmatization and marginalization, we conclude by providing recommendations for research, clinical work, and policy. First, with the growing and ever-changing anti-immigrant sentiment across the United States, more comprehensive research examining the experiences of immigrants is needed. The dynamic nature of anti-immigrant sentiment is particularly salient in the context of the COVID-19 pandemic, which has manifested new microaggressions, such as those related to contamination, against Asian immigrants and Asian Americans. Future empirical research should continue to explore heterogeneous experiences of immigrants by race, ethnicity, and other identities while being intentional in considering history, generation, and citizen and documentation status. Furthermore, additional research is needed to detangle the complex inter- and intragroup relations and shared identities among ethnic minority populations. For example, as noted throughout the chapter, second-generation immigrants may experience microaggressions from U.S.-born White Americans, immigrants from their ethnic group, or both; first-generation immigrants may also experience microaggressions from more Americanized immigrants and the 1.5, second, and later generations.

Regarding clinical work, it is important for psychotherapists to be culturally competent in working with racial minority immigrants (Sue et al., 2019). They must develop knowledge of the diverse experiences of immigrants, people of color, and people who identify as both. They must also develop awareness of how their own cultural identities influence their clients' abilities to trust in the therapy process. For example, research indicates that some communities of color have a cultural mistrust of psychologists and mental health practitioners, especially White therapists, because of the historic oppression of their racial and ethnic groups (David, 2010). As a result, therapists must be aware that others may not initially trust them and may be actively wary, cautious, or distrustful. Finally, therapists must also attain the skills to manage microaggressions that occur in the therapy—by acknowledging that they occur; by comfortably discussing meanings, intents, and impacts of microaggressions; and by assisting clients in coping with microaggressions as they occur.

It is also crucial for psychologists and mental health practitioners to consider and integrate perspectives and experiences of racial minority immigrants in their policies and procedures. For instance, educational institutions can be intentional in providing support for international and undocumented students. Training programs can be more inclusive of international perspectives, and workplace environments can facilitate microaggressions and implicit bias trainings to ensure that employees on all levels are aware of their biases. Systems and institutions across all sectors can be proactive in providing disaggregated data about immigrant experiences so that community members are aware of the specific issues that affect each community. Hospitals, schools, and government agencies can collect and publicize disaggregated data, which can lead to the creation of new and culturally appropriate programs and services.

Finally, it is necessary for psychologists and other practitioners to acknowledge that addressing issues such as microaggressions, discrimination, and oppression is an ethical responsibility and that their obligation is to avoid harming their clients (Nadal, 2017). As such, because psychologists recognize the documented and empirically supported effects of oppression—including systemic and institutional oppression, interpersonal discrimination, and microaggressions—they must do what they can to advocate for humanity and justice in research, practice, and training. In doing so, they create more inclusive environments for all, making society a more just place for all people to live and thrive.

REFERENCES

Ahluwalia, M. K., & Pellettiere, L. (2010). Sikh men post-9/11: Misidentification, discrimination, and coping. *Asian American Journal of Psychology, 1*(4), 303–314. https://doi.org/10.1037/a0022156

Beirich, H., & Buchanan, S. (2018, February 19). 2017: The year in hate and extremism. *Southern Law Poverty Center.* https://www.splcenter.org/fighting-hate/intelligence-report/2018/2017-year-hate-and-extremism

Camarota, S. A., & Zeigler, K. (2018, September). *Record 44.5 million immigrants in 2017.* Center for Immigration Studies. https://cis.org/Report/Record-445-Million-Immigrants-2017

Collingwood, L., Lajevardi, N., & Oskooii, K. A. (2018). A change of heart? Why individual-level public opinion shifted against Trump's "Muslim Ban." *Political Behavior, 40*(4), 1035–1072. https://doi.org/10.1007/s11109-017-9439-z

David, E. J. R. (2010). Cultural mistrust and mental health help-seeking attitudes among Filipino Americans. *Asian American Journal of Psychology, 1*(1), 57–66. https://doi.org/10.1037/a0018814

David, E. J. R., & Okazaki, S. (2006). The Colonial Mentality Scale (CMS) for Filipino Americans: Scale construction and psychological implications. *Journal of Counseling Psychology, 53*(2), 241–252. https://doi.org/10.1037/0022-0167.53.2.241

Dominguez, T. P., Strong, E. F., Krieger, N., Gillman, M. W., & Rich-Edwards, J. W. (2009). Differences in the self-reported racism experiences of US-born and foreign-born Black pregnant women. *Social Science & Medicine, 69*(2), 258–265. https://doi.org/10.1016/j.socscimed.2009.03.022

Dong, L. (Ed.). (2019). *25 events that shaped Asian American history: An encyclopedia of the American mosaic.* ABC-CLIO.

Eberhardt, J. L. (2005). Imaging race. *American Psychologist, 60*(2), 181–190. https://doi.org/10.1037/0003-066x.60.2.181

Fuertes, J. N., Gottdiener, W. H., Martin, H., Gilbert, T. C., & Giles, H. (2012). A meta-analysis of the effects of speakers' accents on interpersonal evaluations. *European Journal of Social Psychology, 42*(1), 120–133. https://doi.org/10.1002/ejsp.862

Gluszek, A., & Dovidio, J. F. (2010). Speaking with a nonnative accent: Perceptions of bias, communication difficulties, and belonging in the United States. *Journal of Language and Social Psychology, 29*(2), 224–234. https://doi.org/10.1177/0261927X09359590

Hall, S. P., & Carter, R. T. (2006). The relationship between racial identity, ethnic identity and perceptions of racial discrimination in an Afro-Caribbean descent sample. *The Journal of Black Psychology, 32*(2), 155–175. https://doi.org/10.1177/0095798406287071

Hill, N. E., & Torres, K. (2010). Negotiating the American dream: The paradox of aspirations and achievement among Latino students and engagement between their families and schools. *Journal of Social Issues, 66*(1), 95–112. https://doi.org/10.1111/j.1540-4560.2009.01635.x

Huber, L. P., & Cueva, B. M. (2012). Chicana/Latina testimonios on effects and responses to microaggressions. *Equity & Excellence in Education, 45*(3), 392–410. https://doi.org/10.1080/10665684.2012.698193

Johnston, M. P., & Nadal, K. L. (2010). Multiracial microaggressions: Exposing mono-racism in everyday life and clinical practice. In D. W. Sue (Ed.), *Microaggressions and marginality: Manifestation, dynamics, and impact* (pp. 123–144). John Wiley & Sons.

Jost, J. T., Banaji, M. R., & Nosek, B. A. (2004). A decade of system justification theory: Accumulated evidence of conscious and unconscious bolstering of the status quo. *Political Psychology, 25*(6), 881–919. https://doi.org/10.1111/j.1467-9221.2004.00402.x

Judd, C. M., & Park, B. (1988). Out-group homogeneity: Judgments of variability at the individual and group levels. *Journal of Personality and Social Psychology, 54*(5), 778–788. https://doi.org/10.1037/0022-3514.54.5.778

Kassin, S., Fein, S., & Markus, H. R. (2018). *Social psychology* (10th ed.). Cengage.

Kim, S., & Kim, R. (2010). Microaggressions experienced by international students attending U.S. institutions of higher education. In D. W. Sue (Ed.), *Microaggressions and marginality: Manifestation, dynamics, and impact* (pp. 171–192). John Wiley & Sons.

Linton, J. M., Griffin, M., Shapiro, A. J., & the Council on Community Pediatrics. (2017). Detention of immigrant children. *Pediatrics, 139*(5), e20170483. https://doi.org/10.1542/peds.2017-0483

Louis, D. A., Thompson, K. V., Smith, P., Williams, H. M. A., & Watson, J. (2017). Afro-Caribbean immigrant faculty experiences in the American academy: Voices of an invisible Black population. *The Urban Review, 49*(4), 668–691. https://doi.org/10.1007/s11256-017-0414-0

Lovato, K., Lopez, C., Karimli, L., & Abrams, L. S. (2018). The impact of deportation-related family separations on the well-being of Latinx children and youth: A review of the literature. *Children and Youth Services Review, 95*, 109–116. https://doi.org/10.1016/j.childyouth.2018.10.011

Moody, A. T., & Lewis, J. A. (2019). Gendered racial microaggressions and traumatic stress symptoms among Black women. *Psychology of Women Quarterly, 43*(2), 201–214.

Nadal, K. L. (2017). "Let's get in formation": On becoming a psychologist–activist in the 21st century. *American Psychologist, 72*(9), 935–946. https://doi.org/10.1037/amp0000212

Nadal, K. L. (2018). *Microaggressions and traumatic stress: Theory, research and practice.* American Psychological Association. https://doi.org/10.1037/0000073-000

Nadal, K. L., Escobar, K. M. V., Prado, G. T., David, E. J. R., & Haynes, K. (2012). Racial microaggressions and the Filipino American experience: Recommendations for counseling and development. *Journal of Multicultural Counseling and Development, 40*(3), 156–173. https://doi.org/10.1002/j.2161-1912.2012.00015.x

Nadal, K. L., Griffin, K. E., Hamit, S., Leon, J., Tobio, M., & Rivera, D. P. (2012). Subtle and overt forms of Islamophobia: Microaggressions toward Muslim Americans. *The Journal of Muslim Mental Health, 6*(2), 15–37. https://doi.org/10.3998/jmmh.10381607.0006.203

Nadal, K. L., Griffin, K. E., Wong, Y., Hamit, S., & Rasmus, M. (2014). The impact of racial microaggressions on mental health: Counseling implications for clients of color. *Journal of Counseling and Development, 92*(1), 57–66. https://doi.org/10.1002/j.1556-6676.2014.00130.x

Nadal, K. L., Issa, M.-A., Griffin, K., Hamit, S., & Lyons, O. (2010). Religious micro-aggressions in the United States: Mental health implications for religious minority groups. In D. W. Sue (Ed.), *Microaggressions and marginality: Manifestation, dynamics, and impact* (pp. 287–310). John Wiley & Sons.

Nadal, K. L., Mazzula, S. L., Rivera, D. P., & Fujii-Doe, W. (2014). Microaggressions and Latina/o Americans: An analysis of nativity, gender, and ethnicity. *Journal of Latina/o Psychology, 2*(2), 67–78. https://doi.org/10.1037/lat0000013

Nadal, K. L., Wong, Y., Sriken, J., Griffin, K., & Fujii-Doe, W. (2015). Racial micro-aggressions and Asian Americans: An exploratory study on within-group differences and mental health. *Asian American Journal of Psychology, 6*(2), 136–144. https://doi.org/10.1037/a0038058

Nienhusser, H. K., Vega, B. E., & Carquin, M. C. S. (2016). Undocumented students' experiences with microaggressions during their college choice process. *Teachers College Record, 118,* 1–33.

O'Keefe, V. M., Wingate, L. R., Cole, A. B., Hollingsworth, D. W., & Tucker, R. P. (2015). Seemingly harmless racial communications are not so harmless: Racial microaggressions lead to suicidal ideation by way of depression symptoms. *Suicide & Life-Threatening Behavior, 45*(5), 567–576. https://doi.org/10.1111/sltb.12150

Pew Research Center. (2013). *Second-generation Americans: A portrait of the adult children of immigrants.* https://www.pewsocialtrends.org/2013/02/07/second-generation-americans/

Pierce, C., Carew, J., Pierce-Gonzalez, D., & Willis, D. (1978). An experiment in racism: TV commercials. In C. Pierce (Ed.), *Television and education* (pp. 62–88). Sage.

Rivera, D. P., Forquer, E. E., & Rangel, R. (2010). Microaggressions and the life experience of Latina/o Americans. In D. W. Sue (Ed.), *Microaggressions and marginality: Manifestation, dynamics, and impact* (pp. 59–83). John Wiley & Sons.

Shenoy-Packer, S. (2015). Immigrant professionals, microaggressions, and critical sensemaking in the U.S. workplace. *Management Communication Quarterly, 29*(2), 257–275. https://doi.org/10.1177/0893318914562069

Stroink, M. L., & Lalonde, R. N. (2009). Bicultural identity conflict in second-generation Asian Canadians. *The Journal of Social Psychology, 149*(1), 44–65. https://doi.org/10.3200/socp.149.1.44-65

Sue, D. W. (2010). *Microaggressions and marginality: Manifestation, dynamics, and impact.* John Wiley & Sons.

Sue, D. W., Bucceri, J., Lin, A. I., Nadal, K. L., & Torino, G. C. (2009). Racial microaggressions and the Asian American experience. *Asian American Journal of Psychology, S*(1), 88–101. https://doi.org/10.1037/1948-1985.S.1.88

Sue, D. W., Capodilupo, C. M., Torino, G. C., Bucceri, J. M., Holder, A. M., Nadal, K. L., & Esquilin, M. (2007). Racial microaggressions in everyday life: Implications for clinical practice. *American Psychologist, 62*(4), 271–286. https://doi.org/10.1037/0003-066X.62.4.271

Sue, D. W., Sue, D., Neville, H. A., & Smith, L. (2019). *Counseling the culturally diverse: Theory and practice.* John Wiley & Sons.

Torino, G. C., Rivera, D. P., Capodilupo, C. M., Nadal, K. L., & Sue, D. W. (Eds.). (2019). *Microaggression theory: Influence and implications.* John Wiley & Sons.

Torres, L., & Taknint, J. T. (2015). Ethnic microaggressions, traumatic stress symptoms, and Latino depression: A moderated mediational model. *Journal of Counseling Psychology, 62*(3), 393–401. https://doi.org/10.1037/cou0000077

Tuan, M. (2002). Second-generation Asian American identity: Clues from the Asian ethnic experience. In P. G. Min (Ed.), *The second generation: Ethnic identity among Asian Americans* (pp. 209–237). Alta Mira.

Waters, M. C. (1994). Ethnic and racial identities of second-generation Black immigrants in New York City. *The International Migration Review, 28*(4), 795–820. https://doi.org/10.1177/019791839402800408

II

SPECIFIC FORMS OF TRAUMA IN IMMIGRANT COMMUNITIES

6

"Forever Foreigners"

Intergenerational Impacts of Historical Trauma From the World War II Japanese American Incarceration

Donna K. Nagata and Reeya A. Patel

Japanese immigrants arriving in the United States in the late 19th century worked hard to establish their lives in a new country despite facing significant discrimination and challenges (Daniels, 2004). On December 7, 1941, however, Japan's military attack on Pearl Harbor, Hawaii, marked the beginning of a particularly powerful and historic racial trauma. Within weeks of declaring war against Japan, the U.S. government portrayed all people of Japanese ancestry living along the Western mainland as potential threats to national security because of their proximity to Japan and ordered them into incarceration[1] camps. Under President Roosevelt's Executive Order 9066 (EO9066), more than 117,000 Japanese Americans[2] were confined in the desolate camps for up to 4 years (United States Commission on Wartime Relocation of Civilians [USCWRIC], 1997). Two thirds were U.S.-born citizens, and although the country was also at war with Germany and Italy, neither German nor Italian Americans were targeted for mass incarceration. Furthermore,

---

[1]The wartime imprisonment of Japanese Americans is often referred to as an internment. However, "internment" is a misnomer since it legally refers to the detention of enemy aliens during times of war. In contrast, most of those affected by the government's wartime actions were U.S. citizens, and the term "incarceration" is now considered a more accurate term (Densho, n.d.). Accordingly, members of the incarceration camps are referred to as "incarcerees" in this chapter.

[2]This chapter uses the term "Japanese American" broadly to refer to Americans of Japanese descent, regardless of citizenship.

Reeya A. Patel's contribution to this work was supported by the Intramural Research Program of the Eunice Kennedy Shriver National Institute of Child Health and Human Development.

https://doi.org/10.1037/0000214-007
Trauma and Racial Minority Immigrants: Turmoil, Uncertainty, and Resistance,
P. Tummala-Narra (Editor)

the government's rationale was contradictory. On one hand, removal and imprisonment was said to be necessary because coastal Japanese Americans lived relatively near to Japan. On the other hand, there was no mass incarceration of Japanese in Hawaii, which was geographically even closer (USCWRIC, 1997).

Those affected by EO9066 suffered tremendous economic losses, the suspension of their constitutional rights while imprisoned, and the burden of living under a shadow of suspected disloyalty. Impacts from these traumas reverberated within their families and communities for decades (Nagata et al., 2015, 2019; USCWRIC, 1997). Forty years later, however, a congressional commission fully investigated the circumstances of the wartime decision. It concluded that the incarceration of Japanese Americans was unjustified and based in race prejudice and wartime panic rather than military necessity (USCWRIC, 1997).

This chapter provides an examination, on the basis of historical and cultural trauma theories, of the extended consequences of the incarceration. *Historical trauma* is trauma shared by a group of people that impacts multiple generations across time (Mohatt et al., 2014), while *cultural trauma* is defined as "when members of a collectivity feel they have been subjected to a traumatic event that leaves indelible marks upon their group consciousness, making memories forever and changing their future identity" (Alexander, 2004, p. 1). We begin with a history of Japanese immigration to the United States as a context for the incarceration decision. Next, we describe the traumatic stressors encountered by individuals who were imprisoned and their intergenerational impacts. Following this, the chapter highlights Japanese Americans' strategies of individual and collective resilience. Finally, implications of the WWII incarceration for the minority and immigrant experience in the United States are discussed.

IMMIGRATION HISTORY AS A CONTEXT FOR WARTIME INCARCERATION

The attack on Pearl Harbor launched the United States into war with Japan, but the subsequent mass incarceration of Japanese Americans was the culmination of decades of prior discrimination and xenophobia. Discrimination against persons of Chinese descent in the late 19th and early 20th centuries set the historical prelude to discrimination faced by the Japanese. Similar to immigrants of other nationalities, Chinese and Japanese immigrants coming to the United States maintained ties to their homelands; this relationship intensified when they encountered barriers to American citizenship. Both groups faced greater discrimination than European immigrants did. Despite their distinct ethnic roots, "all Asian immigrants seemed alike and alike seemed to present a threat to the American standard of living and to the racial integrity of the nation" (Daniels, 2004, p. 4).

Chinese immigrants initially moved to the United States because of Sacramento's gold rush and to take labor jobs in the construction of California's transcontinental railroad line (Daniels, 2004; USCWRIC, 1997). As their presence grew, they were perceived as economic competitors and became the target of anti-immigration activity. These actions included the Naturalization Act of 1790, which was revised to exclude Asian alien residents from citizenship; legalized discrimination against Chinese mine workers (Daniels, 2004; USCWRIC, 1997); and the Chinese Exclusion Act of 1882, which prohibited Chinese laborers from immigrating to the United States (National Archives, 1989). The prohibition of Chinese immigration allowed for a significant growth in Japanese arrivals during the late 19th century. From just 3,000 immigrants in 1890, Japanese immigration grew to 275,000 persons by 1924, with the heaviest concentrations in California (Daniels, 2004). Several factors contributed to this trend, including stronger relations between Japan and the United States and increased labor opportunities with the ban on Chinese immigration (USCWRIC, 1997). Although they never comprised more than 2.1% of California's population (and represented an even smaller percentage of the total U.S. population), the successes of Japanese immigrants in agriculture and fishing raised animosity among labor movements and political groups (Daniels, 2004; USCWRIC, 1997).

By 1919, Japanese farmers in California had control of more than 10% of the total value of the state's harvest (Daniels, 2004). An anti-Japanese movement rooted in economic anxiety took hold and encouraged the prohibition of Japanese immigration. The Japanese were already ineligible for citizenship due to the Naturalization Act of 1790, and additional efforts to limit immigration developed. Starting in 1913 in California and later in other Western states, laws restricted Japanese agricultural success by limiting land ownership (Daniels, 2004; USCWRIC, 1997). While these efforts reduced the amounts of land owned by Japanese (Iwata, 1992), in some cases, *Issei*[3] (i.e., first-generation Japanese immigrants), who were not eligible for citizenship, used the Fourteenth Amendment as a legal loophole and transferred agricultural properties to their children who were U.S. citizens by birth (Daniels, 2004). The anti-Japanese movement escalated after the end of World War I and eventually led to the Immigration Act of 1924, which prohibited any immigration from Japan to the United States (tenBroek et al., 1968; USCWRIC, 1997).

Although governed largely by economic anxiety, the anti-Japanese activity in the decades leading up to EO9066 also reflected fears of a "yellow peril." Popularized by newspapers, this term implied that Asian immigration rates were threatening and uncontrollable. It was first used for propaganda against Chinese immigrants and later against those from Japan. Both groups were perceived to be a "single racial threat" (USCWRIC, 1997, p. 37). As early as 1900, political leaders such as Mayor James Duval Phelan in San Francisco supported anti-Japanese activity because of perceived cultural differences: "Personally we have nothing against Japanese, but as they will not assimilate

---

[3]Japanese Americans identify specific generations based on immigration from Japan. *Issei* are the first generation to immigrate. *Nisei* are the second generation of Japanese in the United States and the first U.S.-born generation. *Sansei* and *Yonsei* are third- and fourth-generation Japanese Americans, respectively.

with us and their social life is so different from ours, let them keep at a respectful distance" (Daniels, 2004, p. 10). Popular films and books promoted similar sentiments (USCWRIC, 1997).

From the beginning of the 20th century, deterioration of relations between the United States and Japan led to increased fear of war with Japan and of unrestricted Japanese population growth on the Pacific West Coast (USCWRIC, 1997). In reality, fears of Japanese overpopulation were unfounded and based on a severe overestimation of population and birth rates of Japanese immigrants (Daniels, 2004; USCWRIC, 1997). The fact that Japan and the United States were on opposite sides during WWII was used as justification for the involuntary "relocation" of Japanese communities to incarceration camps. While war might have heightened tensions against Japanese individuals in the United States, it was a matchstick added to an already-burning flame of discrimination and racism.

INCARCERATION AND TRAUMATIC STRESS

Japanese Americans faced a range of traumatic stressors associated with their wartime incarceration. Immediately following the attack on Pearl Harbor, the government targeted prominent Issei who headed civic and religious organizations. Considered high-risk individuals, these men were rounded up without warning and sent to Immigration and Naturalization Service internment camps for enemy aliens, leaving their families to fend on their own at a time of fear and uncertainty. The absence of elder Issei leaders also created a void in community leadership and reduced the likelihood of organized resistance. In the post-Pearl Harbor climate, Japanese Americans experienced racial harassment, violence, discrimination, and ostracism. With no information about what was unfolding, rumors spread that the government would take all Japanese Americans to a remote area to be shot. The constant shadow of suspicion by non-Japanese and by the government led families to burn photographs and heirlooms from Japan, items they worried would be seen as evidence of loyalty to the enemy. U.S.-born, second-generation Japanese Americans, the *Nisei*, experienced anxiety around the uncertainty of their future and safety and had concerns about whether they would be separated from their Issei parents, who were considered enemy aliens and prohibited from citizenship. Shocked, worried, scared, and confused were prominent emotions Nisei former incarcerees recalled about their experiences soon after Pearl Harbor (Nagata et al., 2012).

Notification that removal would occur in less than 2 weeks created additional stress. Because of the sudden "evacuation,"[4] Japanese Americans

---

[4]The government used euphemistic language throughout the incarceration (i.e., referring to camp inmates as "evacuees," camps as "relocation centers," detention centers as "assembly centers," and U.S. citizens as "non-aliens"), which minimized the severity of what occurred (Ishizuka, 2006).

experienced abrupt and painful separations from non-Japanese friends, neighbors, and colleagues and were forced to leave behind family pets without knowing about the possibility of a return. Packing was especially difficult since Japanese Americans were allowed to take only what they could carry and given no information about where they were being sent or how long they would be gone. Forced to dispose of life belongings and close businesses within 10 days, Japanese Americans also were vulnerable to bargain hunters and swindlers (Weglyn, 1976). Cars and farming equipment were abandoned or put into storage with churches or White friends they hoped could be trusted. For the Issei immigrants, "the rewards of a lifetime of zealous perseverance evaporated within a frenzied fortnight" (Weglyn, 1976, p. 77). Income and property losses, in 1983 dollars adjusted for inflation, were estimated to be between $810 million and $2 billion (USCWRIC, 1997).

Added to these stressors was the government's impersonal treatment of Japanese Americans during the process. Families were not identified by name but instead were assigned numbered tags that they were required to wear. "I lost my identity," testified one Nisei who appeared before the postwar government commission investigating the incarceration. "At that time, I didn't even have a Social Security number but the WRA (War Relocation Authority) gave me an I.D. number. That was my identification. I lost my privacy and my dignity" (Testimony of Betty Matsuo, as cited in USCWRIC, 1997, p. 135).

Most of those affected endured two different moves. Because the government implemented rapid removal to address public and political anti-Japanese pressure before the camps were complete, Japanese Americans were first sent to temporary detention centers for an average of 3 months (USCWRIC, 1997). The centers consisted of hastily converted horse stalls at racetracks, large livestock pavilions, and stockades, all of which were surrounded by armed guards and barbed wire. Life in the detention centers was strenuous. Thousands were housed together under physically challenging conditions: Communal toilets lacked partitions, lack of insulation led to extreme heat and dust, and weeds grew up between floorboards (USCWRIC, pp. 138–139). One Nisei woman noted,

> The building was constructed with cheap lumber, so they had a lot of knots in there. Men would pop the knots so you'd always see some eye looking in, peeking at you. . . . The privacy was absolutely none. Taking showers where they used to wash the horses. (Nagata & Takeshita, 1998, pp. 591–592)

In the largest of the centers, Santa Anita Race Track, which housed more than 18,000 people, 75% of reported illnesses stemmed from living in horse stalls that had been scraped but not covered with flooring (Weglyn, 1976). All meals were taken in communal mess halls, and there were food shortages as well as outbreaks of food poisoning at two of the centers (USCWRIC, 1997). A serious lack of medical facilities and staff compounded the problems (Fiset, 1999; USCWRIC, 1997). "We were depressed," another Nisei recalled, "It was a period where we were all sad and upset and didn't know what to do. . . . We felt like prisoners" (Nagata & Takeshita, 1998, p. 591).

Japanese Americans were moved a second time from the detention centers to one of 10 permanent incarceration camps. This meant another round of separations and forced relocation. A Nisei woman vividly recalled her experience as a young girl, stating, "I was . . . mad that they would just kind of haul us around like animals. We made best friends in assembly center (detention center) and then all of a sudden we were separated again" (Nagata & Takeshita, 1998, p. 589). Once in the camps, they remained under the watch of armed guard towers and enclosed by barbed wire. Harsh weather was an ongoing challenge because the camps were located in deserts and swamplands. Although no longer confined to horse stalls and livestock pavilions, Japanese Americans now lived in uninsulated army-style barracks constructed with wooden planks covered with tarpaper. Entire families lived in a single room ranging from 20 by 16 to 20 by 25 feet in size, furnished with a pot-bellied stove, a light bulb hanging from the ceiling, and canvas cots or cotton mattresses. Each group of approximately 12 to 14 barracks composed a block, and each block had a communal mess hall, toilets, bathing facilities, laundry, and recreation hall (USCWRIC, 1997). A severe shortage of medical care continued, as exemplified by one incarceree's report that the Jerome camp had just seven physicians for 10,000 incarcerees (USCWRIC, 1997). The need for medical care was exacerbated by the inadequate barracks and locations that "exposed the internees to environmental and endemic health conditions" (Nakayama & Jensen, 2011, p. 360).

Food was provided in the camps, although meals were unappetizing (e.g., wieners, dried fish, pickled vegetables, macaroni; USCWRIC, 1997), and instances of malnutrition and food poisoning continued to occur (Dusselier, 2002). Mess-hall dining with large groups of incarcerees disrupted the nuclear family as children gravitated toward eating and socializing with peers rather than their parents (Morishima, 1973). In addition, tensions among incarcerees regarding who might be an informant for the camp administration led to beatings. At the Manzanar camp, such conflicts resulted in military police killing two inmates and wounding nine others (USCWRIC, 1997). The majority of Japanese Americans were able to cope at the time with the multiple incarceration stressors. However, some suffered severe psychiatric consequences. Especially sobering is the estimation that recorded suicides within the camps were 4 times greater than the rates for Japanese Americans before the war (Jensen, 1997).

The psychological impacts on identity were particularly powerful for the U.S.-born Nisei. With an average age of approximately 18 years at the beginning of the war (Fugita & O'Brien, 1991), the Nisei were in a critical period of identity and worldview formation (Erikson, 1968). They had been raised with Japanese values and customs by their immigrant parents, but they led bicultural lives and gravitated toward speaking English and adopting the dress and popular trends of European Americans (Fugita & O'Brien, 1991; Yoo, 2000). The Nisei had experienced job discrimination and restricted access to housing and public facilities (Yoo, 2000), but they hoped that citizenship and hard work would affirm their status as Americans. The incarceration directly contradicted that worldview and invalidated their American identity. "No other second-generation group," noted Yoo (2000), "has had to face the questions of its place in America under the extraordinary conditions that the Nisei encountered" (p. 9).

Questions about how to define the terms "American" and "loyal" were, in themselves, a source of traumatic stress. A mandatory mass registration of all camp inmates 17 years and older conducted in January 1943 brought into relief issues of both national identity and ethnic identity (Nagata et al., 2019). Two questions associated with the registration caused the greatest distress. One, for draft-aged males, was "Are you willing to serve in the armed forces of the United States on combat duty, wherever ordered?" Issei and women were asked to indicate willingness to serve in WACS or Army Nurse Corps. The second question was "Will you swear unqualified allegiance to the United States of America and faithfully defend the United States from any and all attack by foreign or domestic forces, and forswear any form of allegiance or obedience to the Japanese emperor, or any other foreign government, power or organization?" (USCWRIC, 1997, p. 192). The majority of incarcerees, including young Nisei men who wanted to express their patriotism and establish eligibility to join the U.S. military, answered "yes–yes." These men were among the 33,000 Japanese Americans who volunteered to serve or were drafted into segregated units during the war. Nisei who fought in Europe went on to become "the most decorated and distinguished combat unit of World War II" (USCWRIC, 1997, p. 3).

At the same time, the loyalty questions raised significant concerns. Some Nisei were outraged at being asked to swear allegiance to and to fight for a country that unjustly imprisoned them. Others worried that the immigrant Issei, who were barred from becoming U.S. citizens, would be stateless if they answered "yes" to a question asking them to forswear allegiance to Japan. Conflicts between incarcerees regarding how to respond led to tensions within families and escalated to riots in some camps (USCWRIC, 1997). More than 5,000 incarcerees answered "no" to one or both questions, and 4,600 more refused to answer or qualified their responses. These individuals were segregated from other incarcerees into more restrictive conditions within the Tule Lake camp (USCWRIC, 1997). Of the "no–no" group, 20,000 applied to go to Japan, disillusioned· and bitter about their treatment under incarceration, although most did not actually leave (USCWRIC, 1997). A separate group of Nisei incarcerees resisted the draft orders they received while in camp, citing the unconstitutionality of the incarceration. Those convicted of draft evasion were sent to federal prisons for nearly 3 years (Muller, 2001).

Positive responses to the loyalty oath were used not only to determine military eligibility but also to grant early clearance for Nisei who wanted to apply to leave the camps before the end of the war to take positions away from the West Coast (return to the West Coast was still prohibited). With $25, nominal per diem, and a one-way bus or train ticket, eligible Nisei applicants who answered "yes–yes" to the oath and were cleared by the government moved a third time to areas in the Midwest and East where they worked in low-status jobs such as domestics or farmhands (Okihiro, 2013). Most eventually returned to the West Coast to rejoin their Issei parents and relatives who had remained in the camps until the war ended, although sizeable groups remained in their resettled communities.

LONG-TERM AND INTERGENERATIONAL IMPACTS OF THE INCARCERATION

Following the closing of the last camp in 1946 (USCWRIC, 1997), Japanese Americans faced anti-Japanese hostility and discrimination in employment and housing while attempting to rebuild their postwar lives (Loo, 1993; Yoo, 2000). The majority of Issei had lost their life savings and possessions and were too old to restart their livelihoods. Nisei children, in turn, had few resources to establish their adult lives and needed to support their Issei parents (Daniels, 1993). Most Nisei eventually achieved socioeconomic success and were held up as a "model minority" group who overcame the hardships of the incarceration (Nakanishi, 1993), but they continued to face its psychological impacts: "The camp experience carried a stigma that no other American suffered" (USCWRIC, 1997, p. 11). Even as the Nisei resettled, they were instructed by the government to avoid congregating with each other in public. "When I would see a Japanese American approaching me on the street," testified one Nisei, "I would turn and walk away or dash into a nearby store" (p. 300). A key message from the beginning of their imprisonment through to resettlement was that Japanese ethnicity was a liability and put them at risk in mainstream U.S. society.

The congressional commission that investigated the incarceration identified a range of Nisei postwar responses: self-blame and feelings of racial inferiority and avoidance; keeping a low profile; proving themselves to broader U.S. society; distrusting White America and preferring to associate with other Japanese Americans or, conversely, identifying with White America and avoiding associations with Japanese Americans (USCWRIC, 1997). Some even shunned products made in Japan; for example, they only bought American cars (Inouye, 2016; Nagata et al., 2019). At the same time, Nisei also demonstrated a strong push toward achievement that was fueled by both the practical need to move forward and a Japanese sense of *giri* (i.e., obligation) to "clear their name of insult and shame" (Weglyn, 1976, p. 273).

After the war ended, Japanese Americans did not talk about their incarceration experiences with each other or with those outside of their community for decades, reflecting what Kashima (1980) termed a "social amnesia" (p. 113). Part of the silence was shaped by a Japanese cultural stance of *shikata ga nai*, which translates into "it cannot be helped" and reflects an adaptive acceptance of things as they are and an ability to move forward without dwelling on the past. However, the postwar silence can also be seen as avoidance and detachment associated with posttraumatic stress (Nagata et al., 2019). The negative impacts of this internalized stress have been hypothesized to lead to postwar psychosomatic ulcers and peptic ulcers (Mass, 1976) and an increased risk for cardiovascular disease, mortality, and premature death among former incarcerees (Jensen, 1997; Nagata, 1993).

It is important to note the variation and individual differences associated with incarceration-related experiences and responses (Nagata & Takeshita, 1998). Those with higher socioeconomic status and more resources before the war experienced greater economic losses than those with a lower socioeconomic status. Fugita and Fernandez (2004) found that Nisei whose fathers had more prestigious occupations before the war rated their own incarceration experience more negatively, although they were able to articulate both positive and negative camp memories. In contrast, Nisei from families with fewer prewar resources recalled primarily negative memories. From this, the researchers hypothesized that greater prewar resources might have had some beneficial impacts, despite the negative experience of status decrement under incarceration.

Research focusing on age shows that younger Nisei tended to report less-negative impacts (Fugita & Fernandez, 2004; Nagata & Takeshita, 1998) and recall more positive social memories (Fugita & Fernandez, 2004) than older Nisei. One Nisei interviewee who was 11 years old at the time recalled it as "almost an adventure—that you're not going to have school and so therefore no books. . . . It was kind of a fun, scary experience" (Nagata et al., 2012, p. 108). Older Nisei were more likely to have experienced education and career disruptions, to be aware of the injustice, and to hold more negative memories (Fugita & Fernandez, 2004; Nagata & Takeshita, 1998). As one Nisei shared, "Being labeled as an enemy alien and incarcerated in a concentration camp was the most traumatic experience of my life. There is still a feeling of bitterness which I will have the rest of my life" (Nagata et al., 2015, p. 360).

Nisei interviewees also reported varied reflections on their incarceration experiences from the vantage point as older adults. Some noted fewer negative emotions with age: "As you get older, it's one of those things that happened and things have changed for minorities over the years. I'm not as bitter about it now as in my teens" (Nagata & Takeshita, 1998, p. 601). In contrast, others felt greater upset with age: "The older I get the more disturbed I am regarding this whole situation because then I realize how it was for my parents, you know, as you grow older" (Nagata et al., 2012, p. 110).

Gender affected postwar incarceration experiences as well. Too old to reestablish their lives after the camps, many Issei men became reliant on their children. The loss of face and sense of shame from camp imprisonment led some to suicide, a tragic outcome that was most prevalent among more isolated elderly Issei bachelors who lacked familial supports (USCWRIC, 1997). Younger Nisei men, who faced an uncertain future, the burdens of ethnoracial stigma, and gendered expectations to be family breadwinners, seem to have been especially at risk for negative health consequences. In one study (Nagata, 1993), 95 Sansei reported the age at which their father had died. Of the fathers who had been in a camp, 41% had died before the age of 60, compared with 19% of the fathers who had not been in a camp. Similarly, Nisei men from California, most of whom were incarcerated, were 1.6 times more likely to have died from heart disease and suicide and were 1.3 times more likely to die before age 60 than similar-aged Japanese American men from Hawaii, where few were incarcerated (Jensen, 1997). Additionally, the incarceration memories of Nisei men are more likely than those of the women to include difficulties with confinement, prejudice, and discrimination (Fugita & Fernandez, 2004). These findings are consistent with previous literature on Holocaust survivors, suggesting that male survivors fared worse than females because they experienced helplessness that disrupted the male role as protector and provider (Danieli, 1982; Nadler & Ben-Shushan, 1989).

For women, the absence of a private home kitchen disrupted a primary way in which they had contributed to their families before the war. Mothers faced multiple trips daily to wash diapers and bathe young children in communal laundries and found it challenging to provide nutritious food (Nakano, 1990). However, because they were freed of many domestic responsibilities, women could engage in hobbies such as arts and crafts or could take on new opportunities through camp work (Matsumoto, 1984) that furthered their employment options after the war (Nagata, 1999).

The effects of long-term incarceration extended to the Sansei (i.e., third generation) Japanese Americans born after the war. Because of the economic losses of the Issei and Nisei, there were no nest eggs of wealth to inherit (Nagata, 1993; USCWRIC, 1997). There was sadness and mourning as well for the unfulfilled career dreams of their parents (Nagata & Takeshita, 1998). Sansei perceived a familial distance between themselves and their parents due to the latter's reluctance to discuss the incarceration (Nagata, 1993; Nagata et al., 2015). In a large-scale survey study, adult Sansei reported having spoken to their parents about the camps for a total of only 15 to 30 minutes in their lifetime. The noticeable evasion of camp discussions created a gap in the Sansei's personal history (Nagata, 1993).

The incarceration also contributed to weakened cultural ties. In an attempt to prevent their offspring from experiencing potential negative consequences, Nisei did not pass on Japanese language to their Sansei children, raised them to blend into the majority culture, and minimized Japanese traditional practices (Nagata, 1993; USCWRIC, 1997). Noted one Sansei interviewee, "A lot of people (Sansei) didn't even grow up like they were Japanese and it was conscious, you know" (Nagata, 1993, p. 138). Sansei also experienced parental pressure to achieve as a way of showing their worth to the broader society. At the same time, they were aware that such efforts at acculturation and achievement would not have protected their parents and grandparents from the incarceration. Survey data revealed that Sansei maintained a sense of vulnerability into their 20s and 30s. Those who had a parent in camp reported significantly less confidence in their rights as American citizens compared with Sansei who had neither parent incarcerated. More than 40% agreed that an incarceration could happen again to Japanese Americans (Nagata, 1993).

Interestingly, Sansei perspectives on the incarceration changed across their development. An initial sense of childhood confusion and curiosity about their parents' silence changed during adolescence and young adulthood to feelings of anger about the injustice and frustration that Japanese Americans did not resist the removal orders. As they moved into middle adulthood, they developed a greater sense of respect and understanding about reasons for minimal resistance to incarceration (USCWRIC, 1997). Additionally, despite negative intergenerational impacts, the Sansei have been able to find inspiration from their parents' experiences. Some felt a sense of determination to fulfill their parents' unfulfilled dreams and deliberately entered the careers their parents were unable to pursue because of the wartime disruption. Others pursued careers in law or political activism to address future injustices. Also positive is the Sansei's pride in the strength and resilience of their parents and grandparents (Nagata, 1993).

Little research exists on the impacts among fourth-generation Yonsei Japanese Americans, who are the Nisei's grandchildren. Case study data indicate that, similar to the Sansei, the Yonsei experience anger over the incarceration and pride in their families' resilience during the war (Yamano, 1994). Although communications about the incarceration remained minimal in the families of those who participated in research thus far, Yonsei expressed a desire to know more about their grandparents' cultural trauma (Mayeda, 1995; Yamano, 1994). As the fourth generation in the United States, the Yonsei are likely to have weakened ties to Japanese culture and increased assimilation to mainstream American culture. However, Tsuda (2015) noted that they also appear to be undergoing an "ethnic revival" (p. 601) and reconnecting with their Japanese heritage. He suggested possible explanations for this desire to connect with cultural roots as including increased global value of diversity and multiculturalism, increased American interest in Japanese pop culture, and continued racialization of Yonsei as "Japanese" rather than "American" by mainstream American society. Like their Sansei parents, Yonsei children are still asked, "Where are you really from?" (Tsuda, 2014), a reminder that others still perceive a racial difference based on their phenotype.

Incarceration effects extended beyond individuals and families and into the broader Japanese American community. The 4-year removal during the war diminished major Japanese ethnic enclaves that had been important sources of support before the war. The resettlement process that required Nisei leaving the camps to move to areas of the Midwest and East also led to a dispersion of Japanese Americans away from the West Coast. In addition, divisions due to differing expressions of loyalty continued to plague the community for decades after the war, even creating bitterness among family members and tensions regarding who should be acknowledged on Japanese

American incarceration memorials (Murray, 2008; Nagata et al., 2019). Those who answered "no" to the government's loyalty questions while in camp were shunned in the community long after the war ended. Their stance was seen as unpatriotic and having created negative impressions of Japanese Americans to the outside world. Draft resisters were also ostracized by other Japanese Americans, who negatively contrasted their refusal to serve in the military to the willingness of Nisei to risk their lives in combat to prove their American loyalty. Additional postwar intracommunity conflicts have centered on the role of the Japanese American Citizens League (JACL). Founded in 1929, the JACL served as "the most influential Nisei organization before and after World War II" (Fugita & Fernandez, 2004, p. 32). It urged full compliance with the government's wartime executive order, and some JACL members within the camps were seen viewed as spies who identified fellow incarcerees who might cause trouble. Divisions between those who resent the JACL for its accommodationist stance during the war and those who support it have persisted. In 2000, 55 years after the end of WWII, heated controversy emerged among Japanese Americans regarding whether to include a quote from Mike Masaoka, a former leader of the JACL who had urged full cooperation with the government during the war. The quote, based on a creed he wrote in 1940, stated, "I am proud that I am American of Japanese ancestry. I believe in this nation's institutions, ideals, and traditions; I glory in her heritage; I boast of her history; I trust in her future" (Murray, 2008, p. 420). More than 700 individuals signed a resolution to eliminate his name and inscription. In the end, the quote remained as part of the national memorial (Murray, 2008), and the JACL broadened its scope to address the human and civil rights of all Americans, particularly in relation to Asian Pacific American communities. It remains active as the largest Asian American civil rights organization in the country (see https://jacl.org/about/).

RESILIENCE IN RESPONSE TO THE INCARCERATION

Throughout the multiple trials and hardships associated with the incarceration, Japanese Americans have responded with resilience. Meiji-era[5] Japanese values that Issei brought to the United States stressed interpersonal harmony and conflict avoidance and set an important foundation for coping with adversity (Fugita & Fernandez, 2004; Fugita & O'Brien, 1991). Two central values, *gaman* (i.e., to suppress emotions and persevere in the face of hardship) and *shikata ga nai* (i.e., an acceptance of things as they are; Kitano, 1969), encouraged making the best of negative circumstances. The centrality of the family, another key Japanese value, emphasized a commitment to support

---

[5]The Meiji-era Restoration period began in 1868 as Japan shifted from a feudal society to an imperial structure that emphasized interpersonal harmony, obligation and duty, and filial piety (Fugita & Fernandez, 2004).

each other, and the phrase *kodomo no tame ni* (i.e., for the sake of the children) stressed the importance of creating an environment as nurturing and calm as possible while in camp (Nakano, 1990). Efforts to normalize life (Takezawa, 1995) included establishing organized sport teams, scouting, social dances, and other recreational activities.

Structures organized by incarcerees inside the camps supported individual and community resilience. Japanese Americans played a critical role running schools in both the temporary detention centers and the permanent camps, despite the constant hindrance of insufficient supplies (James, 1987; USCWRIC, 1997). They set up cooperatives that assisted small businesses in the camps, coordinated agricultural projects, and published newspapers (Bearden, 1989). Music within the camps also served as "an important means for creating hope, cohesion, resistance, and a sense of identity" (Waseda, 2005, p. 172). There was a revitalization of Japanese music as well as a promotion of American popular music through individual and organized performances (within the high-security Tule Lake camp, however, Japanese music was viewed as a form of resistance against by camp authorities and discouraged; Waseda, 2005). Gardens, both big and small, supported individual resilience. The larger ones were organized projects that reflected cooperative efforts to better the community. Camp gardens, noted Tamura (2004), "were an antithesis to the incarceration experience and military ordered setting; they were places of adoration, symbols of strength and capacity, and testaments to a human connection to place forged out of prison-like landscapes" (p. 20). Some were even constructed to provide relief for incarcerees as they waited in the hot sun 3 times a day for their mess hall meals. Religion, which played an important role in the prewar lives of Japanese Americans, also contributed to their resilience within the camps. Buddhist temples and Christian churches inside the camps aided Japanese Americans by offering them meaning, comfort, and hope and by assisting those transitioning into camp life (USCWRIC, 1997).

Resilience also emerged in the form of resourcefulness (Nagata & Takeshita, 1998). Incarcerees produced art that depicted camp life (Gesensway & Roseman, 1987), crafted jewelry and woodcarvings from the scarce materials around them, and cultivated crops from the desert soil (Dusselier, 2002). Older Nisei who had obtained their medical degree before the war provided extraordinary professional care under the inadequate and underresourced detention centers and camps, even as their own families struggled to deal with the ongoing incarceration challenges (Nakayama & Jensen, 2011). Acts of resistance reflected resilience as well. In addition to resistance around the loyalty oath and military draft, Nisei in the Santa Anita detention center who were making camouflage nets for the government held a sit-down strike to protest poor food and work conditions (USCWRIC, 1997).

Nisei resilience continued after the war through focused efforts on establishing a productive life despite the lack of resources and continued discrimination. Their responses also reflected an ability to construe personal adversity in positive ways, another aspect of resilience (Werner, 1984). For example, individuals who had been incarcerated noted how the policies mandating that they resettle away from the West Coast allowed them to broaden their horizons to the Midwest and Eastern regions of the country and forced them to mature quickly (Nagata & Takeshita, 1998).

SEEKING REDRESS AS A FORM OF COMMUNITY RESILIENCE

Most Nisei and Issei avoided discussing their incarceration following their release from camp (Nagata et al., 2015; Nagata et al., 2019). However, third-generation Sansei, most of whom were born after the war, were positioned to bring attention to the past injustice as they reached college age and learned more about what had happened. Inspired by the Black Power movement, increased attention to civil rights, and knowledge gained through the emergence of ethnic studies, the Sansei were outraged by the government's wartime actions and sought to resurrect the issue of the incarceration (Nagata et al., 2015; Nakanishi, 1993). They began taking pilgrimages to former camp sites and urged older generations to speak about the wartime traumas. By the late 1970s, spurred on by activist Nisei and Sansei, Japanese American communities also started holding annual Day of Remembrance gatherings on or near February 19th, the date on which EO9066 was signed (Loo, 1993). These efforts increased awareness of incarceration traumas and injustice, and proposals to seek financial redress and judicial action gained traction.

Disagreements arose over the best way to rectify the wartime injustice, whether legally through a class action suit or through a governmental commission (Murray, 2008; Takezawa, 1995). Ultimately, however, the congressional committee approach moved forward and led to the establishment of the 1980 bipartisan Commission on Wartime Relocation and Internment of Civilians. The commission investigated the circumstances of the wartime removal and detention of Japanese Americans by reviewing hundreds of documents and hearing testimonies from more than 750 witnesses (USCWRIC, 1997). Many who spoke were former incarcerees who emotionally shared, for the first time, the pain and suffering they had endured. The conclusion in the commission's final report was that there was no military justification for the incarceration and that Japanese Americans had suffered "a grave personal injustice" (USCWRIC, 1983, p. 5). It additionally recommended that there be a formal governmental apology and a one-time compensatory payment of $20,000 to each surviving incarceree. Assisted by the efforts of Nisei senators and representatives in Washington, D.C. who had either served in combat during World War II or were incarcerated as youth, Congress approved the recommendations and passed the Civil Liberties Act of 1988. Issuance of reparation checks began in 1990, 45 years after the war's end (Murray, 2008).

The redress movement exemplifies the importance of viewing resilience across time and generations. The Sansei shared the same visible racial difference and ethnic heritage as their parents and grandparents. However, as a generation not directly burdened by impacts from the camps and growing up more fully embedded in U.S. society, they were positioned to voice their anger and break the silence within their communities. The convergence of Sansei and Nisei efforts enabled a community-wide processing of cultural trauma and mobilization to seek redress from the government:

> Through this cultural reconstruction of the past . . . both generations came to redefine the past and the present, that is, what it means to be Japanese American and what it means to be a minority in American society. (Takezawa, 1995, p. 190)

PRESENT-DAY IMPLICATIONS AND RECOMMENDATIONS

The U.S. government justified their World War II incarceration policies by portraying all Japanese Americans as foreigners and dangers to national security. Decades after the war, issues of racism continue to impact the lives of Japanese Americans. Unlike White immigrants, Japanese American individuals are often perceived as Asian first and American second. Although both Sansei and Yonsei are born in the United States, they are asked questions such as "How long have you lived in the USA?" based solely on physical appearance (Tsuda, 2014). The sobering pattern, noted Yoo (2000), is that "though Asian Americans have been part of the nation for approximately 150 years, they remain perpetual foreigners—strangers in their own country—in public perceptions" (p. 9).

Reactions from mainstream society continue to disregard the unique ethnicity of Japanese Americans and identify them only as "Asian," based on physical appearance. Nearly a century ago, Chinese and Japanese immigrants were considered a single threat (i.e., "the yellow peril"). In 1992, Vincent Chin, a Chinese American, was murdered because he was thought to be Japanese (U.S. Commission on Civil Rights, 1992). Chin's death resulted from White autoworkers directing their anger about Japanese companies overtaking the American auto industry toward someone they erroneously perceived to be Japanese. The tragedy exemplifies, once again, Japanese in the United States being blamed for the actions of their heritage country as well as a failure to distinguish between Asian American ethnic groups.

COVID-19 is a present-day example elucidating how issues similar to those leading to the Japanese American incarceration continue to affect Asian individuals in the United States. Public health officials from the Centers for Disease Control and Prevention and the World Health Organization have discouraged the use of the phrase "Chinese coronavirus" to refer to COVID-19 amid concerns of resultant xenophobia and stigma and in acknowledgment of the fact that the virus is not limited to China or to Asian individuals (Gsalter, 2020; Wise, 2020). However, several government officials, including President Trump and members of Congress, have continued to use terms such as "Wuhan virus" and "Chinese virus" to describe the novel coronavirus (Forgey, 2020; Yam, 2020). Furthermore, a Wisconsin judge compared state-mandated stay-at-home orders created to combat COVID-19 to Japanese

American internment during World War II (Cole, 2020), a comparison JACL rebuked and called a "false equivalency" that "denigrates the history and experience of Japanese Americans" (JACL, 2020b). Physical and verbal harassment faced by Asian Americans have increased as the pandemic continues (Yan et al., 2020; Zhou, 2020), and according to a Federal Bureau of Intelligence report, hate crimes against Asian Americans are also likely to increase (Margolin, 2020). Additionally, Asian restaurants, particularly Chinese eateries, experienced a substantial decrease in business, something purported to be a result of racist fears rooted in concerns about the spread of the virus (Jackson, 2020; Lane, 2020). These events and attitudes indicate a continuation of a deeply rooted tendency to blame Asians for fears arising during national crises; just as Asians were scapegoated for economic fears in the United States in the late 1800s and early- to mid-1900s, Asians are being blamed for the spread of COVID-19. This is concerning, especially since similar underlying attitudes contributed to the fears of espionage that led to Japanese American internment; continued anti-Asian discrimination during COVID-19 could have negative consequences for the community in the future. These recent events have been condemned by JACL (2020a) and are indicative of Asian individuals in the United States continuing to be perceived as "forever foreigners."

The experiences of Japanese Americans during WWII have parallels today. Blame and suspicion continue to be directed toward entire immigrant groups who are perceived as foreign. Arab American and Muslim American communities were quickly targeted as possible threats to national security after the terrorist attacks on September 11, 2001. Members of these communities wondered if they would be incarcerated, similar to the treatment of Japanese Americans after Pearl Harbor (Groves & Hayasaki, 2001). In 1942, EO9066 was presented as necessary for the country's safety against foreign threats, yet it specifically targeted Japanese Americans. Similarly, in 2017, Executive Order No. 13769 (EO13769) cited the danger of terrorism associated with allowing foreign nationals to enter the United States but specifically banned individuals from seven majority-Muslim countries. Recognizing the similarities with the trauma faced by their own families, Japanese Americans in the United States have lent support to these groups. For example, JACL argued that the use of national security as justification for EO9066 paralleled the justification used for EO13769 (JACL, 2017). Japanese Americans were targeted solely because their families originated from Japan, and Muslim Americans today deal with being viewed collectively as a threat due to their national origin and religious beliefs.

Current government policies reminiscent of the incarceration continue to affect groups attempting to immigrate to the United States. In response to a significant increase in migration to the United States through the U.S.–Mexico border, the U.S. Immigration and Customs Enforcement agency has created facilities to hold captured migrants. News reports have suggested that these immigrant detention centers have terrible conditions, including expired food, "dilapidated bathrooms," "lack of provisions," unjustified strip searches, and children separated from parents (Alvarez, 2019; Arnold, 2018). To show solidarity at the U.S.–Mexico border, Japanese Americans have peacefully protested the migrants' detention (Varner, 2019).

The Trump administration has cited national security to justify the detention centers. The administration also recently decided to detain current migrant children at an army base formerly used to incarcerate Japanese Americans during World War II (Hennigan, 2019), a decision immediately opposed by the JACL (2019). The war-years attitudes that the Japanese are too different to assimilate into American culture are similar to ones that members of the current administration have expressed about migrants and other immigrants. For example, John Kelly, who was the White House Chief of Staff at the time of his comment and formerly the secretary of the Department of Homeland Security, remarked that

> the vast majority of people that move illegally into the United States are not bad people . . . but they're also not people that would easily assimilate into the United States into our modern society. They don't integrate well; they don't have skills. (Stacqualursi, 2018)

Kelly's remarks can be seen as parallel to the comments, noted early in this chapter, made by San Francisco Mayor James Phelan about the Japanese in the early 1900s.

The experiences of Japanese Americans suggest several implications for understanding minority and immigrant experiences in the United States. First, the role of Japanese cultural values in shaping their incarceration resilience points to the importance of researching how heritage cultural values and protective factors allow immigrants and minorities to be resilient in the face of discrimination. This knowledge can inform future coping interventions. Second, the documented long-term impacts of the incarceration suggest the importance of empirical investigations into the intergenerational effects of cultural trauma, many of which are covert, within other immigrant communities.

Public education about different cultures is key to preventing race-based discrimination. Muslim Americans, Latinx Americans, and Japanese Americans, among others, have been targets of ignorance in part because the country as a whole lacked knowledge about their cultures. Training programs are encouraged to include course content on historical trauma. Clinical assessments can extend beyond an individual's current life context and attend to potential long-term multigenerational impacts of racism experienced by immigrant populations, keeping in mind that each generation encounters distinct effects of the past (e.g., incarceration impacts for the Sansei are different than those for the Nisei). More broadly, course content at various levels of the education system should also include information on the history of legal barriers and policies that immigrant groups in the United States have encountered and continue to face. Efforts created to combat anti-Asian discrimination such as Stop AAPI Hate (Asian Pacific Policy & Planning Council, n.d.) exemplify how grassroots initiatives can be mobilized to increase community awareness and support other minority and immigrant groups.

Furthermore, the COVID-19 crisis illustrates the need for government officials to be aware of the negative effects of discriminatory language. The past contributions of elected officials in advancing the redress movement (Nagata, 2019) and current efforts condemning anti-Asian discrimination during COVID-19 (Yam, 2020) demonstrate how politicians can have a critical role in reminding the government about the negative consequences of past and ongoing discriminatory actions linked to xenophobia.

Finally, the treatment of Japanese Americans highlighted in this chapter reflects a greater national tendency to perceive Asians as "forever foreigners" instead of Americans. Japanese Americans, regardless of U.S. citizenship or whether they had ever been to Japan, were incarcerated during World War II because of the actions of Japan. Today, Asian Americans, particularly Chinese Americans, are perceived as a threat and face discrimination because COVID-19 originated in China. This pattern of discrimination, in which certain groups of Americans are unfairly linked to the issues in the countries they or their ancestors came from, has also been witnessed in other minority communities, such as Muslim Americans and migrants attempting to enter the United States. As such, these concerns warrant monitoring and attention.[1]

CONCLUSION

During World War II, more than 117,000 Japanese individuals living in the United States, the majority of whom were U.S. citizens, were ordered into incarceration camps based solely on their shared heritage with the country of Japan. Their incarceration was the culmination of decades of discrimination against Japanese communities on the Pacific West Coast. Although the government later acknowledged that the action was unjustified, overt and covert long-term, multigenerational impacts of the incarceration continued after the war ended. Ethnic minority immigrants continue to face ethnoracial discrimination and nonacceptance in the United States, reflective of the same issues underlying discrimination faced by Japanese Americans nearly a century ago. An examination of the Japanese American wartime imprisonment illustrates the powerful intergenerational impacts of historical and cultural trauma linked to racially discriminatory governmental policies as well as sources of resilience that emerge in the face of adversity.

REFERENCES

Alexander, J. C. (2004). Toward a theory of cultural trauma. In J. C. Alexander, E. Eyerman, B. Giesen, N. J. Smelser, & P. Sztompka (Eds.), *Cultural trauma and collective identity* (pp. 1–30). University of California Press. https://doi.org/10.1525/california/9780520235946.003.0001

Alvarez, F. N. (2019). *Exclusive: DHS watchdog finds expired food, dilapidated bathrooms amid "egregious" conditions at ICE facilities in 2018.* CNN. https://www.cnn.com/2019/06/06/politics/ice-detention-center-ig-report/index.html

Arnold, A. (2018). *What to know about the detention centers for immigrant children along U.S.–Mexico border.* The Cut. https://www.thecut.com/2018/06/immigrant-children-detention-center-separated-parents.html

Asian Pacific Policy & Planning Council. (n.d.). *Stop AAPI hate.* http://www.asianpacificpolicyandplanningcouncil.org/stop-aapi-hate/

Bearden, R. (1989). Life inside Arkansas's Japanese-American relocation centers. *The Arkansas Historical Quarterly, 48*(2), 169–196. https://doi.org/10.2307/40030791

Cole, D. (2020, May 5). *Wisconsin Supreme Court justice invokes internment of Japanese-Americans in debate over stay-at-home order.* CNN. https://www.cnn.com/2020/05/05/politics/wisconsin-supreme-court-coronavirus-hearing-japanese-american-internment/index.html

Danieli, Y. (1982). Families of survivors and the Nazi Holocaust: Some short and long-term effects. In C. D. Spielberger, I. G. Sarason, & N. Milgram (Eds.), *Stress and anxiety* (Vol. 8, pp. 405–423). Hemisphere.

Daniels, R. (1993). *Concentration camps: North America. Japanese in the United States and Canada during World War II.* Krieger.

Daniels, R. (2004). *Prisoners without trial: Japanese Americans in World War II.* Macmillan.

Densho. (n.d.). *Terminology.* https://densho.org/terminology/

Dusselier, J. (2002). Does food make place? Food protests in Japanese American concentration camps. *Food & Foodways, 10*(3), 137–165. https://doi.org/10.1080/07409710213923

Erikson, E. H. (1968). *Identity, youth, and crisis.* Norton.

Fiset, L. (1999). Public health in World War II assembly centers for Japanese Americans. *Bulletin of the History of Medicine, 73*(4), 565–584. https://doi.org/10.1353/bhm.1999.0162

Forgey, Q. (2020, March 18). *Trump on "Chinese virus" label: "It's not racist at all."* The Politico. https://www.politico.com/news/2020/03/18/trump-pandemic-drumbeat-coronavirus-135392

Fugita, E. H., & Fernandez, M. (2004). *Altered lives, enduring communities: Japanese Americans remember their World War II incarceration.* University of Washington Press.

Fugita, S. S., & O'Brien, D. J. (1991). *Japanese American ethnicity: The persistence of community.* University of Washington Press.

Gesensway, D., & Roseman, M. (1987). *Beyond words: Images from America's concentration camps.* Cornell University Press.

Groves, M., & Hayasaki, E. (2001, September 26). Reaction reopens wounds of WWII for Japanese Americans. *Los Angeles Times.* https://www.latimes.com/archives/la-xpm-2001-sep-26-me-50006-story.html

Gsalter, M. (2020, March 19). *WHO official warns against calling it "Chinese virus," says "there is no blame in this."* The Hill. https://thehill.com/homenews/administration/488479-who-official-warns-against-calling-it-chinese-virus-says-there-is-no

Hennigan, W. J. (2019). Trump administration to hold migrant children at base that served as WWII Japanese internment camp. *Time Magazine.* https://time.com/5605120/trump-migrant-children-fort-sill/

Inouye, K. M. (2016). *The long afterlife of Nikkei wartime incarceration.* Stanford University Press. https://doi.org/10.11126/stanford/9780804795746.001.0001

Ishizuka, K. L. (2006). *Lost and found: Reclaiming the Japanese American incarceration.* University of Illinois Press.

Iwata, M. (1992). *Planted in good soil: A history of the Issei in the United States agriculture: Vol. 2. American University studies.* Peter Lang.

Jackson, K. (2020, March 10). *Amid coronavirus panic, Chinese restaurants in the US are emptier than ever.* Today. https://www.today.com/food/amid-coronavirus-panic-chinese-restaurants-us-are-emptier-ever-t175326

James, W. (1987). *Exile within: The schooling of Japanese Americans 1942–1945.* Harvard University Press.

Japanese American Citizens League. (2017, January 30). *JACL strongly objects to recent executive orders on immigration.* https://jacl.org/jacl-strongly-objects-to-recent-executive-orders-on-immigration/

Japanese American Citizens League. (2019, June 12). *JACL opposes expanded incarceration of children at Fort Sill.* https://jacl.org/jacl-opposes-expanded-incarceration-of-children-at-fort-sill/

Japanese American Citizens League. (2020a, April 2). *JACL joins Congress in condemning all forms of anti-Asian sentiment as related to COVID-19.* https://jacl.org/jacl-joins-congress-in-condemning-all-forms-of-anti-asian-sentiment-as-related-to-covid-19/

Japanese American Citizens League. (2020b, May 6). *JACL rebukes 2020 Wisconsin justice's comparisons to Japanese American experience.* https://jacl.org/jacl-rebukes-2020-wisconsin-justices-comparisons-to-japanese-american-experience/

Jensen, G. M. (1997). *The experience of injustice: Health consequences of the Japanese American internment* [Unpublished doctoral dissertation]. University of Colorado, Boulder.

Kashima, T. (1980). Japanese American internees: Return, 1945–1955: Readjustment and social amnesia. *Phylon, 41*(2), 107–115. https://doi.org/10.2307/274964

Kitano, H. H. L. (1969). *Japanese Americans: The evolution of a subculture.* Prentice Hall.

Lane, S. (2020, March 4). *Philadelphia fed: "Unfounded fears" harming city's "Asian restaurants and shops."* The Hill. https://thehill.com/policy/finance/485993-philadelphia-fed-unfounded-fears-harming-citys-asian-restaurants-and-shops

Loo, C. M. (1993). An integrative-sequential treatment model for posttraumatic stress disorder: A case study of the Japanese American internment and redress. *Clinical Psychology Review, 13*(2), 89–117. https://doi.org/10.1016/0272-7358(93)90036-L

Margolin, J. (2020, March 27). *FBI warns of potential surge in hate crimes against Asian Americans amid coronavirus.* ABC News. https://abcnews.go.com/US/fbi-warns-potential-surge-hate-crimes-asian-americans/story?id=69831920

Mass, A. I. (1976). Asians as individuals: The Japanese community. *Social Casework, 57*(3), 160–164. https://doi.org/10.1177/104438947605700306

Matsumoto, V. (1984). Japanese American women during world war II. *Frontiers, 8*(1), 6–14. https://doi.org/10.2307/3346082

Mayeda, K. A. (1995). *Generational and transgenerational issues of the Japanese American internment: A phenomenological study* [Unpublished doctoral dissertation]. University of North Texas.

Mohatt, N. V., Thompson, A. B., Thai, N. D., & Tebes, J. K. (2014). Historical trauma as public narrative: A conceptual review of how history impacts present-day health. *Social Science & Medicine, 106*, 128–136. https://doi.org/10.1016/j.socscimed.2014.01.043

Morishima, J. K. (1973). The evacuation: Impact on the family. In S. Sue & N. N. Wagner (Eds.), *Asian Americans: Psychological perspectives* (pp. 13–19). Science and Behavior Books.

Muller, E. L. (2001). *Free to die for their country: The story of the Japanese American draft resisters in World War II.* University of Chicago Press.

Murray, A. Y. (2008). *Historical memories of the Japanese American internment and the struggle for redress.* Stanford University Press.

Nadler, A., & Ben-Shushan, D. (1989). Forty years later: Long-term consequences of massive traumatization as manifested by Holocaust survivors from the city and the Kibbutz. *Journal of Consulting and Clinical Psychology, 57*(2), 287–293. https://doi.org/10.1037/0022-006X.57.2.287

Nagata, D. K. (1993). *Legacy of injustice: Exploring the cross-generational impacts of the Japanese American internment.* Plenum Press. https://doi.org/10.1007/978-1-4899-1118-6

Nagata, D. K. (1999). Expanding the internment narrative: Multiple layers of Japanese American women's experiences. In M. Romero & A. J. Stewart (Eds.), *Women's untold stories: Breaking silence, talking back, voicing complexity* (pp. 71–82). Routledge.

Nagata, D. K. (2019). Japanese American identity, collective memory, and the World War II incarceration. In S. Mukherjee & P. S. Salter (Eds.), *History and collective memory from the margins: A global perspective* (pp. 285–298). Nova Science.

Nagata, D. K., Cheng, W. J. Y., & Nguyen, T. U. (2012). Recollections of historical injustice: A qualitative investigation of emotions in Japanese American incarceration memories. In D. K. Nagata, L. Kohn-Wood, & L. A. Suzuki (Eds.), *Qualitative strategies for ethnocultural research* (pp. 103–118). American Psychological Association. https://doi.org/10.1037/13742-006

Nagata, D. K., Kim, J. H. J., & Nguyen, T. U. (2015). Processing cultural trauma: Intergenerational effects of the Japanese American incarceration. *Journal of Social Issues, 71*(2), 356–370. https://doi.org/10.1111/josi.12115

Nagata, D. K., Kim, J. H. J., & Wu, K. (2019). The Japanese American wartime incarceration: Examining the scope of racial trauma. *American Psychologist, 74*(1), 36–48. https://doi.org/10.1037/amp0000303

Nagata, D. K., & Takeshita, Y. J. (1998). Coping and resilience across generations: Japanese Americans and the World War II internment. *Psychoanalytic Review, 85*(4), 587–613.

Nakanishi, D. T. (1993). Surviving democracy's mistake: Japanese Americans and the enduring legacy of Executive Order 9066. *Amerasia Journal, 19*(1), 7–36. https://doi.org/10.17953/amer.19.1.xu217p1k01521170

Nakano, M. (1990). *Japanese American women: Three generations 1890–1990.* Mina Press.

Nakayama, D. K., & Jensen, G. M. (2011). Professionalism behind barbed wire: Health care in World War II Japanese-American concentration camps. *Journal of the National Medical Association, 103*(4), 358–363. https://doi.org/10.1016/S0027-9684(15)30317-5

National Archives. (1989). *Teaching with documents: Using primary sources from the National Archives.* National Archives and Records Administration.

Okihiro, G. Y. (2013). Resettlement. In G. Y. Okihiro (Ed.), *Encyclopedia of Japanese American internment* (pp. 160–162). Greenwood.

Stacqualursi, V. (2018). *Kelly says undocumented immigrants "don't have the skills" to assimilate into US society.* CNN. https://www.cnn.com/2018/05/11/politics/john-kelly-immigration-education/index.html

Takezawa, Y. I. (1995). *Breaking the silence: Redress and Japanese American ethnicity.* Cornell University Press. https://doi.org/10.7591/9781501720215

Tamura, A. (2004). Gardens below the watchtower: Gardens and meaning in World War II Japanese American incarceration camps. *Landscape Journal, 23*(1), 1–21. https://doi.org/10.3368/lj.23.1.1

tenBroek, J., Barnhart, E. N., & Matson, F. W. (1968). *Prejudice, war and the constitution: Causes and consequences of the evacuation of the Japanese Americans in World War II.* University of California.

Tsuda, T. (2014). "I'm American, not Japanese!": The struggle for racial citizenship among later-generation Japanese Americans. *Ethnic and Racial Studies, 37*(3), 405–424. https://doi.org/10.1080/01419870.2012.681675

Tsuda, T. (2015). Recovering heritage and homeland: Ethnic revival among fourth-generation Japanese Americans. *Sociological Inquiry, 85*(4), 600–627. https://doi.org/10.1111/soin.12095

U.S. Commission on Civil Rights. (1992). *Civil rights issues facing Asian Americans in the 1990s.* U.S. Government Printing Office.

U.S. Commission on Wartime Relocation and Internment of Civilians. (1983). *Personal justice denied: Part 2: Recommendations Report of the Commission on Wartime Relocation and Internment of Civilians.* U.S. Government Printing Office.

U.S. Commission on Wartime Relocation and Internment of Civilians. (1997). *Personal justice denied: Report of the Commission on Wartime Relocation and Internment of Civilians.* University of Washington Press.

Varner, N. (2019). *Immigrant detention centers are a grim reminder of Japanese American history.* PRI. https://www.pri.org/stories/2019-04-05/immigrant-detention-centers-are-grim-reminder-japanese-american-history

Waseda, M. (2005). Extraordinary circumstances, exceptional practices: Music in Japanese American concentration camps. *Journal of Asian American Studies, 8*(2), 171–209. https://doi.org/10.1353/jaas.2005.0044

Weglyn, M. (1976). *Years of infamy: The untold story of America's concentration camps.* Morrow Quill.

Werner, E. E. (1984). Resilient children. *Young Children, 40*(1), 68–72.

Wise, J. (2020, March 10). *CDC Chief says it's wrong to call COVID-19 a "Chinese virus."* The Hill. https://thehill.com/homenews/administration/486920-cdc-chief-says-its-wrong-to-call-covid-19-a-chinese-virus

Yam, K. (2020, March 12). *GOP lawmakers continue to use "Wuhan virus" or "Chinese coronavirus."* NBC News. https://www.nbcnews.com/news/asian-america/cdc-chief-spurns-term-chinese-coronavirus-used-gop-lawmakers-n1156656

Yamano, T. K. (1994). *Brooding silence: A cross-sectional study of informal learning, socialization, and child-rearing practices in a Japanese American family* [Unpublished doctoral dissertation]. University of California, Los Angeles.

Yan, H., Chen, N., & Naresh, D. (2020, February 21). *What's spreading faster than coronavirus in the US? Racist assaults and ignorant attacks against Asians.* CNN. https://www.cnn.com/2020/02/20/us/coronavirus-racist-attacks-against-asian-americans/index.html

Yoo, D. K. (2000). *Growing up Nisei: Race, generation, and culture among Japanese Americans of California, 1924–1949.* University of Illinois Press.

Zhou, L. (2020, April 21). *How the coronavirus is surfacing America's deep-seated anti-Asian biases.* Vox. https://www.vox.com/identities/2020/4/21/21221007/anti-asian-racism-coronavirus

7

Sociopolitical Trauma

Ethnicity, Race, and Migration

Lillian Comas-Díaz

Give me your tired, your poor, Your huddled masses yearning to breathe free . . .
—EMMA LAZARUS'S *THE NEW COLOSSUS*
(POEM MOUNTED AT THE STATUE OF LIBERTY)

People have been immigrating since the beginning of humankind. They migrate to secure food, safety, and a dependable way of living. In addition, many people of color leave their countries to escape oppressive sociopolitical and economic systems. The United States offers both dreams and nightmares to racial minority immigrants. The nation's motto, "E pluribus, unum" (i.e., "From many, one"), has guided the country's immigration policy. However, as a nation of immigrants, the United States has an ambivalent history with immigrants (Schwartz, 2017). To illustrate, during the turn of the last century, immigrants from the south of Italy, Greeks, Slavs, Jews, and Chinese were considered inferior (Schrag, 2010). Moreover, those arriving to Ellis Island in 1914 were labeled "simple minded foreigners," mostly due to their lack of English language skill, and were perceived as criminals (Perrotti, 2016). Interestingly, studies document that compared with native-born people, immigrants are less likely to commit serious crimes, and high rates of immigration are associated with lower rates of violent crimes (Ewing et al., 2015). In 2020, however, negative assumptions continue to prevail regarding many racial minority immigrants. Indeed, the history of U.S. immigration laws documents

https://doi.org/10.1037/0000214-008
Trauma and Racial Minority Immigrants: Turmoil, Uncertainty, and Resistance,
P. Tummala-Narra (Editor)

the racial exclusion of Chinese, Japanese, Mexicans, Haitians, and other people of color (Johnson, 1998). Currently, the bulk of the immigrants to the United States are people of color, originating from Asia, Latin America, and the Caribbean (APA Presidential Task Force on Immigration, 2012). A major difference between past and current immigration is that most racial minority immigrants currently come from unpredictable and unsafe sociopolitical situations (Haines, 2010). As non-White individuals, racial minority immigrants "darken" the White American identity. Therefore, many White Americans fear that this process may create a cultural and racial Babel Tower. As a result, a nativist, xenophobic, racist, and anti-immigration climate results in sociopolitical trauma for many racial minority immigrants. Since immigration from Central America is increasing, I focus on this population.

This chapter offers valuable information to psychologists and other mental health professionals working with racial minority immigrants. First, I present a theoretical framework of sociopolitical trauma and its intersection with racial trauma. Then, I discuss the distress and trauma that numerous people of color experience during their migration process. Afterwards, I examine the effects of coloniality, colonial mentality, and cultural imperialism on racial minority immigrants, then discuss liberation and decolonization approaches to address sociopolitical trauma. Finally, I present a case vignette and conclude the chapter with recommendations.

SOCIOPOLITICAL TRAUMA: THEORETICAL AND EMPIRICAL FRAMEWORK

I use the term *racial minority immigrants* to designate people of color who are immigrants. However, the term *racial minority* when used to refer to people of color is a misnomer. Because of the current transnational nature of immigration, it is important to note that racial minorities are not minorities in the global and geopolitical scenario; rather, they are the majority in the world. I employ the term *racial minority immigrants* for consistency with other chapters in this edited book.

Many racial minority immigrants are exposed to sociopolitical trauma. *Sociopolitical trauma* refers to the insidious distress that marginalized individuals experience while living in a racist, heterosexist, classist, ableist, homophobic, and transphobic oppressive society (Burstow, 2003). Because racism causes trauma (Comas-Díaz et al., 2019), many racial minority immigrants experience racial trauma. *Racial trauma* refers to the cumulative attacks that ethnic and racial minority individuals receive within an oppressive society. Specifically, racial trauma entails people of color responding to real or perceived experiences of discrimination, including threats of harm and injury, as well as witnessing harm to other racial minority individuals (Comas-Díaz et al., 2019). To maintain power over people of color, racial trauma perpetrators promote their interpretation of the racial attacks, contributing to a societal response of blaming the victim (Craig-Henderson & Sloan, 2003). Given the historical connection between dark skin color and oppression and subjugation, sociopolitical trauma and racial trauma constitute two aspects of the same reality.

Sociopolitical trauma shares similarities with posttraumatic stress disorder (PTSD). However, sociopolitical trauma is unique in that victims experience constant and cumulative microaggressions due to social, political, and systemic factors. Likewise, racial trauma is unique in that victims suffer from historical, intergenerational, and contemporary racial microaggressions and attacks. Therefore, the application of a medical model of trauma to sociopolitical and racial trauma is limited because of its social, political, and systemic roots (Comas-Díaz et al., 2019). Moreover, the field of trauma is infused with medical, psychiatric, and diagnostic categories (Tseris, 2013), without consideration of the social, political, and systemic contexts. Therefore, when we medicalize a sociopolitical trauma, we fail to recognize the central roles that historical, social, political, and institutional power differentials have on this type of trauma. For these reasons, migration to the United States exposes people of color to sociopolitical trauma.

MIGRATION AND SOCIOPOLITICAL TRAUMA

Immigration can be traumatic for marginalized people of color (Comas-Díaz, 2016). A significant number of immigrants of color are exposed to traumatic events during their premigration, in-transit journey, and postmigration stages. This section presents immigrants' exposure to sociopolitical trauma throughout their diverse stages of migration.

Premigration Trauma

The number of immigrants from the Northern Triangle countries (i.e., El Salvador, Guatemala, and Honduras) to the United States via Mexico is rapidly increasing. These countries experience widespread violence due to decades of civil wars, massacres, kidnappings, murders, and other types of violence. Illegal drug traffic has added to the violence and the extreme poverty. As a result, the continuous violence and insecurity in these countries are main reasons for migration (Beltran, 2017). Consequently, the road from Central America to the United States is dangerous, resulting in the traumatization of people of color before they arrive to the United States. Moreover, premigration stress is associated with postmigration adjustment (Jasinskaja-Lahti & Yijälaä, 2011). The numbers of female and unaccompanied youth migrating to the United States are increasing (Dash, 2020). Numerous young females world-wide are forced to leave their countries to avoid gendered violence; sexual abuse and violence is a main reason why young Central Americans leave their countries (Ramirez & Ream, 2014). As a result, there is a surge in female immigration to the United States (APA Presidential Task Force on Immigration,

2012). Sadly, Latin America, and particularly Central America, has the highest rate of femicide (United Nations Women, 2017). The premigration of Flor (a composite of several people) provides an example.[1]

Flor is a 17-year-old Salvadorian adolescent girl. She is Indigenous (Pipil) and lives in the countryside with her mother, father, and older brother. One day, while attending to the family goats, three gang members of the Mara Salvatrucha (MS-13) called her a "dirty Indian" while raping her. Sexual abuse of females is a common attack against enemies in war-torn countries (APA, 2019). After Flor's attack, her father hired a *coyote* (i.e., illegal human smuggler) to help her immigrate to the United States. Because Flor's paternal aunt Beatriz lived in the United States and was married to Tom, an African American man, the family planned that Flor would reside with them. Before leaving, Flor consulted Xochil, a Pipil healer, who performed a *limpia* (i.e., spiritual cleansing)—a Latinx shamanistic ritual for balancing body, mind, and spirit.

Peri-Migration: In-Transit Journey

The in-transit migration of some people of color may be simple, such as taking a plane and having relatives or friends waiting for them at the airport. However, many Latinx, especially Central Americans, find a treacherous path on their way to the United States. Because of the devastating situation in Central America, many experience a traumatic peri-migration. Unaccompanied Latinx youth and females become victims of violent acts such as robberies, murders, accidents, physical and sexual abuse, and others, during their peri-migration. Many coyotes abuse and traumatize Latinx during their peri-migration, especially while traveling the Mexico–U.S. border, an area fraught with drug violence (Torres Fernandez & Torres Rivera, 2014). Numerous Central Americans travel in overcrowded cars, vans, trains, and boats, with limited water and food (Comas-Díaz, 2019). As an illustration, Flor traveled by land in a van with six Salvadorians. She kept to herself and hardly socialized with others. During her journey, she was exposed to racial discrimination, being called a "dirty Indian" many times. Moreover, she became very anxious after she witnessed the coyote sexually abusing a 15-year-old adolescent girl. Unfortunately, immigration difficulties involve experiencing physical and/or sexual attacks, witnessing violence toward loved ones (APA Presidential Task Force on Immigration, 2012), and other traumatic events during the immigration process.

Postmigration

Racial minority immigrants struggle with separation from family and culture, acculturative stress, and racial and ethnic discrimination during their

---

[1]All case material has been altered to protect confidentiality.

postmigration (Brabeck & Xu, 2010). Upon arrival, many are subjected to xenophobia, racism, sexism, and gendered racism. To illustrate, immigrant women are frequently targeted for sexual violence. Sadly, the sex trafficking and sexual exploitation of transnational and immigrant females has attained epidemic numbers in the United States (APA Presidential Task Force on Immigration, 2012). Additionally, lesbian, gay, bisexual, transgender, and queer immigrants of color are targeted for hate crimes because of their intersectional identities (APA Presidential Task Force on Immigration, 2012).

A pervasive anti-immigration climate infuses some Americans, including governmental employees, with prejudice toward immigrants. Many unaccompanied young immigrants are held in custody amidst appalling conditions. Indeed, numerous young immigrants housed in government facilities have reported being sexually abused while in Immigration and Customs Enforcement (ICE) custody (Screenivasan, 2018). Consequently, they reexperience their traumatic migration (American Immigration Lawyers Association, 2015). Unfortunately, previous traumatic experiences increase racial minority immigrants' vulnerability to retraumatization (APA Presidential Task Force on Immigration, 2012). Many marginalized racial minority immigrants cope with extreme poverty, crime-plagued communities, racism, family separation, culture shock, and conflict with the police during their postmigration (Smokowski & Bacallao, 2007). Because of their high acculturation stress, undocumented Latinx with low socioeconomic status experience reduced family cohesion (Dillon et al., 2013). Moreover, numerous racial minority immigrants use nicotine and alcohol to cope with decreased family functioning (Lorenzo-Blanco et al., 2017). Many racial minority immigrants become victims of xenophobia and are questioned about their legal status. These circumstances affect racial minority immigrants' health, leading to anxiety, depression, somatic complaints, sleep problems, impulsivity, hypervigilance, hopelessness, PTSD symptoms (Flores et al., 2010), and other mental health problems.

MIGRATION AND RESILIENCE

When your roots are deep, there is no reason to fear the wind.
—AFRICAN PROVERB

Notwithstanding migration challenges, many racial minority immigrants are resilient (Valdez et al., 2013). They embody *cultural resilience*—a set of strengths, values, and practices that promote functional strategies for coping with traumatic oppression (Elsass, 1992). As an illustration, Latinx immigrants have strong traditional values that nurture their cultural resilience, in addition to religiosity and spirituality, which provide a source of hope and hardiness during adversity (Hunter-Hernández et al., 2015). In this way, many Latinx immigrants not only survive, they thrive (Comas-Díaz, 2019).

Even more, Latinx's cultural wealth helps them to flourish amidst adversity. *Cultural wealth* is a compendium of knowledge, skills, behaviors, and abilities that allows Latinx to cope and resist oppression (Yosso, 2006). Some of the Latinx cultural wealth values include (a) determination to survive; (b) hope that things will turn out positively; (c) adaptability to cope and thrive in adversity; (d) a strong work ethic; (e) *connectedness*, defined as having emotional, physical, and spiritual connection to others; (f) collective emotional expression by sharing emotions with others; and (g) resistance by having willpower and courage to stand for beliefs and ideals (Adames & Chavez-Dueñas, 2017). Additionally, Indigenous people exhibit intergenerational resilience (Hearts of our people: Native women artists, 2019). As an illustration, Latinx cultural wealth nurtures children and adolescents' mental health (Marín & García-Vázquez, 2012). Indeed, many second-generation Latinx exhibit cultural wealth when they aim to thrive in order to achieve their immigrant family's dreams (Ceja, 2004). Moreover, research found that a positive ethnic identity increased resilience to racial discrimination and prejudice among ethnic minority adolescents (Romero et al., 2014). Finally, the immigration journey imparts resilience to many Latinxs (Johnson-Motoyama et al., 2012). An operational definition of resilience among Latinx immigrants is the Hispanic health paradox. This concept refers to the research documenting that Latinx immigrants tend to have better health than non-Hispanic White Americans (Morales et al., 2002). Unfortunately, second-generation Latinxs (i.e., born and raised in the United States) do not benefit from the Hispanic health paradox because of the effects of racial discrimination on their health.

Flor's experience illustrates this concern. Flor arrived at the Mexico–U.S. border and was interviewed by a patrol officer. She met the requirements for asylum because she had experienced sexual abuse and was an Indigenous Latinx female minor, and thus she was released under Beatriz's custody. Flor went to live with Tom and Beatriz, but she became scared of the inner-city area where they lived. Consequently, Flor developed sleeping difficulties due to the excessive noise in the neighborhood. Since living in overcrowded and noisy neighborhoods affects adolescents' health (Garcia et al., 2014), Flor developed eating problems and lost significant amounts of weight. Unfortunately, she continued to encounter more stress during her postmigration journey. While looking through the window of her bedroom, Flor witnessed a female neighbor being sexually attacked on the street and was retraumatized. Flor's psychological treatment is discussed in a later section of this chapter. The next section presents a discussion of the effects of colonial mentality and cultural imperialism on racial minority immigrants.

COLONIALITY: COLONIAL MENTALITY AND CULTURAL IMPERIALISM

Most immigrants of color have a history of colonization. This is also true for numerous Americans of color. To illustrate, the first president of color for the American Psychological Association, Kenneth B. Clark (1989), compared

African Americans' condition with that of colonized people. Indeed, Fanon (1967) identified racism as a form of colonization, in which oppressors impose a subordinate mentality to the oppressed. As a sign of colonization, skin color connects many racial minorities, transcending gender, sexual orientation, class, religion, and other identities. Coloniality imposes racial privilege and results in designating people of color as inferior individuals (Comas-Díaz, 1994). In this way, dark skin bears the mark of subjugation.

Trauma populates the U.S. history regarding people of color. To illustrate, the American Indian historical trauma reduced Native Americans to immigrants in their own land. Moreover, the enslavement of Africans and African Americans, the U.S. war against Mexico plus the annexation of Mexican territories, and the U.S. colonization of Hawaii, Guam, the Philippines, and Puerto Rico promoted an "us (White Americans) and them (people of color)" mentality (Comas-Díaz, 2012). Additionally, the U.S. history of political conflict and wars with Japan, Korea, and Vietnam resulted in an ambivalent relationship with Asian Americans. Furthermore, the attacks on September 11, 2001, generated fear and suspiciousness against Muslims and those perceived to be Muslims (e.g., Arab Americans, South Asian Americans) as well as a resurgence of Islamophobia (Haque et al., 2019).

Sadly, a history of colonization, subordination, and oppression persists through coloniality. *Coloniality* refers to the dominant group's systemic organization and distribution of power through the control of resources. According to Quijano (2000), *coloniality of power* refers to how the colonizing systems of control, power, and privilege prevalent during colonization continue to influence individuals with a colonial history, exposing them to neocolonization. Lugones (2008) developed the concept of *coloniality of gender* to describe how the coloniality of power ranks women as inferior to men. Similarly, Comas-Díaz (1994) conceived the concept of coloniality of color as a major factor in sociopolitical trauma. Within this framework, *coloniality of color* refers to the designation of people of color as colonized entities, promoting a racial consciousness that equates dark skin color with subjugation (Comas-Díaz, 2007). *Colorism*—the preference for light-skin-color individuals, as opposed to darker-skin-color persons (Monk, 2015)—is a vestige of colonialism. Colorism negatively affects the lives of many people of color. Indeed, research documented that Latinx females with dark skin color felt less attractive than Latinx females with lighter skin color, wanted their skin color to be lighter, and expressed negative self-perceptions (Telzer & Vazquez-Garcia, 2009). As an instrument of internalized racism, colorism reinforces power differentials among many people of color.

Colonial Mentality

The worldwide politics of domination and subordination reinforce the effects of coloniality in every aspect of society (Grosfoguel & Georas, 2010). Coloniality permeates the cultures, hearts, and minds of the colonized

(Maldonado-Torres, 2007). *Colonial mentality* refers to the belief that the colonized is inferior to the colonizer (David & Okazaki, 2006). Since the colonizer exerts control over the minds and bodies of the colonized (Said, 1994), a colonial mentality diminishes agency and efficacy among the colonized (Moane, 1999). Consequently, individuals suffering from a colonized mentality tend to internalize negative stereotypes about themselves, become estranged from their original culture, and develop a desire to be more like the colonizer (Freire, 1970).

A colonial mentality continues to affect individuals long after the conclusion of the political domination. For instance, David and Okazaki (2010) found that many Filipinx Americans endorsed an unconscious colonial mentality. In a subsequent study, David and Nadal (2013) found that Filipinx American immigrants' experiences of ethnic and cultural denigration in the Philippines, as well as in the United States, may have contributed to the development of a colonial mentality and thus to the development of negative mental health.

Cultural Imperialism

Cultural imperialism—the imposition of mainstream White culture as dominant and superior—colonizes the minds of people of color (Comas-Díaz, 2000). Cultural imperialism reinforces coloniality of color, power, and gender. Moreover, it promotes *neocolonization*—a situation in which a country is identified as superior in order to justify exercising dominion over its marginalized members (Said, 1994). That is, cultural imperialism imposes the dominant group's values, experiences, and culture as the norm. To illustrate, cultural imperialism designates individualistic values such as self-agency, internal locus of control, and meritocracy as normative while excluding people of color's collectivistic values. In this fashion, cultural imperialism infuses powerlessness and learned helplessness among the oppressed. Unfortunately, individuals subjected to cultural imperialism compromise their cultural worth (Said, 1994). Particularly, cultural imperialism affects immigrants of color because it interferes with the retention of their native culture during their acculturation process. In other words, pressured by cultural imperialism, some racial minority immigrants could perceive the dominant culture as superior to their own. Such negative perceptions are grounded in a sociopolitical designation of racial minority immigrants' cultures as deviant and inferior to the dominant culture (Comas-Díaz, 2000).

DECOLONIAL, LIBERATION, AND CULTURALLY RESPONSIVE PSYCHOLOGICAL APPROACHES

Many racial minority immigrants enter the United States because they suffer. Sadly, they continue to suffer from sociopolitical trauma past their arrival. Many develop trauma symptoms that require healing. However, a deficit-oriented model to treat trauma is limited in this population given the societal roots of sociopolitical and racial trauma. Moreover, the coloniality of power imposes Eurocentric values into the definitions of trauma, traumatic stress, and trauma treatment (Hernández-Wolfe, 2013). Consequently, working with immigrants who suffer from sociopolitical and racial trauma requires decolonial, liberation, and culturally responsive psychological approaches.

Decolonial Psychological Approaches

Decolonial approaches nurture the emergence of new narratives to resist oppression and to uncover innovative opportunities for decolonization and healing (Hook, 2005). According to Mignolo (2009), a colonial history classifies regions and people around the globe as underdeveloped, both economically and mentally. Mignolo argued that decolonial options relate to the principle that regeneration of life needs to prevail over the production of goods at the cost of life. In this vein, decolonial therapists aim to promote awareness of the negative effects of colonial mentality and cultural imperialism. Therefore, they help clients recognize that the imposition of Eurocentric values maintains systems of oppression that recreate a dominance pattern. Moreover, they foster the reevaluation of taken-for-granted constructs of psychological functioning.

Since cultural imperialism subjugates the knowledge of the oppressed, decolonial therapists redefine empowerment as an insurrection of subjugated knowledge (Pease, 2002). They support geopolitical (i.e., Global South) sources of knowledge (Mignolo, 2009). Consequently, decolonial therapists support oppressed clients' subjugated and discounted knowledge as a decolonization effort (Watkins & Shulman, 2008). In other words, they promote decolonization by helping clients recognize their history, recover their ancestral memory, and critically understand their oppressive circumstances. Moreover, decolonial therapists focus on identifying racial minority immigrants' survivalist and resilient responses to oppression. Within this context, they nurture clients' border thinking—a skill born out of living at the borderlands of cultures (Anzaldúa, 1987)—to examine power differentials, create new ways of knowledge, and uncover innovative paths of action (Mignolo, 2011).

To decolonize themselves, therapists can engage in self-reflection. For example, decolonial therapists use critical pedagogy (Freire, 1970) to decolonize their mindsets. In this fashion, they can ask critical questions such as Who benefits from sociopolitical oppression? Who benefits from nativism, racism, and xenophobia? Whose knowledge is represented in therapy? Does Eurocentric therapy address immigrants of color's psychological and health needs? Do Eurocentric therapies help to maintain the sociopolitical status quo?

Therapists with a history of colonization can engage in autoethnography as a self-decolonization method (Popova, 2016). Additionally, they can explore their colonized mentality through Zabala's (2017) 50 signs of colonial mentality. For instance, some of these signs are hating the dark color of their skin, using whitening products to lighten their skin, and looking down on people with dark skin.

In previous work (Comas-Díaz, 1994), I proposed a decolonization process from the perspective of the colonized. First, I recommended an increased awareness of the presence of colonized mentality, coupled with an understanding of the effects of colonization. Then, I suggested the correction of cognitive schemas and beliefs held by the individuals experiencing colonization, including the ambivalence they feel toward the colonizers. From this orientation, decolonization entails reclaiming positive cultural identities, leading to a sense of mastery, agency, and autonomous dignity. A self-transformation emerges through the release of the colonization effects, leading to the development of a solid sense of self and community. This decolonization approach can be applied to individuals with a legacy of colonization as well as to those experiencing cultural imperialism and neocolonization.

Liberation Psychology

A decolonial approach is grounded in *liberation psychology*. Liberation psychology provides resistance to colonization (Varas-Díaz & Serrano-García, 2003). It involves the use of psychological approaches to understand and address oppression among individuals and groups (Martín-Baró, 1994). Through this lens, liberation therapists conceptualize oppression as the interaction of intrapsychic factors with systemic factors, such as power differentials and sociopolitical injustice. Therefore, they promote healing and transformation through empowerment, critical consciousness, cultural ancestry recovery, and sociopolitical action (Comas-Díaz, 2000).

Liberation therapists aim to promote awareness of oppression, nurture clients' strengths and cultural identities, and foster sociopolitical change to decrease suffering and improve lives (Martín-Baró, 1994). Moreover, they help clients to reformulate their ethnocultural and racial identities, engage in critical consciousness, develop sociopolitical consciousness, and engage in personal and collective transformation (Comas-Díaz et al., 1998). For these reasons, liberation therapists integrate dominant psychotherapy, ethnic indigenous healing, and diverse disciplines into their practice. Furthermore, they help clients to examine the effects of cultural imperialism and coloniality while paying attention to the effects of racism, trauma, and sociopolitical oppression. To accomplish these goals, liberation therapists use culturally relevant forms of healing. For instance, they examine clients' ethnic psychology healing and, when appropriate, integrate these approaches into therapy. The integration of ethnic indigenous healing in psychotherapy promotes self-healing (Comas-Díaz, 2012). Within this context, liberation therapists provide a cultural holding environment to help immigrants of color recover from sociopolitical and racial trauma, increase resilience, reconnect with their original cultures, foster sociopolitical transformation, and nurture psychospiritual development (Comas-Díaz, 2016, 2020).

Liberation therapists nurture clients' voices in the form of *testimonio*. Born in Latin America, testimonio is a healing and empowering narrative method in which the person narrates their experience with marginalization, oppression, and trauma (Cienfuegos & Monelli, 1983). Testimonio gives voice to the voiceless and nurtures agency, posttraumatic meaning making, and self-healing (Brabeck, 2003). Moreover, it reduces depression, anxiety, and PTSD (Agger et al., 2012). As such, testimonio is a culturally relevant and trauma-informed psychotherapy for racial minority immigrants. Liberation therapists listen without judging their clients' testimonios. They hold the place while bearing witness to clients' painful narratives (Comas-Díaz, 2020). Likewise, immigrants of color can use autoethnography as a therapeutic tool to cope with life transitions resulting from migration (Wright, 2009).

Even though the liberation psychotherapy relationship shares similarities with the mainstream psychotherapy relationship, it is unique in several ways. To illustrate, liberation psychotherapists aim to relate to their clients in a heart-to-heart fashion through cultural humility (i.e., other-oriented therapeutic relationship stand; Hook et al., 2013), cultural empathy, and accompaniment and by nurturing psychospiritual development (Comas-Díaz, 2020). Radical humility entails a capacity to feel the pain of the sufferer. Liberation therapists accompany their clients by listening, witnessing, advocating, and opening a space to develop innovative knowledge (Watkins & Shulman, 2008). This approach helps therapists to demonstrate humility, compassion, respect, altruism, and positive regard toward their clients. Furthermore, therapists examine power differentials in society and conduct power differential analyses (Worell & Remer, 2003) between themselves and their clients.

Liberation therapists foster clients' creativity because expressive arts can heal sociopolitical stress and trauma (Shapiro & Alcántara, 2016). Indeed, art therapy has been used successfully to treat sociopolitical trauma (Karcher, 2017). Similarly, given liberation psychology's promotion of social justice action, liberation therapists foster *artivism*—art created to promote social justice action (Sandoval & Latorre, 2008)—as a healing and social justice method. Forms of artivism include street art, Indigenous murals, hip hop music, spoken word, altar making, and several others. Furthermore, as a feminist artivism, *autohistoria* (i.e., self-history using multiple media) helps to integrate people of color's fractured identity (Anzaldúa, 1987).

Liberation psychology has been effective in addressing the needs of Latinx immigrants. To illustrate, Chavez-Dueñas and colleagues (2019) developed HEART (i.e., Healing Ethno and Racial Trauma), a healing framework integrating liberation psychology, intersectionality theory, and trauma-informed care into psychotherapy with Latinx immigrants. The goals of the program were to create awareness and coping with systemic oppression by increasing resistance to sociopolitical and ethnoracial trauma. Composed of four phases, each HEART phase helped clients to become aware and cope with systemic oppression and to develop resistance to the external forces that caused the sociopolitical trauma. Likewise, Torres Fernandez and Torres Rivera (2014) successfully treated Latinx children suffering from trauma due to the violence on the U.S.–Mexico border with liberation psychology approaches such as

Indigenous healing, experiential exercises, and narrative therapy to foment critical consciousness.

Liberation therapists promote community empowerment to address sociopolitical trauma. For example, Watts et al. (1999) developed a program to foster sociopolitical consciousness as an antidote to oppression among young urban African American males. Following a liberation psychology model, they included artivism such as rap music, videos, and films to foster the development of critical consciousness. As another community liberation illustration, THRIVE is an empowering healing approach for adolescent girls of color that is both culturally relevant and gender relevant (Bryant-Davis & Rajan, 2019). This approach effectively combines group therapy, psychoeducation, expressive art, mindfulness (e.g., prayer, meditation, reflection), and community empowerment. Organized by the acronym THRIVE, this 6-week group program included Touchstones, Healing Hearts, Road to the Future, Intimate Issues, Voice, and Empowerment (Bryant-Davis & Rajan, 2019).

TREATMENT ILLUSTRATION: LA FLOR DE IZOTE (THE *IZOTE* FLOWER)

You don't heal the wound, the wound heals you.

—GLORIA ANZALDÚA

As previously indicated, Flor began to lose weight after her arrival to the United States. Flor's aunt Beatriz took her to an internist, who recommended mental health treatment. Beatriz scheduled an appointment at a community mental health clinic. Dr. Esperanza Fuentes (a composite case), a Latina therapist with experience working with immigrants, saw Flor. Flor requested that Beatriz accompany her to the first therapy session. At the end of the session, Dr. Fuentes asked Flor if she could be alone during the next session. Flor was ambivalent but agreed to do so. During the second therapy session, Beatriz accompanied Flor, but she stayed in the reception area. Dr. Fuentes asked Flor about her home in El Salvador. Flor's eyes widened, and she spoke about the beauty of her country. Suddenly, Flor began to shake and became anxious. Dr. Fuentes taught her deep breathing exercises. After a while, Flor calmed down and said, "Can you teach me more ways to calm myself?" "Yes, I can help you connect with your inner healer," Dr. Fuentes replied. The culturally relevant intervention initiated the development of rapport. In subsequent sessions, Flor learned several soothing techniques, namely acupressure and the eye movement desensitization and reprogramming (EMDR) butterfly hug (Shapiro, 1995). "You can call me Esperanza, if you wish," Dr. Fuentes told Flor, exercising the cultural concept of *familismo*—a Latinx warm supportive personal relational style. "I don't know," Flor replied in a soft voice. She added, "But, I like your name Esperanza." "I like it too," Dr. Fuentes said. They both smiled, noting the emergence of a positive therapeutic alliance.

To know Flor better, Dr. Fuentes suggested an exercise of looking into the four directions. "I'm familiar with the four directions concept," Flor stated. Dr. Fuentes used Ayeli, a Native American psychospiritual assessment in which East represents belonging, South is related to mastery, West is associated with independence, and North is related to generosity (Garrett & Garrett, 1994). The exercise revealed Flor's pain, strengths, and the need to envision a life purpose. In other words, Flor described her pain as having a lump in her throat. She identified spirituality as her strength, but she could not name her purpose in life.

Flor began to feel grounded after completing the Ayeli exercise. Dr. Fuentes suggested that she visualize a healing energy entering her throat. After several practices of the visualization, Flor's appetite returned, and she slowly regained weight. Additionally, Dr. Fuentes suggested that Flor try yoga as a complement to the trauma-informed therapy (van der Kolk et al., 2014). Flor followed the advice and initiated a yoga practice; Beatriz joined her.

Flor agreed to accompany Beatriz to her *promotora* (i.e., a Latinx community health advocate) neighborhood work. Flor took English lessons and demonstrated an ability for languages. She felt better, but she continued to experience sleeping difficulties. Dr. Fuentes suggested EMDR, and Flor agreed to try it. However, when they initiated the EMDR, Flor began to shake. Fortunately, Flor calmed herself with a butterfly hug. Dr. Fuentes did not continue the EMDR. Instead, she invited Flor to write her testimonio.

Flor spent several months completing her testimonio. In the meantime, therapy focused on nurturing Flor's self-care. When Flor finished her testimonio, Dr. Fuentes asked her to read it during therapy. Flor agreed, and she invited Beatriz to the session. A significant aspect of her testimonio was a traumatic image of one MS-13 member holding her throat while he raped her. "He had a spiderweb tattoo on his upper right arm," Flor said. Consequently, she disclosed having recurrent nightmares of being caught in a spider web. After reading her testimonio, Flor reported a decrease in her nightmares. However, one day, when Flor was accompanying Beatriz in her community work, a Latinx man called Flor a "dirty Indian." She processed the incident in therapy. Dr. Fuentes suggested an ethnic healing, Feeding Your Demons, a Buddhist psychology method based on a shamanistic practice (Allione, 2008). In this approach, the therapist guides the sufferer into a trance-like state to name the demon (i.e., problem), ask what it needs, feed the demon with an elixir, and finally transform the demon into an ally. Flor identified her demon as fear and recognized love as what the demon needed. Therefore, Flor fed her fear with love and transformed her demon into an ally. In processing the exercise, Flor said, "I realized that my real wound is that I don't have self-love because I see myself as a dirty Indian." Dr. Fuentes worked with Flor to address her internalized racism in order to heal her sociopolitical and racial trauma. She helped Flor to develop critical consciousness and asked critical questions (Freire & Macedo, 2000), such as "Who benefits from racism? Who benefits from calling you a dirty Indian?" Moreover, to promote decolonization,

Dr. Fuentes helped Flor to develop an awareness of the concepts of coloniality of power, gender, and color. She invited Flor to reconnect with her Pipil culture and language. Sadly, the Pipil language (Nawat) was almost banished as a result of a racial war in El Salvador against the Pipil people (http://www.native-languages.org/pipil.htm) and as a neocolonization method. Flor became interested and joined an online group promoting the Pipil language.

Flor worked in therapy for 3 years. During that time, she became fluent in English, completed her high school diploma, and was accepted at a community college. At her last therapy session, Flor said: "The *izote* (Lord's candle) is our national flower." She then took off her sweater and uncovered a tattoo of izote flowers on her upper right arm. "The izote flower has a bitter taste, but when it is cooked with other ingredients, it makes delicious meals." Dr. Fuentes moved her chair closer to Flor to admire the tattoo. "My trauma is like the izote flower," Flor said. "It brought bitterness into my life, but it was transformed during therapy." Flor smiled and said, "As a result, I learned to love myself."

RECOMMENDATIONS

One doesn't ask of one who suffers: What is your country and what is your religion? One merely says, you suffer, this is enough for me, you belong to me and I shall help you.
—LOUIS PASTEUR

Mental health professionals working with racial minority immigrants may want to become familiar with decolonial and liberation psychology approaches. Moreover, they can engage in cultural self-assessments to examine their power differentials with their immigrant clients. Specifically, clinicians need to examine their conscious, preconscious, and unconscious attitudes toward racial minority immigrants. For example, some therapists may harbor a political countertransference (Chung, 2005), leading to a belief that all racial minority immigrants are undocumented, rapists, and/or criminals.

Given that state institutions are responsible for the creation of sociopolitical trauma, therapists need to implement radical solutions, such as radical education (Burstow, 2003). Therefore, it is important that psychologists working with racial minority immigrants keep informed of the changing sociopolitical contexts, immigrant policies, and legal contexts as well as new developments in sociopolitical and trauma treatments (Dash, 2020). Indeed, because of the intersectionality of race, ethnicity, gender, sexuality, and class among oppressed communities, mental health services are required to be trauma informed (Berger & Quiros, 2014) as well as culturally and gender responsive.

Needless to say, psychologists need to exhibit cultural humility and flexibility in their roles when working with racial minority immigrants. For example, they can help immigrants of color to connect with social support networks to get emotional support, information, and advocacy (Ayón, 2011). Finally, psychologists can work to help align the U.S. laws and immigration policies with international laws to discontinue the cycles of trauma and to establish feasible means of sustainable development for immigrant children and second-generation individuals who experience traumas such as parental deportation (Rojas-Flores et al., 2019).

CONCLUSION

You have witnessed my descent. Now watch my rising.

—RUMI

Numerous racial minority immigrants suffer from sociopolitical trauma throughout their migration journey. Unfortunately, they are exposed to more sociopolitical and racial trauma after their arrival to the United States. For these reasons, racial minority immigrants require decolonial, liberation, culturally relevant, gender-informed, and trauma-informed treatment. However, trauma experiences can lead to resilience, and many immigrants from Asia, Europe, Latin America, and other regions have exhibited immigrant resilience (American Psychological Association [APA] Presidential Task Force on Immigration, 2012). Certainly, numerous therapists have witnessed their clients' sociopolitical trauma before witnessing their resilience. Working with racial minority immigrants requires that a psychologist transcend the professional role in order to advocate for racial minority immigrants. Indeed, professionals working with immigrants of color can ameliorate their clients' suffering by committing to work against all types of oppression—nationally, transnationally, and globally.

REFERENCES

Adames, H. Y., & Chavez-Dueñas, N. Y. (2017). *Cultural foundations and interventions in Latino/a mental health: History, theory, and within group differences.* Routledge.

Agger, I., Igreja, V., Kiehle, R., & Polatin, P. (2012). Testimony ceremonies in Asia: Integrating spirituality in testimonial therapy for torture survivors in India, Sri Lanka, Cambodia, and the Philippines. *Transcultural Psychiatry, 49*(3–4), 568–589. https://doi.org/10.1177/1363461512447138

American Immigration Lawyers Association. (2015). *Declaration from Karen Lucas (AILA) and Lindsey Harris (the American Immigration Council) regarding complaints filed with DHS, CRCL, and ORG on deplorable medical conditions and psychological impact of detention, along with declarations from attorneys Kim Hunter, Laura Litcher, and Katherine Park.* https://www.americanimmigrationcouncil.org/sites/default/files/research/a_guide_to_children_arriving_at_the_border_and_the_laws_and_policies_governing_our_response.pdf

Allione, T. (2008). *Feeding your demons: Ancient wisdom for resolving inner conflict.* Little, Brown and Company.

American Psychological Association. (2019). *Guidelines for psychological practice with girls and women.* https://www.apa.org/practice/guidelines/girls-and-women

American Psychological Association Presidential Task Force on Immigration. (2012). *Presidential Task Force on Immigration Report: Crossroads: The psychology of immigration in the new century*. American Psychological Association. https://www.apa.org/topics/immigration/executive-summary.pdf

Anzaldúa, G. (1987). *Borderlands/La Frontera: The new Mestiza*. Spinster/Aunt Lute Publishers.

Ayón, C. (2011). Latino families and the public child welfare system: Examining the role of social support networks. *Children and Youth Services Review, 33*(10), 2061–2066. https://doi.org/10.1016/j.childyouth.2011.05.035

Beltran, A. (2017). *Children and families fleeing the violence in Central America*. Washington Office of Latin America. https://www.wola.org/analysis/people-leaving-central-americas-northern-triangle/

Berger, R., & Quiros, L. (2014). Supervision for trauma-informed practice. *Traumatology, 20*(4), 296–301. https://doi.org/10.1037/h0099835

Brabeck, K. (2003). Testimonio: A strategy for collective resistance, cultural survival, and building solidarity. *Feminism & Psychology, 13*(2), 252–258. https://doi.org/10.1177/0959353503013002009

Brabeck, K., & Xu, Q. (2010). The impact of detention and deportation on Latino immigrant children and families: A quantitative exploration. *Hispanic Journal of Behavioral Sciences, 32*(3), 341–361. https://doi.org/10.1177/0739986310374053

Bryant-Davis, T., & Rajan, I. (2019). Next steps: An integrated model for conducting feminist therapy. In T. Bryant-Davis (Ed.), *Multicultural feminist therapy: Helping adolescent girls of color to thrive* (pp. 189–207). American Psychological Association. https://doi.org/10.1037/0000140-007

Burstow, B. (2003). Toward a radical understanding of trauma and trauma work. *Violence Against Women, 9*(11), 1293–1317. https://doi.org/10.1177/1077801203255555

Ceja, M. (2004). Chicana college aspirations and the role of parents: Developing educational resiliency. *Journal of Hispanic Higher Education, 3*(4), 338–362. https://doi.org/10.1177/1538192704268428

Chavez-Dueñas, N. Y., Adames, H. Y., Perez-Chavez, J. G., & Salas, S. P. (2019). Healing ethno-racial trauma in Latinx immigrant communities: Cultivating hope, resistance, and action. *American Psychologist, 74*(1), 49–62. https://doi.org/10.1037/amp0000289

Chung, R. C.-Y. (2005). Women, human rights, and counseling: Crossing international boundaries. *Journal of Counseling and Development, 83*(3), 262–268. https://doi.org/10.1002/j.1556-6678.2005.tb00341.x

Cienfuegos, A. J., & Monelli, C. (1983). The testimony of political repression as a therapeutic instrument. *American Journal of Orthopsychiatry, 53*(1), 43–51. https://doi.org/10.1111/j.1939-0025.1983.tb03348.x

Clark, K. B. (1989). *Dark ghetto: Dilemmas in social power* (2nd ed.). Wesleyan University Publishers.

Comas-Díaz, L. (1994). An integrative approach. In L. Comas-Diaz & B. Greene (Eds.), *Women of color: Integrating ethnic and gender identities in psychotherapy* (pp. 287–318). Guilford Press.

Comas-Díaz, L. (2000). An ethnopolitical approach to working with people of color. *American Psychologist, 55*(11), 1319–1325. https://doi.org/10.1037/0003-066X.55.11.1319

Comas-Díaz, L. (2007). Ethnopolitical psychology: Healing and transformation. In E. Aldarondo (Ed.), *Promoting social justice in mental health practice* (pp. 91–118). Lawrence Erlbaum Associates.

Comas-Díaz, L. (2012). *Multicultural care: A clinician's guide to cultural competence*. American Psychological Association. https://doi.org/10.1037/13491-000

Comas-Díaz, L. (2016). Racial trauma recovery: A race-informed therapeutic approach to racial wounds. In A. N. Alvarez, C. T. H. Liang, & H. A. Neville (Eds.), *Contextualizing the cost of racism for people of color: Theory, research, and practice* (pp. 341–375). American Psychological Association. https://doi.org/10.1037/14852-012

Comas-Díaz, L. (2019). Latina adolescents at the cultural borderlands. In T. Bryant-Davis (Ed.), *Multicultural feminist therapy: Helping adolescent girls of color to thrive* (pp. 155–187). American Psychological Association. https://doi.org/10.1037/0000140-006

Comas-Díaz, L. (2020). Liberation psychotherapy. In L. Comas-Díaz & E. Torres Rivera (Eds.), *Liberation psychology: Theory, method, practice, and social justice* (pp. 169–185). American Psychological Association.

Comas-Díaz, L., Hall, G. N., & Neville, H. A. (2019). Racial trauma: Theory, research, and healing: Introduction to the special issue. *American Psychologist, 74*(1), 1–5. https://doi.org/10.1037/amp0000442

Comas-Díaz, L., Lykes, M. B., & Alarco-n, R. D. (1998). Ethnic conflict and the psychology of liberation in Guatemala, Peru, and Puerto Rico. *American Psychologist, 53*(7), 778–792. https://doi.org/10.1037/0003-066X.53.7.778

Craig-Henderson, K., & Sloan, L. (2003). Helping psychologists help victims of racist hate crime. *Clinical Psychology: Science and Practice, 10*(4), 481–490. https://doi.org/10.1093/clipsy.bpg048

Dash, G. F. (2020). Ethical considerations in providing psychological services to unaccompanied immigrant children. *Ethics & Behavior, 30*(2), 83–96. https://doi.org/10.1080/10508422.2019.1623031

David, E. D. R., & Okazaki, S. (2010). Activation and automaticity of colonial mentality. *Journal of Applied Social Psychology, 40*(4), 850–887. https://doi.org/10.1111/j.1559-1816.2010.00601.x

David, E. J., & Nadal, K. L. (2013). The colonial context of Filipino American immigrants' psychological experiences. *Cultural Diversity & Ethnic Minority Psychology, 19*(3), 298–309. https://doi.org/10.1037/a0032903

David, E. J., & Okazaki, S. (2006). Colonial mentality: A review and recommendation for Filipino American psychology. *Cultural Diversity & Ethnic Minority Psychology, 12*(1), 1–16. https://doi.org/10.1037/1099-9809.12.1.1

Dillon, F. R., De La Rosa, M., & Ibañez, G. E. (2013). Acculturative stress and diminishing family cohesion among recent Latino immigrants. *Journal of Immigrant and Minority Health, 15*(3), 484–491. https://doi.org/10.1007/s10903-012-9678-3

Elsass, P. (1992). *Strategies for survival: The psychology of cultural resilience in ethnic minorities.* New York University Press.

Ewing, W., Martinez, D. E., & Rumbaut, R. G. (2015, July 13). *The criminalization of immigration in the United States.* American Immigration Council. https://www.americanimmigrationcouncil.org/research/criminalization-immigration-united-states

Fanon, F. (1967). *Black skin, White masks.* Grove Press, Inc.

Flores, E., Tschann, J. M., Dimas, J. M., Pasch, L. A., & de Groat, C. L. (2010). Perceived racial/ethnic discrimination, posttraumatic stress symptoms, and health risk behaviors among Mexican American adolescents. *Journal of Counseling Psychology, 57*(3), 264–273. https://doi.org/10.1037/a0020026

Freire, P. (1970). *Pedagogy of the oppressed.* Continuum.

Freire, P., & Macedo, D. (2000). *The Paulo Freire reader.* Continuum.

Garcia, C., Zhang, L., Holt, K., Hardeman, R., & Peterson, B. (2014). Latina adolescent sleep and mood: An ecological momentary assessment pilot study. *Journal of Child and Adolescent Psychiatric Nursing, 27*(3), 132–141. https://doi.org/10.1111/jcap.12082

Garrett, J. T., & Garrett, M. W. (1994). The path of good medicine: Understanding and counseling Native American Indians. *Journal of Multicultural Counseling and Development, 22*(3), 134–144. https://doi.org/10.1002/j.2161-1912.1994.tb00459.x

Grosfoguel, R., & Georas, C. S. (2010). "Coloniality of power" and racial dynamics: Notes toward a reinterpretation of Latino Caribbeans in New York City. *Identities (Yverdon), 7*(1), 85–125. https://doi.org/10.1080/1070289X.2000.9962660

Haines, D. W. (2010). *Safe heaven? A history of refugees in America.* Kumarian Press.

Haque, A., Tubbs, C. Y., Kahumoku-Fessler, E. P., & Brown, M. D. (2019). Microaggressions and Islamophobia: Experiences of Muslims across the United States and clinical implications. *Journal of Marital and Family Therapy, 45*(1), 76–91. https://doi.org/10.1111/jmft.12339

Hearts of our people: Native women artists [Exhibition]. (2019, June 2–August 18). Minneapolis Institute of Art, Minneapolis, MN, United States. https://new.artsmia.org/hearts-of-our-people-native-women-artists/

Hernández-Wolfe, P. (2013). *A borderlands view on Latinos, Latin Americans, and decolonization: Rethinking mental health.* Jason Aronson.

Hook, D. (2005). A critical psychology of the postcolonial. *Theory & Psychology, 15*(4), 475–503. https://doi.org/10.1177/0959354305054748

Hook, J. N., Davis, D. E., Owen, J., Worthington, E. L., Jr., & Utsey, S. O. (2013). Cultural humility: Measuring openness to culturally diverse clients. *Journal of Counseling Psychology, 60*(3), 353–366. https://doi.org/10.1037/a0032595 (Correction published 2015, *Journal of Counseling Psychology, 62*(1), pp. iii–v. https://doi.org/10.1037/a0038582)

Hunter-Hernández, M., Costas-Muñíz, R., & Gany, F. (2015). Missed opportunity: Spirituality as a bridge to resilience in Latinos with cancer. *Journal of Religion and Health, 54*(6), 2367–2375. https://doi.org/10.1007/s10943-015-0020-y

Jasinskaja-Lahti, I., & Yijälaä, A. (2011). The model of pre acculturative stress: A pre-migration study of potential migrants from Russia to Finland. *International Journal of Intercultural Relations, 35*(4), 499–510. https://doi.org/10.1016/j.ijintrel.2010.11.003

Johnson, K. I. (1998). Race, the immigration laws, and domestic race relations: A "magic mirror" into the heart of darkness. *Indiana Law Journal, 73*(4), 2. http://www.repository.law.indiana.edu/ilj/vol73/iss4/2

Johnson-Motoyama, M., Dettlaff, A. J., & Finno, M. (2012). Parental nativity and the decision to substantiate: Findings from a study of Latino children in the Second National Survey of Child and Adolescent Well-being (NSCAW). *Children and Youth Services Review, 34*(11), 2229–2239. https://doi.org/10.1016/j.childyouth.2012.07.017

Karcher, O. P. (2017). Sociopolitical oppression, trauma, and healing: Moving toward a social justice art therapy framework. *Art Therapy, 34*(3), 123–128. https://doi.org/10.1080/07421656.2017.1358024

Lorenzo-Blanco, E. I., Meca, A., Unger, J. B., Romero, A., Szapocznik, J., Piña-Watson, B., Cano, M. Á., Zamboanga, B. L., Baezconde-Garbanati, L., Des Rosiers, S. E., Soto, D. W., Villamar, J. A., Lizzi, K. M., Pattarroyo, M., & Schwartz, S. J. (2017). Longitudinal effects of Latino parent cultural stress, depressive symptoms and family functioning on youth emotional well-being and health risk behaviors. *Family Process, 56*(4), 981–996. https://doi.org/10.1111/famp.12258

Lugones, M. (2008). The coloniality of gender. *Worlds & Knowledge Otherwise, 2*(2), 1–17. https://globalstudies.trinity.duke.edu/sites/globalstudies.trinity.duke.edu/files/file-attachments/v2d2_Lugones.pdf

Maldonado-Torres, N. (2007). On the coloniality of being: Contributions to the development of a concept. *Cultural Studies, 21*(2–3), 240–270. https://doi.org/10.1080/09502380601162548

Marín, M. R., & García-Vázquez, E. (2012). The intersection of family and community resilience to enhance mental health among Latino children, adolescents, and families. *Committee on Children, Youth, and Families Newsletter.* http://www.apa.org/pi/families/resources/newsletter/2012/07/family-community.aspx

Martín-Baró, I. (1994). *Writings for a liberation psychology: Ignacio Martín-Baró* (A. Aron & S. Corne, Eds. & Trans.). Harvard University Press.

Mignolo, W. (2009). Epistemic disobedience, independent thought, and decolonial freedom. *Theory, Culture & Society, 26*(7–8), 159–181. https://doi.org/10.1177/0263276409349275

Mignolo, W. (2011). Geopolitics of sensing and knowing: On (de)coloniality, border thinking and epistemic disobedience. *Postcolonial Studies, 14*(3), 273–283. https://doi.org/10.1080/13688790.2011.613105

Moane, G. (1999). *Gender and colonialism. A psychological analysis of oppression and liberation.* Palgrave.

Monk, E. P., Jr. (2015). The cost of color: Skin color, discrimination, and health among African Americans. *American Journal of Sociology, 121*(2), 396–444. https://doi.org/10.1086/682162

Morales, L. S., Lara, M., Kington, R. S., Valdez, R. O., & Escarce, J. J. (2002). Socio-economic, cultural, and behavioral factors affecting Hispanic health outcomes. *Journal of Health Care for the Poor and Underserved, 13*(4), 477–503. https://doi.org/10.1353/hpu.2010.0630

Pease, B. (2002). Rethinking empowerment: A postmodern reappraisal for emancipatory practice. *British Journal of Social Work, 32*(2), 135–147. https://doi.org/10.1093/bjsw/32.2.135

Perrotti, M. (2016). *The oppression of immigrants in America: A plan of action.* https://prezi.com/wc15uerbt6uy/the-oppression-of-immigrants-in-america-a-plan-of-action/

Popova, D. (2016). Decolonizing the self. In G. A. Tilley-Lubbs & S. Bénard Calva (Eds.), *Retelling our stories: Critical autoethnographic narratives* (pp. 173–185). Springer. https://doi.org/10.1007/978-94-6300-567-8_13

Quijano, A. (2000). Coloniality of power, Eurocentrism and Latin America. *Nepantla, 1*(3), 533–580. https://doi.org/10.1177/0268580900015002005

Ramirez, M., & Ream, A. K. (2014, July 24). Migrant children are fleeing a region rife with sexual violence. *The New Republic.* https://newrepublic.com/article/118820/sexual-violence-major-cause-immigration-us

Rojas-Flores, L., Koo, J. H., & Vaughn, J. M. (2019). Protecting U.S. children whose Central American parents have temporary protected status. *International Perspectives in Psychology: Research, Practice, Consultation, 8*(1), 14–19. https://doi.org/10.1037/ipp0000100

Romero, A. J., Edwards, L. M., Fryberg, S. A., & Orduña, M. (2014). Resilience to discrimination stress across ethnic identity stages of development. *Journal of Applied Social Psychology, 44*(1), 1–11. https://doi.org/10.1111/jasp.12192

Said, E. W. (1994). *Culture and imperialism.* Vintage Books.

Sandoval, C., & Latorre, G. (2008). Chicana/o artivism: Judy Baca's digital work with youth of color. In A. Everett (Ed.), *Learning race and ethnicity: Youth and digital media.* MIT Press.

Schrag, P. (2010, September 13). *The unwanted: Immigration and nativism in America.* American Immigration Council. https://www.americanimmigrationcouncil.org/research/unwanted-immigration-and-nativism-america

Schwartz, J. (2017, February 2). *U.S., a nation of immigrants but ambivalent about immigration.* AP News. https://apnews.com/d984a89f25ea41aab1993990bffafcdc

Screenivasan, H. (2018, July 22). *While in ICE custody, thousands of migrants reported sexual abuse.* PBS News Hour Weekend. Available from https://www.pbs.org/newshour/show/while-in-ice-custody-thousands-of-migrants-reported-sexual-abuse

Shapiro, E., & Alcántara, D. (2016). *Mujerista* creativity: Latin@ sacred arts as life-course developmental resources. In T. Bryant-Davis & L. Comas-Díaz (Eds.), *Womanist and mujerista psychologies: Voices of fire, acts of courage* (pp. 195–216). American Psychological Association. https://doi.org/10.1037/14937-009

Shapiro, F. (1995). *Eye movement desensitization and reprocessing: Basic principles, protocols, and procedures.* Guilford Press.

Smokowski, P. R., & Bacallao, M. L. (2007). Acculturation, internalizing mental health symptoms, and self-esteem: Cultural experiences of Latino adolescents in North Carolina. *Child Psychiatry and Human Development, 37*(3), 273–292. https://doi.org/10.1007/s10578-006-0035-4

Telzer, E. H., & Vazquez-Garcia, H. A. (2009). Skin color and self-perceptions of immigrant and U.S.-born Latinas. *Hispanic Journal of Behavioral Sciences, 31*(3), 357–374. https://doi.org/10.1177/0739986309336913

Torres Fernandez, I., & Torres Rivera, E. (2014). Moving though trauma and grief in children impacted by the violence on the U.S.–Mexico border: A liberation psychology approach. In M. T. Garrett (Ed.), *Youth and adversity: Understanding the psychology and influences of child adolescent resilience and coping* (pp. 209–226). Nova Science Publishers.

Tseris, E. J. (2013). Trauma theory without feminism? Evaluating contemporary understandings of traumatized women. *Affilia, 28*(2), 153–164. https://doi.org/10.1177/0886109913485707

United Nations Women. (2017, February 15). *Take five: Fighting femicide in Latin America.* http://www.unwomen.org/en/news/stories/2017/2/take-five-adriana-quinones-femicide-in-latin-america

Valdez, C. R., Lewis Valentine, J., & Padilla, B. (2013). "Why we stay": Immigrants' motivations for remaining in communities impacted by anti-immigration policy. *Cultural Diversity & Ethnic Minority Psychology, 19*(3), 279–287. https://doi.org/10.1037/a0033176

van der Kolk, B. A., Stone, L., West, J., Rhodes, A., Emerson, D., Suvak, M., & Spinazzola, J. (2014). Yoga as an adjunctive treatment for posttraumatic stress disorder: A randomized controlled trial. *The Journal of Clinical Psychiatry, 75*(6), e559–e565. https://doi.org/10.4088/JCP.13m08561

Varas-Díaz, N., & Serrano-García, I. (2003). The challenge of a positive self-image in a colonial context: A psychology of liberation for the Puerto Rican experience. *American Journal of Community Psychology, 31*(1–2), 103–115. https://doi.org/10.1023/A:1023078721414

Watkins, M., & Shulman, H. (2008). *Toward psychologies of liberation.* Palgrave/McMillan. https://doi.org/10.1057/9780230227736

Watts, R. J., Griffith, D. M., & Abdul-Adil, J. (1999). Sociopolitical development as an antidote for oppression—Theory and action. *American Journal of Community Psychology, 27*(2), 255–271. https://doi.org/10.1023/A:1022839818873

Worell, J., & Remer, P. (2003). *Feminist perspectives in therapy* (2nd ed.). John Wiley & Sons.

Wright, J. K. (2009). Autoethnography and therapy writing on the move. *Qualitative Inquiry, 15*(4), 623–640. https://doi.org/10.1177/1077800408329239

Yosso, T. J. (2006). *Critical race counterstories along the Chicana/Chicano educational pipeline.* Routledge Taylor & Francis Group.

Zabala, S. A. (2017, June 8). *50 possible signs you may have colonial mentality.* https://thoughtcatalog.com/sade-andria-zabala/2017/06/50-possible-signs-you-may-have-colonial-mentality/

8

Racial Stress and Racialized Violence Among Black Immigrants in the United States

Marisol L. Meyer, Monique C. McKenny, Esprene Liddell-Quintyn, Guerda Nicolas, and Gemima St. Louis

Historically, immigrants to the United States have experienced social hostility on the basis of race and ethnicity, and this xenophobia continues to persist for many groups in the current political and sociocultural atmosphere (Dominguez et al., 2009; Gee & Ford, 2011). Among the various current immigrant groups that experience these inequitable systems, Black immigrants are particularly understudied. The stress of immigration and acculturation to the United States, compounded by traumatic experiences of racism and discrimination, may lead to racial stress and trauma among Black immigrants. These experiences with racial stress and trauma threaten the health and well-being of this group (Kirmayer et al., 2011). This chapter begins with an overview of the diversity within the Black immigrant population. It then explores various forms of discrimination Black immigrants face upon adjusting to life in the United States and the disparities that systemic racism and discrimination create. The consequences of this continual exposure to racism—racial stress and racialized violence—are summarized. The chapter concludes with a model to better conceptualize racial stress and trauma as experienced by Black immigrants and strategies that this group uses to cope with racism and discrimination while highlighting strengths that enable them to flourish.

This chapter is guided by three theoretical perspectives aimed at providing a better understanding of the ways in which systemic discrimination and prejudice constitute racialized violence (Helms et al., 2012) and how exposure

https://doi.org/10.1037/0000214-009
Trauma and Racial Minority Immigrants: Turmoil, Uncertainty, and Resistance,
P. Tummala-Narra (Editor)

to trauma and stress over a lifetime impacts Black immigrants (Herman, 1992). Herman's (1992) theory on complex trauma posits that "prolonged, repeated trauma" incites and perpetuates the subordination of individuals, with consequences that manifest psychologically, physiologically, economically, and socially (p. 377). While Herman's conceptualization of trauma is undoubtedly important, we also draw upon Helms et al. (2012) to illuminate the unique function of racialized stress and trauma. Helms et al. suggested that understanding racialized trauma requires consideration of the unique function of discrete racial stressors and long-term exposure to racism including trauma-related symptomatology such as "(a) direct cataclysmic racial or ethnic cultural events, (b) vicarious or witnessed cataclysmic events, and (c) racial and cultural microaggressions" (p. 66). Finally, more broadly throughout the chapter we seek to utilize a social-ecological framework to allow for a recognition and deeper understanding of how various systems, institutions, and individuals interact with and constantly expose Black immigrants to racism and discrimination (American Psychological Association [APA] Presidential Task Force on Immigration, 2012). These perspectives together allow for an analysis of the interpersonal impact of racial stress and trauma for Black immigrants along with the larger systemic implications of racialized violence.

BLACK IMMIGRANT POPULATIONS IN THE UNITED STATES: A SOCIOHISTORICAL OVERVIEW

When not explicitly defined, the grossly vague term "Black immigrants" can potentially homogenize groups that are otherwise culturally and ethnically distinct. Whether intentional or not, this homogenization undermines the divergent experiences of the diverse individuals that constitute "Black immigrants" in the United States (Dominguez et al., 2009). In a country where racial identity is often viewed through a binary lens, the sociohistorical Black/White racial paradigm dictates that Black individuals in the United States are often seen as belonging only to a racial group, ignoring intersectional cultural or ethnic group membership (Vickerman, 2007). Black immigrants from diverse ethnic backgrounds may respond differently to this forced binary based on a variety of factors, such as personal characteristics (e.g., skin color, country of origin, age), racial socialization, racial ideologies prior to migration, and perception of the American culture prior to migration (Adjepong, 2018). Ethnicity may be emphasized for various reasons, such as cultural pride or prior familial socialization (Showers, 2015; Vickerman, 2007).

While it may be true that distinct ethnic and cultural groups employ various strategies to cope and thrive within a country that continues to grapple with racial hostility, ultimately, all Black immigrants (regardless of ethnicity and culture) are likely to face experiences of racism and discrimination. Thus, while cultural and ethnic backgrounds may or may not modify experiences with racism and discrimination, it is imperative to recognize the critical role race plays in the experiences of Black immigrants in the United States.

POPULATION

Individuals originating from countries within Africa comprise some of the fastest growing groups immigrating to the United States (Venters & Gany, 2011) and will likely constitute 16.5% of the Black population in the United States by 2060 (Hamilton & Green, 2018). As of 2016, West and Eastern Africa (specifically, Nigeria, Ethiopia, Ghana, Kenya, and Somalia) were the regions of origin for most Africans migrating to the United States (Anderson & López, 2018). This increased presence of African migration to the United States defies historical migration patterns, as immigration from Africa to the United States was virtually nonexistent until the 1960s and did not begin to accelerate until the beginning of the 21st century (Anderson, 2015; Hamilton & Green, 2018).

Black immigrants from the Caribbean (a region also referred to as the West Indies) have historically constituted the highest percentage of Black individuals migrating to the United States (Dominguez et al., 2009). As of 2016, individuals from Jamaica and Haiti made up the largest percentage of Black Caribbean people immigrating to the United States, but a sizeable number of Black immigrants hail from countries such as Trinidad and Tobago and the Dominican Republic (Anderson & López, 2018). The Caribbean is home to one of the most culturally and ethnically distinct Black immigrant groups: Afro Latinx. Specifically, individuals that identify as Afro Latinx may migrate from regions such as Cuba and Puerto Rico. Beyond the Caribbean, this population extends geographically into Central and South America, including regions such as Mexico, Costa Rica, Panama, Columbia, and Guyana (Luis, 2012). While African, Caribbean, and Afro Latinx Black immigrants are regionally, culturally, and ethnically distinct, individuals that migrate to the United States are immigrating to a country with a longstanding history of anti-Black sentiments.

EXPERIENCES WITH RACIAL TRAUMA AND RACIALIZED VIOLENCE

Harrell (2000), in defining the various levels of discriminatory events, conceptualized *race-related stress* as "race-related transactions between individuals or groups and their environment that emerge from the dynamics of racism and that are perceived to tax or exceed existing individual and collective resources or threaten well-being" (p. 14). Researchers such as Carter (2007) and Bryant-Davis and Ocampo (2005) built upon this definition by emphasizing the potentially traumatic nature of racialized incidents. Therefore, *racial stress and trauma* refers to the distress experienced before, during, or after a discriminatory event (Carter, 2007). Both direct and vicarious (i.e., witnessing a discriminatory event online) discriminatory incidents can serve as an impetus for racial stress and trauma. Researchers have linked racial incidents and the resulting stress to clinical symptomology of posttraumatic stress disorder (PTSD; Bryant-Davis & Ocampo, 2005; Carter, 2007): Individuals who experience direct and/or vicarious discriminatory encounters may exhibit symptoms including hypervigilance, anxiety, rumination, and avoidance (Pieterse et al., 2012; Stevenson, 2014; Tynes et al., 2019).

However, racism and discrimination impact individuals beyond inter-personal interactions that are frequently associated with racial stress and trauma. To capture the systemic, omnipresent impact of race in the lives of people of color, scholars have begun to use the term *racialized violence* to call attention to the damage to communities of color that results from large, histor-ically oppressive systems. Specifically, racialized violence refers to "any act that leads to injury, disfigurement, or death of Black people and other people of color because of their race" (Nicolas & Thompson, 2019, p. 588). In alignment with other forms of violence maintained by societal structures, racialized violence is interconnected with other forms of racialized experiences, including racial stress and racial trauma, and can exist at the interpersonal, community, and structural levels. Instances of racialized violence are illustrated in the history of the United States and globally, through the Atlantic slave trade and American slavery, along with the forced colonization of Caribbean nations, where many Black immigrants originate today.

DISCRIMINATION AND DISPARITIES

Black immigrant communities, like many other Black groups within the United States, face unique stressors at the cross section of race and immigra-tion status. Black immigrants can experience racism based on race as well as prejudice based on language and foreign birth (Gee & Ford, 2011). In addition to these interpersonal encounters with discrimination, Black immigrants exist within structural racism that interferes with all aspects of their residence in the United States, including economic mobility, sociocultural acceptance, and access to health and mental health care (Viruell-Fuentes et al., 2012).

Economically, Black immigrants face serious barriers that may include race-based wage inequity and feeling devalued in the workplace (Showers, 2015). For example, Black immigrants, regardless of skin tone, tend to earn less than White individuals with similar educational backgrounds (Vickerman, 2007). For darker skinned immigrants, this disparity is worsened, with darker complex-ioned Black immigrants earning 15% less than their phenotypically lighter counterparts (Vickerman, 2007). Immigrants also frequently report that they work in dangerous, segregated environments for employers that seek to take advantage of their immigrant employees (Gee & Ford, 2011). Structural racism creates and perpetuates these socioeconomic disparities, which have a direct impact on Black immigrants' mental and physical health (Viruell-Fuentes et al., 2012).

An uncritical review of the literature indicates that Black immigrants appear to have better physical and mental health than their native Black American counterparts (Hamilton & Green, 2018). However, this phenomenon is far more complicated, as revealed by scholars asserting that the "healthy immigrant effect" may elucidate why immigrants generally have better health than native members of their host society (Hamilton & Hummer, 2011, p. 1552; see also Acevedo-Garcia et al., 2010). This effect explains the considerable health advantage of immigrants as a product of selective migration, host country selectivity of immigrants granted citizenship, and a disinclination of first-generation immigrants to take up specific unhealthy North American cultural behaviors such as smoking, alcohol use, and poor dietary patterns (Gee & Ford, 2011; Hamilton & Green, 2018; Hamilton & Hummer, 2011; Viruell-Fuentes et al., 2012). While discriminatory immigration policies in the United States may result in the appearance of healthier immigrant populations, these same discriminatory policies and constant exposure to other products of structural racism may erode Black immigrants' mental and physical health over time (Gee & Ford, 2011; Hamilton & Hummer, 2011).

Read and Emerson (2005) put forth the racial context of origin hypothesis to explore more deeply how diverse Black immigrant populations may differentially feel the long-term impacts of exposure to racism. This hypothesis posits that the extent to which Black immigrants faced racism in their country of origin will impact the health outcomes they experience in the United States (Read & Emerson, 2005). Specifically, the longer a person has been exposed to racism (e.g., coming from a predominantly White region), the poorer their health will be throughout the lifespan and therefore in the United States (Hamilton & Hummer, 2011; Read & Emerson, 2005).

Discrimination and racism also impact Black immigrants' mental health. Cultural barriers between mental health specialists and Black immigrants may exacerbate this problem. Culturally, many Black immigrants face stigmas regarding mental illness and an intrapersonal resistance to breach tradition by seeking mental health services (Venters & Gany, 2011). Culturally rooted aversion to mental health services may be compounded by structural racism and systemic barriers that can prevent access to mental health care for Black immigrants. Moreover, many Black immigrants find that some mental health providers are not culturally competent to understand the various ways culture informs manifestations of mental illness (Venters & Gany, 2011). Westernized conceptualizations of mental health often inherently minimize culturally informed beliefs Black immigrants may have about their own experience with mental distress (Eamer et al., 2017). Thus, the language used by practitioners to explicate and treat mental distress may be confusing and frustrating to Black immigrants, regardless of English proficiency (Wafula & Snipes, 2014). For example, Haitian immigrants may experience the culturally informed syndrome of *Se'izisman* (i.e., "seized-up-ness"—a form of paralysis when experiencing volatile emotions; Nicolas et al., 2006). While Western mental health specialists may attempt to act in culturally competent ways when treating clients, there is little space in the Western paradigm for acknowledging culturally bound etiologies for this illness, such as supernatural forces.

Another institutional barrier is a lack of access to health insurance, as Black immigrants are proportionally less likely to be employed by employers mandated to provide health insurance coverage (Venters & Gany, 2011). A socioecological approach allows us to conceptualize the multifaceted and multiplicitous ways Black immigrants face racism and discrimination daily and the disparities created by the long-term exposure to these forces (APA Presidential Task Force on Immigration, 2012). When incorporating complex trauma theory into this conceptualization, it is clear that the long-term exposure to racism and discrimination has a powerful and deleterious impact on Black immigrants' mental health (Helms et al., 2012; Herman, 1992). Given the cumulative impact of racism, discrimination, and acculturation stress encountered by Black immigrants, it is critical to understand the coping mechanisms used by this group to manage those daily stressors.

BEYOND COPING: EFFORTS TO EMPOWER BLACK IMMIGRANTS

Black immigrants cope with racial stress and trauma in a variety of ways. For example, research shows that by maintaining transnational ties, Black immigrants remain connected to cultural practices that serve as buffers against stress (Cobb et al., 2019). Members of this group, when facing discrimination and racial violence, also draw on the values and beliefs from ethnic enclaves in which they live (Araújo Dawson, 2009). Furthermore, when Black immigrants migrate, their cultural values and collectivist culture encourage the reliance on kinship relations for social support that helps them cope with personal difficulties (Taylor et al., 2015). Finally, many Black immigrants rely on religion for hope and solace and use it as a means to cope in times of stress (Agyekum & Newbold, 2016; Butler-Barnes et al., 2018; Chatters et al., 2008).

Although coping amidst challenging situations is critical, using this lens to improve health and well-being for Black immigrants stresses the importance of asking individuals to remain resilient, implying that the individual's lack of resilience is to blame if the individual cannot overcome a problem (McCubbin & Cohen, 2003). Moving beyond coping therefore suggests that immigrants will continue to experience racial discrimination and stress as long as society fails to recognize and challenge systemic injustice and inequity (Vesely et al., 2017). Efforts to build the capacity and empowerment of Black immigrants should take into account internalized oppression and the ways in which it facilitates learned helplessness (McCubbin & Cohen, 2003). Focusing on empowerment means that interventions must reexamine the tendency to focus solely on psychological empowerment (Riger, 1993), which suggests that individuals develop self-efficacy and self-determination skills (Zimmerman, 1995). This form of empowerment exemplifies placing the responsibility on individuals by asking them to pull themselves up by the bootstraps. Reframing empowerment in terms of taking control over resources redirects individuals to become critically aware of the need to redistribute resources that promote unfairness and are associated with racial stress and trauma (Keys et al., 2017; Ocloo & Matthews, 2016). Overall, moving beyond coping calls for scholars and practitioners to identify transformative change, which gives attention to the institutionalized and systemic challenges contributing to racial stress and discrimination among immigrants (Vesely et al., 2017). Shifting our gaze from what is wrong with individuals to examining the ecological factors that remain unchallenged presents opportunities to critically examine policies that disproportionately affect Black immigrants while identifying power differentials in relationships and within various spaces that both implicitly and explicitly maintain oppression of Black immigrants.

A MODEL FOR UNDERSTANDING THE PSYCHOLOGICAL TRAUMA OF RACISM AMONG BLACK IMMIGRANTS

As this review of the literature suggests, racism exists and can be experienced as traumatic by Black immigrants in the United States (Helms et al., 2012). These traumatic experiences profoundly influence the lives of Black immigrants. Figure 8.1 presents a model exploring Black immigrants' experiences with racialized trauma. The following section delineates the various factors that constitute the model.

FIGURE 8.1. Model of Black Immigrants' Traumatic Experiences With Racism

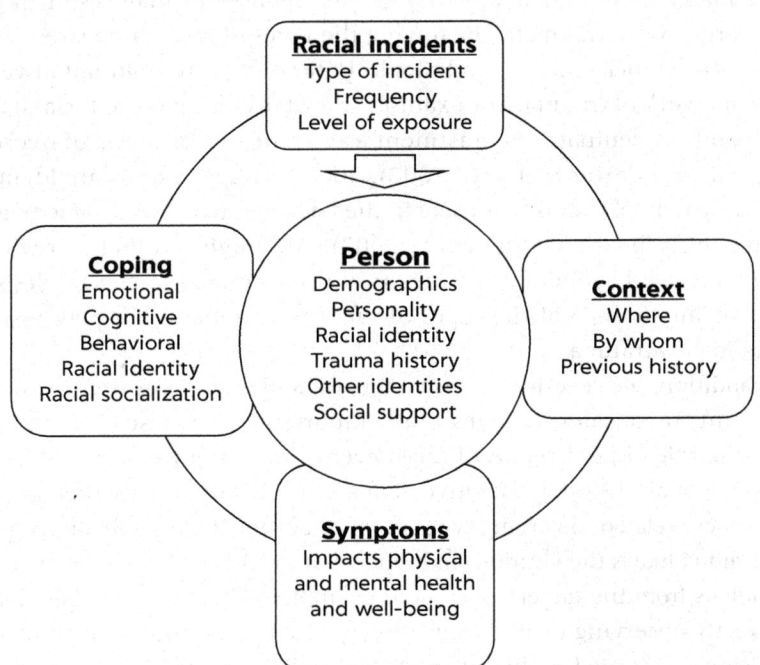

The model recognizes racialized violence as a form of complex trauma and uses a social–ecological framework to explore how various systems, institutions, and individuals interact with and constantly expose Black immigrants to racism and discrimination and the related coping methods, symptoms of trauma, and individual factors (APA Presidential Task Force on Immigration, 2012; Helms et al., 2012; Herman, 1992). It is centered on personal experiences with racism, as informed by the context, and how these experiences inform responses and coping. It should be noted that racism is outside of the individual. While connected to the context, symptoms, and coping process, racism is an external stressor that acts upon a person and significantly impacts that individual from within.

The visual representation of this model is designed to represent the interconnected nature of the domains involved in the psychological experience of racism. The model is not, however, designed to be a stage or process model. Much research is needed to further delineate the directionality and magnitude of the relationships among these variables as well as to further understand each variable's unique and shared contribution to the process of coping with racism and to the mental health outcomes. Beyond that, ongoing research is needed to address the ways in which these important research and practical considerations interact to influence an individual (Brondolo et al., 2009).

Characteristics of the Racial Incident

Carter (2007) explained that racist events that are experienced as negative, memorable, sudden, and uncontrollable lead to posttraumatic stress responses. While many factors outside of the events themselves may result in race-based stress being traumatic, qualifying the types of race-based stressors has been a strong focus in the psychological literature, although not always in the framework of trauma. For example, racial discrimination, racial harassment, and discriminatory harassment are delineated as levels of overtness (Carter, 2007; Carter & Helms, 2002), and microaggressions are identified as consistent, brief events that come in the form of microassaults, microinsults, and microinvalidations (Sue et al., 2007). Although a complete review of this literature is beyond the parameters of this chapter, these examples show the clear importance of the types of racist experiences that may result in psychological trauma.

In addition, the severity, intensity, length, and number of stressors may be important to consider. Perhaps most important is the research that highlights the role of perceptions of racist events, not simply objective measures (McNeilly et al., 1996). Qualitative data are needed to identify themes in the experiences related to varying types of racist events. Beyond the direct impact to the individual is the vicarious influence that racist events may have on other individuals from the target groups. For example, individuals may be impacted by directly observing racist events directed toward another person through television, print media, the internet, and social media (Tynes et al., 2012).

Thus, the racist events may take on many different forms and can target the individual directly or indirectly.

One must also consider that Black immigrants may or may not be migrating from a society in which racism is less prevalent than it is in the United States. More research focusing on how Black immigrants from diverse cultural and geographic backgrounds experience racial encounters upon adjusting to United States society is needed. However, regardless of one's immigration status and despite the forms of the exposure, these events have significant impacts on the well-being of the individual.

The Person Experiencing Racism

At the core of this model is the person experiencing the various racist events. Previous models, including the biopsychosocial model of racism (Clark et al., 1999) and the racial encounter coping appraisal socialization theory (Anderson & Stevenson, 2019), identified the process by which racism leads to or causes coping responses and physical and mental health problems through individual level factors such as racial identity and racial socialization. These frameworks align in their understanding that racist events are experienced differently by different people. For Black immigrant groups, these individual level factors include age of the person, age at which one immigrated, and country of birth. Much more research is needed to identify the individual factors that influence how Black immigrants from diverse backgrounds experience and cope with racist events in the United States, as the majority of the research on this topic has been conducted with U.S.-born populations.

In the present conceptualization, the person is central: Characteristics unique to each individual are crucial to the experience of racist events as traumatic. While personal characteristics are important when considering individual experiences with racism, it should not be misinterpreted that the individual is in any way responsible for racism. Rather, a person experiencing racism is a victim—interpreting the context, experiencing symptoms, and utilizing coping skills in individualized ways. Thus, although all marginalized groups experience some form of racism in their lifetime, the experiences are not the same for all individuals; various factors influence the different experiences from one individual. These factors merit a closer examination by researchers and clinicians.

Countless examples of the personal factors involved in the psychological impacts of racism exist in the literature. Heterosexism and racism have been shown to be interrelated, with gendered racism accompanied by increases in psychological distress among African American women (Thomas et al., 2008). In addition, a person's racial identity has been shown to be an important consideration in the relationship between race-related stress and mental health, with both racial identity and race-related stress predicting mental health (Franklin-Jackson & Carter, 2007). Finally, age and stage of life influence racial identity attitudes (Parham, 1989). Different themes characterize the experiences of racial identity at each life stage. Late adolescence and early adulthood are characterized by an activist-involved lens, whereas middle adulthood is seen as driven by the institutions of which a person is a part and in which the individual seeks to survive. Racial identity in late adulthood is seen as reflective and adjusting to change (Helms, 2007).

Another factor that may affect the response patterns to a racist event is the person's previous history with these experiences; one might respond differently if it is a first-time incident than they would if they have had previous experiences within the same context regarding the same issue. As previously mentioned, Black immigrants may have differentially experienced racism in their countries of origin. More research is needed to delineate other areas that may inform one's experiences with racist events, including the influence of personality factors, social support, spirituality, race-based and other trauma history, acculturation, and the possible additive effects of multiple "isms" for individuals with multiple oppressed identities. Thus, attention needs to be paid to these factors in understanding the overall impact of racist events in the lives of individuals.

Context

In addition to the type and nature of the racist event(s), the context in which the stressor takes place serves to greatly inform the experiences of the oppressed individual. Environments in which racism is unexpected and unprepared for, such as one's home, school, or work, or within a context expected to be friendly may cause a more unexpected, memorable negative experience. A context in which one feels generally safe may serve to reduce the influence of a single racist event, whereas an environment where racism is pervasive may make a similar event take on a different meaning. This is not to say that racism is worse in certain contexts and excusable in others but rather that an individual may perceive racism in different ways based on their context, which informs their psychological experiences. Simply put, a single racist experience at a local store with a stranger may have a different impact than a similar experience with a coworker with whom one must have a professional relationship or more frequent interactions.

The perpetrators and witnesses of racism have meaning, as do other individuals who may be present during, prior to, or following a race-based stressor. For example, if racist comments are made by a person in power, such as one's boss, or by someone who is valued, such as a close friend, teacher, or therapist, the event may take on a different meaning than a seemingly random racist event. Racism can also be individually, institutionally, or culturally perpetrated (Essed, 1991). Furthermore, if family or friends are present during the experience and stand by while it is happening or minimize its meaning, the target's coping mechanisms may be altered. It is important, then, to observe, consider, and measure the contextual factors that influence one's perception and psychological meaning-making of racism.

Symptoms

When understanding the responses and symptoms related to race-based traumatic stress, it is crucial for researchers and practitioners to consider cultural beliefs and practices (Wilson, 2007). Illnesses may be understood in very different ways across cultures, and symptom expression may vary greatly. Furthermore, while research suggests that race-based trauma is similar to PTSD and other traumatic events (Carter, 2007), further study may reveal unique symptom clusters or patterns in various Black immigrant populations may be revealed upon further study. While more research is desperately needed to understand responses to racism, considering the role of racism in one's health responses is clearly a necessary yet all-too-often neglected consideration in research and practice.

It is also important to consider that symptoms may not be directly attributed to the racist traumatic event, particularly because microaggressions are often questioned by the target and others (Sue et al., 2007). In clinical settings, therapists may ask about sexual and physical abuse histories but not inquire about experiences with racism or other oppressive events. Furthermore, while there is a significant body of research regarding racism as a stressor, many in the field as well as much of society may not acknowledge the relevance of racism to one's psychological experiences (McFarlane, 2000). The fact that the source of the symptoms may be blurred or denied may, in fact, be interpreted as pathologizing and diminishing of the person's experience, thus causing an elevation in the symptoms. Gray and Lombardo (2004) demonstrated that individuals exhibiting PTSD symptoms were more likely to have a global and stable attributional style, such that they view racist events as uncontrollable, pervasive, and likely to happen again. This attributional style may be part of the person's characteristics, but racism may also be pervasive and continuously endangering the client. Therefore, the hyperarousal and avoidance typical of PTSD may serve as a necessary coping mechanism.

Coping

Existing research has demonstrated that exposure to and experiences with racism are significant stressors in the lives of individuals, and such stressors (similar to other stressors) can impact the individuals significantly (Brondolo et al., 2011; Kaholokula et al., 2017). Thus, an individual may develop many strategies in an attempt to cope effectively with this type of stressor in their life. The many variations of coping can seemingly be categorized into the major themes of emotional, cognitive, behavioral, and racial identity and racial socialization coping mechanisms. An example of emotional coping is the use of humor or anger. Cognitively, an individual may ruminate on the event in an effort to find a way they might have prevented it, or they may attribute the event to an external source that is unrelated to them. Behaviorally, racism may result in hypervigilance and hypersensitivity, particularly in new or unknown situations (Comas-Díaz & Jacobsen, 2001). Individuals may also behave in conforming ways. That is, they may adhere to cultural norms of the dominant culture in an attempt to avoid racist events.

In response to the threat racial stressors pose to the mental health of Black communities, researchers have investigated culturally relevant coping tools that can be protective against deleterious outcomes. Among these are racial identity and racial socialization. *Racial identity* refers to how an individual views race in relation to their self-concept. Racial identity has been associated with positive outcomes for Black communities, including high self-esteem, low psychological distress, and positive academic outcomes. *Racial socialization* is the method by which individuals learn how to navigate, respond to, and cope with racial stressors. Like racial identity, racial socialization can be a buffer against negative psychosocial outcomes from discrimination (Hughes et al., 2006).

While these protective factors are frequently discussed in the literature on how Black communities cope with, navigate, and challenge racialized violence, few studies distinguish between ethnic subgroups. While likely similar in many ways, racial identity and racial socialization processes are also likely to be unique across culturally and geographically diverse Black immigrant groups. Socialization practices among families who have been immersed in, coped with, and pushed back on racial oppression in the United States for generations will differ from those who recently immigrated to the United States from minority-majority countries.

It is important to recognize the meaning and purpose of coping in this context. Coping allows an individual to manage and survive critical stressors, and it is crucial to a person's survival and emotional health. People of color utilize many forms of culturally relevant coping to deal with the intense stressors of racism. Removing or diminishing coping does not serve to remove symptoms but rather removes the individual's means of dealing with those symptoms and the cause of the symptoms (e.g., racism).

This model highlights how a person will uniquely experience and respond to racism based on not only their individual factors and personal history but also the specific racist incident itself, the context in which the incident occurred, and the coping tools available to the individual. Each of these dimensions will likely impact the remaining dimensions, as racism and discrimination are insidiously transmutable and are therefore experienced based on the variables delineated in the model. More research must focus on the ways in which Black immigrants from various backgrounds uniquely experience and cope with racism in the United States. Furthermore, current and future individuals involved in the field of psychology must learn and remember that racism as a stressor is the problem and that eliminating racism is the ultimate goal. Entrenching ourselves only in reacting to the stressor risks losing sight of the optimal goal of reducing the stressor for the individual. In essence, we must balance coping with present race-based stressors and accept the social responsibility to reduce and eliminate racism.

DISCUSSION AND CONCLUSION

Throughout this chapter, we have highlighted some key summaries of the literature. First, interpersonally and systemically, racism in the United States is a longstanding and continuous problem experienced by Black people who are born in the United States and by those who immigrate to the country. Second, racism and discrimination can and do create significant damages to one's psyche and personality. Finally, an individual's reactions to racial stress and violence may be manifested physiologically, cognitively, behaviorally, and through emotional expression and can be manifested as anxiety, anger, rage, depression, compromised self-esteem, shame, and guilt. Alternatively, the reactions can be adaptive and positive, as reflected in coping strategies that aid in moderating the effects of the race-based traumatic stress among Black immigrants (Ani, 1996).

Knowing what we know about racism as a stressor, the field desperately needs a practical, applied model that moves understanding of race-based traumatic stress for Black immigrants forward while attending to the unique needs of the individual. Here, we present a framework for understanding personal experiences with racism for Black immigrants in the United States This model is crucial for the reinvention of

- *Research.* A model is needed that moves researchers beyond race as a category or construct, instead providing a deeper understanding of how a racialized person and their traumatic experiences with racism are linked to mental health outcomes or other factors (e.g., education).

- *Practice.* A model is needed that informs the development of effective assessments and interventions that explicitly integrate race-based traumatic experiences. Furthermore, this model should also inform clinical training and the creation of tools to incorporate experiences of race-based traumatic experiences into therapy more effectively.

If in fact we are interested in understanding the link between Black immigrants' experiences and factors such as health outcomes, it is imperative that we have a better understanding of their experiences with racism and the various ways that these experiences are impacting their lives. The model presented in this chapter provides a framework for starting such a discourse and encourages all researchers and clinicians to pay closer attention to the experience of Black immigrants in the United States. Through such inquiries, we can expand on this model further, integrate racism experiences in research studies, and develop effective methods to reduce the overall effects of racism on the well-being of individuals.

REFERENCES

Acevedo-Garcia, D., Bates, L. M., Osypuk, T. L., & McArdle, N. (2010). The effect of immigrant generation and duration on self-rated health among U.S. adults 2003–2007. *Social Science & Medicine, 71*(6), 1161e1172.

Adjepong, A. (2018). Afropolitan projects: African immigrant identities and solidarities in the United States. *Ethnic and Racial Studies, 41*(2), 248–266. https://doi.org/10.1080/01419870.2017.1281985

Agyekum, B., & Newbold, B. K. (2016). Religion/spirituality, therapeutic landscape and immigrant mental well-being amongst African immigrants to Canada. *Mental Health, Religion & Culture, 19*(7), 674–685. https://doi.org/10.1080/13674676.2016.1225292

American Psychological Association. (2012). *Crossroads: The psychology of immigration in the new century.* Report of the APA Presidential Task Force on Immigration. https://www.apa.org/topics/immigration/executive-summary.pdf

Anderson, M. (2015). *A rising share of the U.S. Black population is foreign born; 9 percent are immigrants; and while most are from the Caribbean, Africans drive recent growth.* Pew Research Center. https://www.pewsocialtrends.org/2015/04/09/a-rising-share-of-the-u-s-black-population-is-foreign-born/

Anderson, M., & López, G. (2018, January 24). *Key facts about Black immigrants in the U.S.* Pew Research Center. https://www.pewresearch.org/fact-tank/2018/01/24/key-facts-about-black-immigrants-in-the-u-s/

Anderson, R. E., & Stevenson, H. C. (2019). RECASTing racial stress and trauma: Theorizing the healing potential of racial socialization in families. *American Psychologist, 74*(1), 63.

Ani, M. (1996). The Afrikan asili. In J. Ladner & S. Gbadegisin (Eds.), *Ethics, higher education, and social responsibilities* (pp. 1–14). Howard University Press.

Araújo Dawson, B. (2009). Discrimination, stress, and acculturation among Dominican immigrant women. *Hispanic Journal of Behavioral Sciences, 31*(1), 96–111. https://doi.org/10.1177/0739986308327502

Brondolo, E., Gallo, L. C., & Myers, H. F. (2009). Race, racism and health: Disparities, mechanisms, and interventions. *Journal of Behavioral Medicine, 32*(1), 1–8. https://doi.org/10.1007/s10865-008-9190-3

Brondolo, E., ver Halen, N. B., Libby, D., & Pencille, M. (2011). Racism as a psychosocial stressor. In R. J. Contrada & A. Baum (Eds.), *The handbook of stress science: Biology, psychology, and health* (pp. 167–184). Springer.

Bryant-Davis, T., & Ocampo, C. (2005). The trauma of racism: Implications for counseling, research, and education. *The Counseling Psychologist, 33*(4), 574–578. https://doi.org/10.1177/0011000005276581

Butler-Barnes, S. T., Martin, P. P., Copeland-Linder, N., Seaton, E. K., Matusko, N., Caldwell, C. H., & Jackson, J. S. (2018). The protective role of religious involvement in African American and Caribbean Black adolescents' experiences of racial discrimination. *Youth & Society, 50*(5), 659–687. https://doi.org/10.1177/0044118X15626063

Carter, R. T. (2007). Racism and psychological and emotional injury: Recognizing and assessing race-based traumatic stress. *The Counseling Psychologist, 35*(1), 13–105. https://doi.org/10.1177/0011000006292033

Carter, R. T., & Helms, J. E. (2002, September). *Racial discrimination, and harassment: A race based traumatic stress disorder* [Conference paper]. American College of Forensic Examiners Conference, Orlando, FL, United States.

Chatters, L. M., Taylor, R. J., Jackson, J. S., & Lincoln, K. D. (2008). Religious coping among African Americans, Caribbean Blacks and non-Hispanic Whites. *Journal of Community Psychology, 36*(3), 371–386. https://doi.org/10.1002/jcop.20202

Clark, R., Anderson, N. B., Clark, V. R., & Williams, D. R. (1999). Racism as a stressor for African Americans: A biopsychosocial model. *American Psychologist, 54*(10), 805–816. https://doi.org/10.1037/0003-066X.54.10.805

Cobb, C., Branscombe, N., Meca, A., Schwartz, S., Xie, D., Zea, M., Molina, L. E., & Martinez, C. R., Jr. (2019). Toward a positive psychology of immigrants. *Perspectives on Psychological Science, 14*(4), 619–632. https://doi.org/10.1177/1745691619825848

Comas-Díaz, L., & Jacobsen, F. M. (2001). Ethnocultural allodynia. *The Journal of Psychotherapy Practice and Research, 10*(4), 246–252.

Dominguez, T. P., Strong, E. F., Krieger, N., Gillman, M. W., & Rich-Edwards, J. W. (2009). Differences in the self-reported racism experiences of US-born and foreign-born Black pregnant women. *Social Science & Medicine, 69*(2), 258–265. https://doi.org/10.1016/j.socscimed.2009.03.022

Eamer, A., Fernando, S., & King, A. E. (2017). Still on the margins: Migration, English language learning, and mental health in immigrant psychiatric patients. *Diaspora, Indigenous, and Minority Education, 11*(4), 190–202. https://doi.org/10.1080/15595692.2017.1289918

Essed, P. (1991). *Understanding everyday racism: An interdisciplinary theory* (Vol. 2). Sage.

Franklin-Jackson, D., & Carter, R. T. (2007). The relationships between race-related stress, racial identity, and mental health for Black Americans. *The Journal of Black Psychology, 33*(1), 5–26. https://doi.org/10.1177/0095798406295092

Gee, G. C., & Ford, C. L. (2011). Structural racism and health inequities: Old issues, new directions. *Du Bois Review, 8*(1), 115–132. https://doi.org/10.1017/S1742058X11000130

Gray, M. J., & Lombardo, T. W. (2004). Life event attributions as a potential source of vulnerability following exposure to a traumatic event. *Journal of Loss and Trauma, 9*(1), 59–72. https://doi.org/10.1080/15325020490255313

Hamilton, T. G., & Green, T. L. (2018). From the West Indies to Africa: A universal generational decline in health among Blacks in the United States. *Social Science Research, 73*, 163–174.

Hamilton, T. G., & Hummer, R. A. (2011). Immigration and the health of U.S. Black adults: Does country of origin matter? *Social Science & Medicine, 73*(10), 1551–1560.

Harrell, S. P. (2000). A multidimensional conceptualization of racism-related stress: Implications for the well-being of people of color. *American Journal of Orthopsychiatry, 70*(1), 42–57. https://doi.org/10.1037/h0087722

Helms, J. E. (2007). Some better practices for measuring racial and ethnic identity constructs. *Journal of Counseling Psychology, 54*(3), 235–246. https://doi.org/10.1037/0022-0167.54.3.235

Helms, J. E., Nicolas, G., & Green, C. E. (2012). Racism and ethnoviolence as trauma: Enhancing professional and research training. *Traumatology, 18*(1), 65–74. https://doi.org/10.1177/1534765610396728

Herman, J. L. (1992). Complex PTSD: A syndrome in survivors of prolonged and repeated trauma. *Journal of Traumatic Stress, 5*(3), 377–391. https://doi.org/10.1002/jts.2490050305

Hughes, D., Rodriguez, J., Smith, E. P., Johnson, D. J., Stevenson, H. C., & Spicer, P. (2006). Parents' ethnic-racial socialization practices: A review of research and directions for future study. *Developmental Psychology, 42*(5), 747–770.

Kaholokula, J. K., Antonio, M. C. K., Ing, C. K. T., Hermosura, A., Hall, K. E., Knight, R., & Wills, T. A. (2017). The effects of perceived racism on psychological distress mediated by venting and disengagement coping in Native Hawaiians. *BMC Psychology, 5*(2). https://doi.org/10.1186/s40359-017-0171-6

Keys, C. B., McConnell, E., Motley, D., Liao, C. L., & McAuliff, K. (2017). The what, the how, and the who of empowerment: Reflections on an intellectual history. In M. A. Bond, I. Serrano-García, C. B. Keys, & M. Shinn (Eds.), *APA Handbook of community psychology: Theoretical foundations, core concepts, and emerging challenges* (pp. 213–231). American Psychological Association. https://doi.org/10.1037/14953-010

Kirmayer, L. J., Narasiah, L., Munoz, M., Rashid, M., Ryder, A. G., Guzder, J., Hassan, G., Rousseau, C., & Pottie, K. (2011). Common mental health problems in immigrants and refugees: General approach in primary care. *Canadian Medical Association Journal, 183*(12), E959–E967.

Luis, W. (2012). Afro-Latino/a literature and identity. In S. Bost & F. R. Aparicio (Eds.), *The Routledge companion to Latino/a Literature* (pp. 50–61). Routledge.

McCubbin, M., & Cohen, D. (2003). *Empowering practice in mental health social work: Barriers and challenges*. Research Group on Social Aspects of Health and Prevention (GRASP). http://citeseerx.ist.psu.edu/viewdoc/download?doi=10.1.1.199.7629&rep=rep1&type=pdf

McFarlane, A. C. (2000). On the social denial of trauma and the problem of knowing the past. In A. Y. Shalev, R. Yehuda, & A. C. McFarlane (Eds.), *International handbook of human response to trauma* (pp. 11–26). Kluwer. https://doi.org/10.1007/978-1-4615-4177-6_2

McNeilly, M. D., Anderson, N. B., Armstead, C. A., Clark, R., Corbett, M., Robinson, E. L., Pieper, C. F., & Lepisto, E. M. (1996). The Perceived Racism Scale: A multidimensional assessment of the experience of White racism among African Americans. *Ethnicity & Disease, 6*(1–2), 154–166.

Nicolas, G., DeSilva, A. M., Grey, K. S., & Gonzalez-Eastep, D. (2006). Using a multicultural lens to understand illnesses among Haitians living in America. *Professional Psychology, Research and Practice, 37*(6), 702–707. https://doi.org/10.1037/0735-7028.37.6.702

Nicolas, G., & Thompson, C. (2019). Racialized violence in the lives of Black people: Illustrations from Haiti (Ayiti) and the United States. *American Psychologist, 74*(5), 587–595. https://doi.org/10.1037/amp0000453

Ocloo, J., & Matthews, R. (2016). From tokenism to empowerment: Progressing patient and public involvement in healthcare improvement. *BMJ Quality & Safety, 25*(8), 626–632. https://doi.org/10.1136/bmjqs-2015-004839

Parham, T. A. (1989). Cycles of psychological nigrescence. *The Counseling Psychologist, 17*(2), 187–226. https://doi.org/10.1177/0011000089172001

Pieterse, A. L., Todd, N. R., Neville, H. A., & Carter, R. T. (2012). Perceived racism and mental health among Black American adults: A meta-analytic review. *Journal of Counseling Psychology, 59*(1), 1–9. https://doi.org/10.1037/a0026208

Read, J. N. G., & Emerson, M. O. (2005). Racial context, Black immigration and the U.S. Black/White health disparity. *Social Forces, 84*(1), 181–199. https://doi.org/10.1353/sof.2005.0120

Riger, S. (1993). What's wrong with empowerment. *American Journal of Community Psychology, 21*(3), 279–292. https://doi.org/10.1007/BF00941504

Showers, F. (2015). Being Black, foreign and woman: African immigrant identities in the United States. *Ethnic and Racial Studies, 38*(10), 1815–1830. https://doi.org/10.1080/01419870.2015.1036763

Stevenson, H. C. (2014). *Promoting racial literacy in schools: Differences that make a difference*. Teachers College Press.

Sue, D. W., Capadilupo, C. M., Torino, G. C., Bucceri, J. M., Holder, A. M. B., Nadal, K. L., & Esquilin, M. (2007). Racial microaggressions in everyday life: Implications for clinical practice. *American Psychologist, 62*(4), 271–286. https://doi.org/10.1037/0003-066X.62.4.271

Taylor, R. J., Chae, D. H., Lincoln, K. D., & Chatters, L. M. (2015). Extended family and friendship support networks are both protective and risk factors for major depressive disorder and depressive symptoms among African-Americans and Black Caribbeans. *Journal of Nervous and Mental Disease, 203*(2), 132–140. https://doi.org/10.1097/NMD.0000000000000249

Thomas, A. J., Witherspoon, K. M., & Speight, S. L. (2008). Gendered racism, psychological distress, and coping styles of African American women. *Cultural Diversity and Ethnic Minority Psychology, 14*(4), 307–314.

Tynes, B., Willis, H., Stewart, A., & Hamilton, M. (2019). Race-related traumatic events online and mental health among adolescents of color. *The Journal of Adolescent Health, 65*(3), 371–377. https://doi.org/10.1016/j.jadohealth.2019.03.006

Tynes, B. M., Umaña-Taylor, A. J., Rose, C. A., Lin, J., & Anderson, C. J. (2012). Online racial discrimination and the protective function of ethnic identity and self-esteem for African American adolescents. *Developmental Psychology, 48*(2), 343–355. https://doi.org/10.1037/a0027032

Venters, H., & Gany, F. (2011). African immigrant health. *Journal of Immigrant and Minority Health, 13*(2), 333–344. https://doi.org/10.1007/s10903-009-9243-x

Vesely, C. K., Letiecq, B. L., & Goodman, R. D. (2017). Immigrant family resilience in context: Using a community-based approach to build a new conceptual model. *Journal of Family Theory & Review, 9*(1), 93–110. https://doi.org/10.1111/jftr.12177

Vickerman, M. (2007). Recent immigration and race. *Du Bois Review, 4*(1), 141–165. https://doi.org/10.1017/S1742058X07070087

Viruell-Fuentes, E. A., Miranda, P. Y., & Abdulrahim, S. (2012). More than culture: Structural racism, intersectionality theory, and immigrant health. *Social Science & Medicine, 75*(12), 2099–2106. https://doi.org/10.1016/j.socscimed.2011.12.037

Wafula, E. G., & Snipes, S. A. (2014). Barriers to health care access faced by Black immigrants in the U.S.: Theoretical considerations and recommendations. *Journal of Immigrant and Minority Health, 16*(4), 689–698. https://doi.org/10.1007/s10903-013-9898-1

Wilson, J. P. (2007). The lens of culture: Theoretical and conceptual perspectives in the assessment of psychological trauma and PTSD. In J. P. Wilson & C. S. Tang (Eds.), *Cross-cultural assessment of psychological trauma and PTSD* (pp. 3–30). Springer Science. https://doi.org/10.1007/978-0-387-70990-1_1

Zimmerman, M. A. (1995). Psychological empowerment: Issues and illustrations. *American Journal of Community Psychology, 23*(5), 581–599. https://doi.org/10.1007/BF02506983

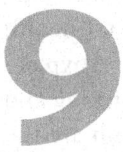

An Examination of Racial Minority Immigrants and the Trauma of Human Trafficking

Indhushree Rajan and Thema Bryant-Davis

Bryant-Davis and Tummala-Narra (2017) noted that intersecting forms of oppression, including racism, sexism, xenophobia, and classism, increase the risk for human trafficking and create barriers to service access in the aftermath of escape. The lived experience of human trafficking is often contextualized by intersectionality, and specifically being a member of multiple marginalized groups, for example, women of color (Oleksy, 2011). Intersectional feminist approaches to theory, practice, and activism aimed at combatting human trafficking also require fighting ethnic hatred, racism, sexism, additional forms of violence against women, educational segregation, poverty, and extreme social exclusion (Schultz, 2012). Crawford (2017) called for an intersectional feminist approach to addressing sex trafficking, which disproportionately affects women; to effectively counter sex trafficking, researchers and practitioners must explore the ways gender intersects with other systems of social dominance, such as caste, tribe, and ethnicity. Intersectional feminist practice, also known as multicultural feminist therapy, centers the experience of the marginalized; resists oppression; celebrates cultural and individual strengths; and pursues the well-being, growth, healing, and thriving of culturally marginalized women (Bryant-Davis & Comas-Díaz, 2016).

This chapter provides an overview of human trafficking by exploring the psychosocial realities of traffickers and victims. To contextualize trafficking from the perspective of intersectional feminism, we discuss the connection between racism and sexism as they impact human trafficking. With an

https://doi.org/10.1037/0000214-010
Trauma and Racial Minority Immigrants: Turmoil, Uncertainty, and Resistance,
P. Tummala-Narra (Editor)

understanding of the macro role of oppression in the lives of trafficking victims, we then provide some key aspects of the legal and mental health care barriers and challenges that trafficking survivors face. We next explain the psychological treatment needs of survivors of both human trafficking and the societal trauma of oppression, along with a case study to illuminate the experience and treatment needs of survivors. Finally, we turn our lens to the experience of Asian immigrant survivors, highlighting the need for helping professionals to attend to the cross-cultural realities of human trafficking as well as culturally specific dynamics. We draw on theoretical, research, and practice conclusions based on the state of the field and our experiences working with trafficking survivors.

OVERVIEW: HUMAN TRAFFICKING, TRAFFICKERS, AND VICTIMS

The United Nations Office on Drugs and Crime (UNODC; 2004) defined *human trafficking* as

> the recruitment, transportation, transfer, harboring or receipt of persons, by means of the threat or use of force or other forms of coercion, of abduction, of fraud, of deception, of the abuse of power or of a position of vulnerability or of the giving or receiving of payments or benefits to achieve the consent of a person having control over another person, for the purpose of exploitation. (p. 42)

Specifically, they explained, "exploitation shall include, at a minimum, the exploitation of the prostitution of others or other forms of sexual exploitation, forced labour or services, slavery or practices similar to slavery, servitude or the removal of organs" (UNODC, 2004, p. 42). Every year, millions of women, children, and men are trafficked and enslaved in the labor and sex trades around the world. "It is estimated that human trafficking generates many billions of dollars of profit per year, second only to drug trafficking as the most profitable form of transnational crime" (U.S. Department of Justice, 2020, para. 3).

The Victims

Victims of human trafficking span all gender identities, ages, races, nationalities, levels of education, and socioeconomic backgrounds. Men, women, and children are lured into sexual and labor-based slavery by desires that drive most human beings: well-paying jobs, the promise of love and marriage, better opportunities for their children, education—essentially the hope of a better life. Vulnerability and risk of trafficking increase based on factors that diminish the likelihood that people will be able to meet these needs for themselves and their families. Factors that tend to increase the risk of being trafficked include poverty, lack of education, the prevalence and normalization of gender-based violence, discrimination based on race, homelessness, histories of sexual assault and domestic violence, and weakened family and community systems.

The exploitation of cultural rites, practices, and traditions is also a common way in which women and children are trafficked. For example, in India, women and girls who are sold into forced sex work and enslavement have long been sourced by Devadasi culture. *Devadasi* or *Devaradiyar* means "servant of God" and refers to a tradition dating back to the 7th century in South India, in which some women are dedicated in marriage to God and forbidden to marry men (Rajam, 2017). These women were free to choose partners, whether single or married, as long as they were not financially dependent on the men that they chose (Rajam, 2017). As companions or courtesans to wealthy men of high status, they could form and continue relationships over short or long periods of time, and these relationships often highlighted forms of entertainment such as singing and classical dance. Devadasi women were also enlisted to perform sacred religious rituals (Hartmann, 2019). Over time, Devadasi traditions became a hotbed for sexual exploitation, and in modern India, these traditions account for a large number of girls involved in forced commercial prostitution. A Reuters report (Nagaraj, 2017) noted that of an estimated 20 million commercial prostitutes living in India, 16 million were female victims of sex trafficking, and many were recruited through Devadasi practices. Since 1988, Devadasi practices have been illegal across India, yet owing to the long association of the Devadasi with higher social status, wealth, and blessings from God, the culture continues to successfully draw thousands of young girls—some as young as 5 or 6 years—into India's sex trade every year (Shingal, 2015).

Superstitious beliefs about the Devadasi also fuel high recruitment of girls into trafficking and prostitution. Such beliefs include the ideas that intercourse with a child is the ultimate curative for disease and that a relationship with a Devadasi girl will bring many blessings to the family of her partner (Levesque, 1999). Parents are also duped into believing that their children are being recruited to live a spiritual life of consecration to God and are learning to sing and dance, as was true in early Devadasi tradition, rather than working as a prostitute (Levesque, 1999). "Making exploitation and abuse a ritual rite of culture or religion is tantamount to *obliging* victims to suffer in the name of spiritual or cultural mandate" (Rajan, 2013, p. 23). Within this context, Grover (2007) noted that "the commitment to the eradication of child prostitution and child sex trafficking [must be made] without deference to traditional cultural practices" (p. 294).

It is also important to emphasize that even though victims of trafficking share many characteristics that mark them as being more vulnerable to trafficking-related exploitation than other groups are, even individuals of high socioeconomic status can be exploited and trafficked. Polaris (2019) noted that although the impoverished and uneducated are at highest risk of being socio-culturally displaced and trafficked, "victims have diverse ethnic and socio-economic backgrounds, varied levels of education, and may be documented or undocumented."

Traffickers

Human traffickers prey on the vulnerable and ensnare them into forced sex and labor trafficking. Traffickers engage in the recruitment, transport, sale, or harboring of victims, and they often use abusive, psychologically manipulative, and threatening means to exploit their targets. The promise of high-paying jobs, romance and seemingly loving relationships, or educational, travel, and marriage opportunities appeal to impoverished, overburdened families, women, men, and children, who in most cases have no prospects for success, much less survival. In other instances, victims are kidnapped, and subdued with drugs and/or physical and sexual violence. Polaris (2019) noted: "Traffickers employ a variety of control tactics, including physical and emotional abuse, sexual assault, confiscation of identification and money, isolation from friends and family, and even renaming [of] victims."

Even more insidious than the horrific physical violence victims are made to endure are the ways in which traffickers psychologically manipulate, control, and break victims. Often, traffickers identify and leverage their victims' vulnerabilities to create dependency. They make promises aimed at addressing the needs of their targets to impose control. As a result, victims become trapped and fear leaving for myriad reasons, including psychological trauma, shame, emotional attachment, and physical threats to themselves or their children's safety (Polaris, 2019). Traffickers even emphasize things they have in common with their victims as a way to bond with them while grooming them, creating confusion and the illusion of a relationship. This in turn can cause victims to feel guilty if they are tempted to be disobedient or disloyal. The National Human Trafficking Hotline (n.d.) noted:

> Often, traffickers and their victims share the same national, ethnic, or cultural background, allowing the trafficker to better understand and exploit the vulnerabilities of their victims. Traffickers can be foreign nationals and U.S. citizens, males and females, family members, intimate partners, acquaintances, and strangers.

IMPACT OF RACISM AND SEXISM ON THE PREVALENCE OF HUMAN TRAFFICKING

Inequity across the landscapes of race, gender, and socioeconomic status create deep divides in societies that feed the growing pandemic of human trafficking worldwide. Racial and gender-based discrimination force the world's most vulnerable populations to suffer disproportionate abuses. Within this context, "race intersects with other forms of subordination including gender, class, and age to push people of color disproportionately into prostitution and keep them trapped in the commercial sex industry," and "intersectional oppression is fueled by the persistence of myths about minority teen sexuality, which in turn encourages risky sexual behavior" (Nelson Butler, 2015, p. 1464).

Victims of trafficking are largely racial and ethnic minorities. In the United States, the Bureau of Justice Statistics (2011) determined that between 2008 and 2010, non-White children accounted for 358 of the 460 cases (i.e., 77.8%) of child sex trafficking investigated by the U.S. Department of Justice, the majority of whom were Black and Latinx. In Thailand, the ethnic minorities are the hill tribes and stateless children who have been denied basic rights and protections, leaving them most vulnerable to trafficking (Keller, 2018). In India, Dalit communities are disproportionately trafficked. Racism lends itself to poverty and exclusion and, in turn, creates pathways into commercial sexual exploitation (Keller, 2018). In addition, religious minorities, migrants, and refugees are vulnerable to enslavement. At particular risk are those fleeing war and armed conflict, such as the Yazidi minority in Iraq and Syria and Myanmar's Muslim Rohingya population (Council on Foreign Relations, n.d.). Furthermore, child prostitutes who are members of racial or ethnic minorities are more likely to be targets of harassment and arrest and are more likely to encounter harsher punishments when arrested (Nelson Butler, 2015).

Perhaps most compelling when considering the impact of racism on the perpetuation of global human trafficking is the notion that racism affects women differently than men; these experiences of gendered racism evoke culturally congruent approaches to coping resistance (Spates et al., 2019). Drawing from Nagel's (2003) notions of sexual citizenship and ethnosexuality, Gutiérrez Chong (2014) wrote, "Racism affects women differently than men. The coinage of 'ethnosexuality' is indeed useful, as sex and sexuality are not detached from the social and cultural implications of race, racism and nationalism" (p. 196). The underlying notion is that women, nationalism, and specifically state building and nation formation embody a brand of racism and ethnicity inherently defined by sexuality, at both the symbolic and objective levels:

> . . . the following themes are interrelated: racist and sexist stereotypes of women are used in the sex industry; traditional patriarchal culture plays a role in reproducing female passivity and submission; racialised and ethnicised groups are prone to experience violence in all its forms, sexual exploitation being one of them. (Gutiérrez Chong, 2014, p. 196)

Indeed, rapid economic industrialization in formerly undeveloped countries and regions, coupled with sociocultural paradigms that oppress women, is a primary facilitator of the sex trade (Bertone, 2000).

HUMAN TRAFFICKING AND BARRIERS RELATED TO INTERNATIONAL LAW AND LAW ENFORCEMENT

Slavery thrives in the absence of a properly functioning system of law enforcement. In developing nations, impoverished conditions contribute to power vacuums and corruption, often abetted by police and other law enforcement authorities. In these kinds of conditions, traffickers are able to operate with little consequence. To complicate matters of law, convoluted power paradigms perpetuate political and legal corruption amidst war-torn countries and communities, perpetuating human trafficking, violence against women and girls, and slavery. Groups that face discrimination, including ethnic and religious minorities, women and children, and migrants and refugees, are vulnerable to enslavement.

At local and global levels, corruption and lack of awareness of the trafficking pandemic and the various practices that perpetuate its growth and power are important issues to address in helping trafficking survivors have better protections. Owing to these issues, people have little to no government or police protection from traffickers (Free the Slaves, n.d.). Whenever the rule of law is weaker in a given society, or those who are meant to protect citizens from exploitation and crime are unaware of the extent and manner of practice of those crimes, people who are vulnerable to being trafficked and enslaved are put in greater danger.

Slavery is also more likely to occur where "corruption is rife. It can also happen to groups of people who are not protected by the law. For example, migrants whose visa status is irregular are easy to blackmail with deportation" (Anti-Slavery International, 2020). Trafficking survivors in the United States face barriers within the legal system, including biases and stigma that judges and lawyers attribute to trafficking survivors as well as members of marginalized communities who are more frequently trafficked; retraumatization of being required to share their story multiple times and often to persons who have not been trained to create a supportive, safe environment; sexual exploitation by agents of the law, such as corrupt police officers; perception and treatment by court officials as consenting criminals instead of victims of violence and abuse; culturally contextualized barriers such as being undocumented, being uninformed of their rights and resources, bias in convictions, and sentencing that disregards the rights and integrity of marginalized community members and trafficking survivors; and distrust of the courts based on primary experiences of injustice as well as intergenerational trauma (Bryant-Davis et al., 2017).

HUMAN TRAFFICKING AND BARRIERS TO MENTAL HEALTH SERVICES

Perhaps one of the biggest barriers to human trafficking survivors receiving mental health care is poverty. The populations most vulnerable to human trafficking in both developed and developing nations are those who live in impoverished communities and are unable to avail themselves of the kinds of jobs and life opportunities that traffickers use as lures; once victimized, they are unable to qualify for or afford health care. Despite decades of substantial progress in boosting prosperity and reducing poverty, the world continues to suffer from substantial inequalities. Among the estimated 780 million illiterate adults worldwide, nearly two thirds are women. Poor people face higher risks of malnutrition and death in childhood and lower odds of receiving key health care interventions (World Bank Group, 2016). Issues of affordability and access to services, as well as responsiveness of those services to the complex needs of survivors, are common issues identified by service providers (Clawson & Dutch, 2008). Providers uniformly point to access to mental health services as a significant challenge for both international and domestic victims.

Beyond the barriers to connecting survivors with appropriate mental health care, the extent of other life needs that survivors often have upon rescue creates multiple barriers to survivors' ability to receive or proactively engage in mental health care. For example, how can a trafficking survivor benefit from therapy, even if it is made available to them, when they have no home, job, or legal recourse if they have been arrested? Clawson and Dutch (2008) pointed out that survivors have a different scope of needs: "While the needs [of survivors] are relatively similar regardless of whether someone is an international or domestic victim, adult or minor, one point is clear—the magnitude of these needs varies for each victim depending on his or her circumstances" (p. 3). In addition, a lack of qualified mental health care providers in poorer countries, as well as pervasive stigma around both human trafficking and mental health issues, often prevent trafficking victims from identifying themselves as such or seeking out mental health services (Aberdein & Zimmerman, 2015).

CLINICAL ISSUES AND RECOMMENDATIONS

In considering the clinical profiles of sex trafficking survivors, it is critical to consider several aspects of trauma and how they are addressed in therapy, including containment/stabilization, cultural impact on treatment, relationship, expression and integration of self or identity, and how this sense of self can be expressed in context to life after human trafficking.

In clinical work with survivors, certain recurring themes and needs tend to surface and prove critical to building trust and a sense of containment and safety. Research has established mental health consequences of sex trafficking, particularly posttraumatic stress disorder (PTSD), depression, and anxiety (Abas et al., 2013; Ottisova et al., 2018; Zimmerman et al., 2011). A critical review of the literature on health consequences of domestic minor trafficking in the United States (Le et al., 2018) identified 27 studies and concluded that sex trafficking survivors experience elevated rates of substance use, suicidal behaviors, PTSD, and depression. Ultimately, these consequences tend to work against safety, trust, and motivation for change within and outside of therapy.

Another issue that is difficult to confront until sufficient trust has been achieved in the therapeutic space is abuse that is repressed because of survivors' internalized pressure to remain silent under the threat of further punishment. The fear of retribution from traffickers is so pervasive that even a partial recounting of abuses that a survivor has endured can trigger a dissociative episode or the presence of a different alter. Forced submission to secrecy in this regard creates barriers to disclosure in traditional talk therapy. Within this context, it becomes important to consider culturally congruent, trauma-informed treatments and interventions that can be effective in helping to increase survivors' chances of remaining in long-term treatment; face and move through dark, painful material; and minimize chances of retraumatization and self-harm. Trauma-informed treatment for trafficking survivors is research informed, assessment driven, strengths based, hopeful, and empowerment/advocacy centered (Elliott et al., 2005; Hopper, 2018; Scott et al., 2019).

A third critical issue is to help survivors overcome their pervasive fear and mistrust of their communities so that they may begin to rebuild their lives and develop a sense of empowered autonomy beyond the therapeutic relationship. Within this context, clinicians and researchers working with survivors need to utilize wraparound treatment services that incorporate agencies, shelters, law enforcement, and others in the community that can cocreate a larger container for survivors' ongoing safety and physical and mental health.

Within this context, certain trauma-focused treatment approaches have been recommended in clinical work with human trafficking survivors. These interventions include but are not limited to cognitive behavioral therapy, mindfulness based therapy, prolonged exposure therapy, expressive arts therapy, eye movement desensitization and reprocessing, cognitive processing therapy, psychodynamic therapy, and narrative psychotherapy (Contreras et al., 2017; Countryman-Roswurm & DiLollo, 2017; Edmond, 2018; Márquez et al., 2020; Robjant et al., 2017; Schrader & Wendland, 2012). These interventions include, to varying degrees, psychoeducation; relaxation training; disclosing the narrative; processing the narrative to disrupt distorted, unhelpful thoughts; teaching and reviewing coping strategies; and psychological, vocational, and educational efforts aimed at preventing a return to trafficking. For survivors of human trafficking, these interventions can provide self-awareness, capacity to connect and build trust, knowledge of the way trauma has shaped their lives, and empowerment through life skills to regulate affect and shift distorted cognitions (Salami et al., 2018). Behavioral therapy focuses on increasing desired behaviors and decreasing problem behaviors through environmental manipulation. Cognitive therapy works to change behaviors and feelings by altering how patients comprehend and understand significant life experiences. Psychodynamic therapy explains behavior and personality as being motivated by inner forces, including past experiences, inherited instincts, and biological drives, and targets patients' unconscious (American Psychological Association, 2008). Providing cultural modifications of these interventions, as well as integrating culturally emergent practices of liberation therapy, multicultural feminist therapy, and womanist and *mujerista* therapies, can heighten consciousness raising, resistance to internalizing the oppressive messages that contributed to the risk of trafficking, and acknowledgment of cultural resources and traditions to cope and heal (Bryant-Davis & Comas-Díaz, 2016; Bryant-Davis & Gobin, 2019). While a detailed examination of each of these interventions is beyond the scope of this chapter, further research on the implementation, potential integration, and evaluation of these approaches is warranted.

HOW DOES CULTURE INFORM THE CLINICAL LENS?

In clinical work with survivors from multicultural and multiethnic backgrounds, it is imperative to adopt a resilience-based perspective, which honors authentic voice and seeks to help survivors recognize choice, agency, and power from within aspects of culture. This process informs their sense of self and empowers healing of self-concept in the larger work of retranslating identity from object to subject, shifting from one solely acted upon to one who has agency. Within this context, understanding spiritual practices, belief systems, and cultural rites and traditions may help to inform survivors' orientations to power dynamics in relationships pertaining to gender roles, familial structure, and attitudes toward sex, sexuality, and related exploitation.

In her study examining aspects of coercion and exploitation between religious belief systems and human trafficking, Heil (2016) considered the potential connection between religion and victim coercion, deepening exploitation of the victim on an interpersonal level through exploiting faith. In a larger sociocultural context, Heil noted that

> the exploitation of religious beliefs as a tool of coercion has been widely studied in the fields of sociology and psychology. Notably, it has been argued that religion is a tool of political authority and oppression, with the political leaders having a divine relationship with God.

It is, however, important to balance this perspective with the notion that survivors also often gain strength and are able to adopt a resiliency perspective regarding their trauma because of their spiritual orientation and faith. Bryant (2016) noted that "themes of the power of faith and spiritual practice resonated in the stories of resilience" and that "even when religious belief was never introduced to them, several women [spoke] of sensing 'someone out there' to whom they begged for freedom." A survivor shared the role of spirituality while she was enslaved: "while being abused as a young girl, she would look out the window and focus on the moon. 'I knew there was something Greater out there than what was happening to me at that moment.' Her ability to latch on to the transcendent kept her soul alive" (Bryant, 2016).

In addressing the impact of family roles and structure on the exploitation and trafficking of girls, de Chesnay (2013) stated:

> Traffickers are expert manipulators who create a new family structure of rigid rules and norms with the girls they exploit. Street pimps might use the "Romeo" approach in which they seduce the girl into loving them, creating a powerful loyalty. Others simply exert control by threatening to harm the girls' families. This technique is particularly effective with young women who come from cultures that value the family above the individual and would do anything to protect their families, even if the parents sold the girl into early marriage or prostitution. (p. 1)

When practitioners allow the treatment lens to be informed by culture, it becomes easier to foster important relationships with individuals and agencies in the community, who form the larger container informing survivor rescue and care. Providing culturally based care is critical to working in collaborative networks that include law enforcement, prosecutors, medical and social services, and the business community (de Chesnay, 2013).

Individuals' ethnicity is often directly related to their worldviews and thus their experiences. Ethnicity can affect how individuals seek assistance, define their problems, attribute psychological difficulties, experience their unique trauma, and perceive future recovery options. Ethnicity can also directly influence patients' outlooks on their pain, expectations of mental health treatment, and beliefs regarding the best course of treatment.

In many cultural contexts, individuals may not differentiate psychological, emotional, and spiritual reactions from more physical reactions; rather, they focus on the impact of trauma on the body as a whole. Additionally, cultural factors influencing individuals' beliefs about threats and response to danger can play an important role in how individuals respond to violent crimes (Office of Refugee Resettlement, 2008).

Health care providers should remember that every culture has a distinct framework or perspective about mental health and, as a result, distinct beliefs about the benefits of seeking mental health services (Office of the Assistant Secretary for Planning and Evaluation, U.S. Department of Health and Human Services, 2010). Counseling, in general, is a predominantly Western practice; in some cultures folk healing, healing rituals, and secret societies are the commonly accepted forms of health care provision (Williamson et al., 2008). Mental health care providers should familiarize themselves with the beliefs, values, and practices of the various cultural contexts of their patients, so that they are able to provide culturally competent care.

CASE STUDY: PATIENCE—CULTURAL ISSUES INFORMING CLINICAL WORK WITH SURVIVORS

Patience was born in West Africa, and her parents died of AIDS.[1] She was being raised by her aunt for a year when her aunt's visa to come to the United States was approved. Her aunt did not have legal status to bring Patience with her, and other family members had either poor health or limited finances. Patience's aunt thus gave Patience to a friend to raise for a year while the aunt worked to bring Patience to the United Status. A few months later, the friend who was raising Patience told her that she was taking her to the United States to meet her aunt. In reality, the guardian was trafficking Patience to the United States. Upon arriving in the United States, Patience was locked in a room with other girls and women from West Africa. They were not allowed to leave the house unaccompanied, they had no access to phones, and they were sexually trafficked daily in one primary location and sometimes taken to other locations. Patience's aunt found out from

---

[1]All case material has been altered to protect confidentiality.

former neighbors that Patience was in the United States. After nearly 2 years, Patience was able to make a phone call, which helped the aunt and police officers locate and rescue her.

Patience presented to psychotherapy with fear of the traffickers finding her and harming her. She was told and believed that they had spiritual powers and could locate her and curse her. She also experienced somatic complaints, PTSD, depression, and dissociation, as well as difficulty trusting others. Treatment required a full assessment, including trauma history, pretrauma developmental history, cultural and spiritual resources and barriers to care, social support, and symptoms of distress.

Treatment utilized an integration of spiritually integrated psychotherapy and mindfulness-based cognitive therapy. These approaches were applied to both the traumatic loss of her parents and the trauma of human trafficking. Additionally, music therapy interventions and storytelling (i.e., narrative therapy) were used in congruence with her cultural heritage. Music therapy interventions included writing testimonial songs, singing cultural and religious songs of inspiration, and expressing various emotions utilizing African instruments. Identity formation was explored as it relates to normative adolescent development, complex trauma, and being an African immigrant living in the United States and facing gendered racism and microaggressions based on her migration status. In addition to individual psychotherapy, recommendations were made for Patience to visit a West African church to build community similar to the community she lost. She joined the church and enjoyed the youth group, but shame and fear of judgment had caused her not to disclose her trauma history with anyone besides her aunt. After 8 months of treatment, Patience demonstrated a decrease in symptoms of distress and evidenced posttraumatic growth.

Patience's treatment reflected intersectional feminism and more specifically womanist therapy, which centers on the experience, dignity, needs, and strengths of women of African descent (Bryant-Davis & Comas-Díaz, 2016). Womanist models of care, as evidenced in Patience's treatment, include exploring the experience, effects, and potential responses to gendered racism, integrating spirituality and the expressive arts, and affirming and empowering survivors to define themselves, build social networks, reclaim their sexuality, and resist internalized oppression.

SPECIAL FOCUS: HUMAN TRAFFICKING TRENDS AND FIGURES FOR ASIAN IMMIGRANTS

Asia has long been a primary global driver and source for human trafficking. It is reported that over two thirds of human trafficking victims worldwide originate from many countries throughout Asia (Asian Century Institute, 2016). In many Asian countries, social and gender biases, violation of legal and economic rights, and poverty combine to make women and girls extremely vulnerable to a lifetime of isolation and abuse (Rajan, 2013). According to Niaz and Hassan (2006),

> Even in the new millennium, women in South Asia are deprived of their socio-economic and legal rights. They live in a system where religious injunctions, tribal codes, feudal traditions and discriminatory laws are prevalent. They are beset by a lifetime of social and psychological disadvantage. . . . They often end up experiencing poverty [and] isolation. (pp. 118–120)

Increases in revenue gained by organized crime syndicates (Rajan, 2011), corruption in government organizations at both local and national levels, and resistance against forming a federal law enforcement agency (Kumar, 2004) make it quite clear that India's attempts to create and enforce laws protecting human trafficking victims have proven not only unsuccessful but quite often insincere (Rajan, 2013). Inefficiencies and corruption surround the enforcement of laws against trafficking and have long perpetuated its practice and growth (Rajan, 2013). For example, the Suppression of Immoral Traffic in Women and Girls Act of 1956 had a loophole that prevented the criminalization of males involved in prostitution and trafficking and punished the women because the law equated "immoral traffic" with women, by definition (Human Rights Watch, 1995).

India: A Major Origin, Portal, and Destination Country

India continues to be a major source, destination, and transit country for men, women, and children subjected to forced labor and sex trafficking. Forced labor constitutes India's largest trafficking problem; men, women, and children in debt bondage—sometimes inherited from previous generations—are forced to work in brick kilns, rice mills, embroidery factories, and agriculture (United Nations High Commissioner for Refugees, 2017). Most of India's trafficking problem is internal, and individuals from the most disadvantaged social strata—lowest caste *Dalits*, members of tribal communities, religious minorities, and women and girls from excluded groups—are most vulnerable. Within India, some are subjected to forced labor in sectors such as construction; steel, garment, and textile industries; wire manufacturing for underground cables; biscuit factories; pickling; floriculture; fish farms; and ship breaking ("India Doesn't Meet Minimum Standards for Curbing Trafficking: US," 2018). Workers within India who mine for sand are potentially vulnerable to human trafficking. Thousands of unregulated work placement agencies reportedly lure adults and children under false promises of employment into sex trafficking or forced labor, including domestic servitude (New Delhi Television Limited, 2018).

Though statistics fluctuate and are often inaccurate owing to under-reporting, approximately 40 million men, women, and children are trafficked and enslaved in forced labor, coerced marriage, and sexual exploitation worldwide (International Labour Organization and Walk Free Foundation, 2017).

One of the world's most lucrative and systematized crimes, human trafficking is estimated to globally generate more than $150 billion a year. Roughly two thirds of its victims are in East Asia and the Pacific, according to the *Global Slavery Index 2016* (Walk Free Foundation, 2016). These figures are only estimates: Because human trafficking remains a shadow crime, its victims are enslaved in the shadows and held fast by fear of reprisals, intimidation, and abuse.

East Asia, Southeast Asia, and the Pacific: Leading Destination Countries

Alarmingly, more than 85% of victims were trafficked from within East Asia and the Pacific (UNODC, 2016). China, Japan, Malaysia, and Thailand are popular destination countries, and within Southeast Asia, Thailand is the leading destination for trafficking victims from Cambodia, Lao P.D.R., and Myanmar (International Labour Organization and Walk Free Foundation, 2017). Malaysia is a destination for victims from Indonesia, the Philippines, and Vietnam. Roughly a third of all trafficking victims in East Asia are children, and 51% are women (UNODC, 2016). Caballero-Anthony (2018) outlined the disproportionate abuses of women and children spanning sexual and labor-based trafficking and exploitation:

> During 2012–14, more than 60 percent of the 7,800 identified victims were trafficked for sexual exploitation. Females are also victims of domestic servitude and other forms of forced labor. In many cases, the women and children are from remote and impoverished communities. Forced marriages of young women and girls are rampant in the Mekong region of Cambodia, China, Myanmar, and Vietnam. (p. 19)

The documented rise in this region's child trafficking is connected to a disproportionate increase in online child pornography, including live streaming of child sexual abuse. It is a lucrative business estimated to generate $3 billion to $20 billion in profit a year; countries such as Cambodia and Thailand have been identified as major suppliers of pornographic material (Caballero-Anthony, 2018). International traffic survivors who have been brought to the United States, as well as survivors who were trafficked domestically often end up at strip clubs, street corners, truck stops, massage parlors, pornography sets, low-cost hotels, and private homes (Contreras & Farley, 2011).

Many Southeast Asian victims migrate because of unemployment but end up being forced into labor in agriculture, fishing, domestic servitude, and construction (Caballero-Anthony, 2018). Most are men who become vulnerable to debt bondage (UNODC, 2018). Forced labor in the fishing industry is dominant in Cambodia, Indonesia, and Thailand; victims are forced to work for 20 or more hours per day and given little if any pay. South Asian trafficking survivors face the realities of poverty, risk of HIV, lack of social support, untrustworthy migration facilitators who are actually traffickers, violence, cultural and religious beliefs that support the exploitation, and sex tourism that consistently seeks out children at younger ages (Silverman et al., 2007). One survivor describes her experience in these words:

> My stepmother never wanted me to go to school. I was a good student and yet I never got a chance to go to school after she married my father. I had two younger sisters and my new mother gave birth to a son that year. She told me that I was the eldest and since my father had lost crops twice in the season, he would like me to take up some job. I knew how to read and write, so I at that time she was asking for my support. I also heard my father talk to the landlord about getting me work in a nearby city. But, I had no idea that they were selling me for money. When I went to Mumbai with six other girls, we were asked to do all kinds of jobs for no money. Money was directly sent to my family. (Jani & Anstadt, 2013)

This survivor's narrative supports the need for an intersectional feminist frame that attends to her multiple oppressed identities, gender roles, family roles, duty/obligation, exploitation, and secrecy. While these oppressive realities must be acknowledged, a practitioner working with this survivor would also need to acknowledge and integrate her individual and cultural strengths.

Impact of Conflicts and Natural Disasters

Human trafficking is widely complicated by the displacement and vulnerability caused by regional wars, conflicts, and natural disasters. As Caballero-Anthony (2018) pointed out, "Typhoons and other natural disasters are becoming more intense and frequent in Southeast Asia because of climate change, adding to the flow of potential victims, including children who are orphaned or separated from their families" (p. 20). A staggering 227.6 million people have been displaced since 2008 (Caballero-Anthony, 2018). One such example of a natural disaster causing displacement is Typhoon Haiyan, which struck the Philippines in 2013. In the aftermath of the storm, survivors widely ended up in forced work as domestic servants, beggars, prostitutes, and laborers. Drought-affected migrants emigrated from Cambodia into Thailand (Calma, 2017; Tesfay, 2015) and were targeted by crime networks because of the unstable and dangerous routes of their travel. Yet despite growing evidence that climate change increasingly drives forced migration, its link with human trafficking remains relatively unexplored. Climate change and natural disasters are "rarely regarded as contributing to human trafficking in global discussions or national-level policy frameworks" (Caballero-Anthony, 2018, p. 20).

Conflicts in Myanmar and the southern Philippines, areas that have large populations of refugees, are another major source of vulnerable refugees. More than 5,000 Rohingya people from Myanmar have been trafficked into Bangladesh (Caballero-Anthony, 2018). Kachin, Shan, Akha, and Lahu women in the region are trafficked for sexual exploitation in Thailand and sold as brides in China. "Armed groups in the Philippines, including Moro rebels and communists, recruit children, at times through force, for combat and non-combat roles" (Caballero-Anthony, 2018, p. 20). Working with human trafficking survivors who are Asian immigrants, or immigrants from other regions necessitates attention to the specific country of origin, a complete trauma history, exposure to cultural oppression, and utilization of cultural resources.

CONCLUSION

Racial minority immigrants face increased risk for human trafficking and face additional barriers to the recovery process. Gendered racism in the lives of immigrants and descendants of intergenerational traumas, such as colonialism, results in specific stigmas and stereotypes that increase vulnerability to poverty, objectification, lack of protection, and sexualization. Intersectional theorists, practitioners, and activists attend to the multiple forms of oppression coexisting in survivors' lives to effectively provide culturally congruent care, safety, and justice. While interventions for survivors of sex trafficking are needed, prevention activities including raising awareness of human trafficking, implementing policies to combat socioeconomic and political oppression, and efforts to address xenophobia are also critical.

REFERENCES

Abas, M., Ostrovschi, N. V., Prince, M., Gorceag, V. I., Trigub, C., & Oram, S. (2013). Risk factors for mental disorders in women survivors of human trafficking: A historical cohort study. *BMC Psychiatry, 13*(1), 204. https://doi.org/10.1186/1471-244X-13-204

Aberdein, C., & Zimmerman, C. (2015). Access to mental health and psychosocial services in Cambodia by survivors of trafficking and exploitation: A qualitative study. *International Journal of Mental Health Systems, 9*, Article 16. https://doi.org/10.1186/s13033-015-0008-8

American Psychological Association. (2008). *Psychology matters: Glossary.* http://www.psychologymatters.org/glossary.html#p

Anti-Slavery International. (2020). *What is modern slavery?* https://www.antislavery.org/slavery-today/modern-slavery/

Asian Century Institute. (2016). *Human trafficking and smuggling in Asia.* https://asiancenturyinstitute.com/society/1120-human-trafficking-and-smuggling-in-asia

Bertone, A. M. (2000). Sexual trafficking in women: International political economy and the politics of sex. *Gender Issues, 18*(1), 4–22. https://doi.org/10.1007/s12147-999-0020-x

Bryant, K. (2016). *Resilience in women survivors.* Global Sisters Report. https://www.globalsistersreport.org/column/trafficking/resilience-women-survivors-37061

Bryant-Davis, T., Adams, T., & Gray, A. (2017). Women, sex trafficking, and the justice system: From victimization to restoration. In C. C. Datchi & J. R. Ancis (Eds.), *Gender, psychology, and justice: The mental health of women and girls in the legal system* (pp. 75–100). New York University Press. https://doi.org/10.18574/nyu/9781479819850.003.0004

Bryant-Davis, T., & Comas-Díaz, L. (2016). Introduction: Womanist and *mujerista* psychologies. In T. Bryant-Davis & L. Comas-Díaz (Eds.), *Womanist and mujerista psychologies: Voices of fire, acts of courage* (pp. 3–25). American Psychological Association. https://doi.org/10.1037/14937-001

Bryant-Davis, T., & Gobin, R. L. (2019). Still we rise: Psychotherapy for African American girls and women exiting sex trafficking. *Women & Therapy, 42*(3–4), 385–405. https://doi.org/10.1080/02703149.2019.1622902

Bryant-Davis, T., & Tummala-Narra, P. (2017). Cultural oppression and human trafficking: Exploring the role of racism and ethnic bias. *Women & Therapy, 40*(1–2), 152–169. https://doi.org/10.1080/02703149.2016.1210964

Bureau of Justice Statistics. (2011). *Most suspected incidents of human trafficking involved allegations of prostitution of an adult or child.* https://www.bjs.gov/content/pub/press/cshti0810pr.cfm

Caballero-Anthony, M. (2018). A hidden scourge: Southeast Asia's refugees and displaced people are victimized by human traffickers, but the crime usually goes unreported. *Finance & Development, 55*(3), 18–21. https://www.imf.org/external/pubs/ft/fandd/2018/09/pdf/human-trafficking-in-southeast-asia-caballero.pdf

Calma, J. (2017, May 2). *Climate change has created a new generation of sex-trafficking victims.* Quartz.

Clawson, H. J., & Dutch, N. (2008). *Addressing the needs of victims of human trafficking: Challenges, barriers, and promising practices.* Office of the Assistant Secretary for Planning and Evaluation, U.S. Department of Health and Human Services. https://aspe.hhs.gov/system/files/pdf/75471/ib.pdf

Contreras, M., & Farley, M. (2011). Human trafficking: Not an isolated issue. In T. Bryant-Davis (Ed.), *Surviving sexual violence: A guide to recovery and empowerment* (pp. 22–36). Rowman & Littlefield.

Contreras, P. M., Kallivayalil, D., & Herman, J. L. (2017). Psychotherapy in the aftermath of human trafficking: Working through the consequences of psychological coercion. *Women & Therapy, 40*(1–2), 31–54. https://doi.org/10.1080/02703149.2016.1205908

Council on Foreign Relations. (n.d.). *Modern slavery.* https://www.cfr.org/interactives/modern-slavery

Countryman-Roswurm, K., & DiLollo, A. (2017). Survivor: A narrative therapy approach for use with sex trafficked women and girls. *Women & Therapy, 40*(1–2), 55–72. https://doi.org/10.1080/02703149.2016.1206782

Crawford, M. (2017). International sex trafficking. *Women & Therapy, 40*(1–2), 101–122. https://doi.org/10.1080/02703149.2016.1206784

de Chesnay, M. (2013). Cultural aspects of treating survivors of sex trafficking. *Hawai'i Journal of Medicine & Public Health: A Journal of Asia Pacific Medicine & Public Health, 72*(8, Suppl. 3), 12.

Edmond, T. (2018). Evidence-based trauma treatments for survivors of sex trafficking and commercial sexual exploitation. In A. J. Nichols, T. Edmond, & E. C. Heil (Eds.), *Social work practice with survivors of sex trafficking and commercial sexual exploitation* (pp. 70–96). Columbia University Press. https://doi.org/10.7312/nich18092-006

Elliott, D. E., Bjelajac, P., Fallot, R. D., Markoff, L. S., & Reed, B. G. (2005). Trauma-informed or trauma-denied: Principles and implementation of trauma-informed services for women. *Journal of Community Psychology, 33*(4), 461–477. https://doi.org/10.1002/jcop.20063

Free the Slaves. (n.d.). *Slavery today.* https://www.freetheslaves.net/our-model-for-freedom/slavery-today/

Grover, S. (2007). Children as chattel of the state: Deconstructing the concept of sex trafficking. *International Journal of Human Rights, 11*(3), 293–306. https://doi.org/10.1080/13642980701443525

Gutiérrez Chong, N. (2014). Human trafficking and sex industry: Does ethnicity and race matter? *Journal of Intercultural Studies, 35*(2), 196–213. https://doi.org/10.1080/07256868.2014.885413

Hartmann, M. (2019, June 19). *The Devadasi: Female slaves in modern India.* The Exodus Road. https://blog.theexodusroad.com/the-devadasi-female-slaves-in-modern-india

Heil, E. (2016). It is God's will: Exploiting religious beliefs as a means of human trafficking. *Critical Research on Religion, 5(1),* 48–61. https://doi.org/10.1177/2050303216676520

Hopper, E. K. (2018). Trauma-informed psychological assessment of human trafficking survivors. In N. M. Sidun & D. L. Hume (Eds.), *A feminist perspective on human trafficking of women and girls: Characteristics, commonalities and complexities* (pp. 6–24). Routledge/Taylor & Francis Group.

Human Rights Watch. (1995). *Rape for profit: Trafficking of Nepali girls and women to India's brothels*. https://www.hrw.org/reports/1995/India.htm

India doesn't meet minimum standards for curbing trafficking: U.S. (2018, June 29). *The Quint*. https://www.thequint.com/news/india/india-human-trafficking-us-report

International Labour Organization and Walk Free Foundation. (2017). *Global estimates of modern slavery: Forced labour and forced marriage*. https://www.ilo.org/global/publications/books/WCMS_575479/lang—en/index.htm

Jani, N., & Anstadt, S. P. (2013). Contributing factors in trafficking from South Asia. *Journal of Human Behavior in the Social Environment, 23*(3), 298–311. https://doi.org/10.1080/10911359.2013.739010

Keller, J. (2018, January 18). *Confronting the beast: Racism's role in human trafficking*. The Freedom Story. https://thefreedomstory.org/confronting-the-beast-racisms-role-in-human-trafficking

Kumar, V. (2004, February 1). *India could lead the fight against human trafficking*. Hindu. http://www.hindu.com/2004/02/01/stories/2004020114221000.htm

Le, P. D., Ryan, N., Rosenstock, Y., & Goldmann, E. (2018). Health issues associated with commercial sexual exploitation and sex trafficking of children in the United States: A systematic review. *Behavioral Medicine, 44*(3), 219–233. https://doi.org/10.1080/08964289.2018.1432554

Levesque, R. J. R. (1999). *Sexual abuse of children: A human rights perspective*. Indiana University Press.

Márquez, Y. I., Deblinger, E., & Dovi, A. T. (2020). The value of trauma-focused cognitive behavioral therapy (TF-CBT) in addressing the therapeutic needs of trafficked youth: A case study. *Cognitive and Behavioral Practice, 27*(3), 253–269. https://doi.org/10.1016/j.cbpra.2019.10.001

Nagaraj, A. (2017, December 13). *Rescued child sex workers in India reveal hidden cells in brothels*. Reuters. https://www.reuters.com/article/us-india-trafficking-brothels-idUSKBN1E71R1

Nagel, J. (2003). *Race, ethnicity, and sexuality: Intimate intersections, forbidden frontiers*. Oxford University Press. http://hdl.handle.net/2027/heb.03513.0001.001

National Human Trafficking Hotline. (n.d.). *Traffickers*. https://humantraffickinghotline.org/what-human-trafficking/human-trafficking/traffickers

NDTV. (2018, June 29). *Action on human trafficking "disproportionately low" in India: US report*. https://www.ndtv.com/india-news/action-on-human-trafficking-disproportionately-low-in-india-us-trafficking-in-persons-report-2018-1875267

Nelson Butler, C. (2015). The racial roots of human trafficking. *UCLA Law Review, 62*(1464).

Niaz, U., & Hassan, S. (2006). Culture and mental health of women in South-East Asia. *World Psychiatry, 5*(2), 118–120.

Office of the Assistant Secretary for Planning and Evaluation, U.S. Department of Health and Human Services. (2010). *Evidence-based mental health treatment for victims of human trafficking*. https://aspe.hhs.gov/report/evidence-based-mental-health-treatment-victims-human-trafficking

Office of Refugee Resettlement. (2008). *Sex trafficking fact sheet*. https://www.acf.hhs.gov/sites/default/files/orr/fact_sheet_sex_trafficking.pdf

Oleksy, E. H. (2011). Intersectionality at the cross-roads. *Women's Studies International Forum, 34*(4), 263–270. https://doi.org/10.1016/j.wsif.2011.02.002

Ottisova, L., Smith, P., & Oram, S. (2018). Psychological consequences of human trafficking: Complex posttraumatic stress disorder in trafficked children. *Behavioral Medicine, 44*(3), 234–241. https://doi.org/10.1080/08964289.2018.1432555

Polaris. (2019). *Human trafficking*. https://polarisproject.org/victims-traffickers

Rajam, K. (2017, April 24). *How Devadasis went from having high social status to being sex slaves and child prostitutes.* YourStory. https://yourstory.com/2017/04/devadasis-india

Rajan, I. (2011). Voices from the void: A depth psychological reconceptualization of sex trafficking in modern-day India. *Psychotherapy and Politics International, 9*(2), 97–102. https://doi.org/10.1002/ppi.238

Rajan, I. (2013). *Speaking self out of darkness: The lived experience of sex trafficking survivors in Kolkata, India* (Accession Order No. 3619411) [Doctoral dissertation, Pacifica Graduate Institute]. ProQuest Dissertations and Theses Global.

Robjant, K., Roberts, J., & Katona, C. (2017). Treating posttraumatic stress disorder in female victims of trafficking using narrative exposure therapy: A retrospective audit. *Frontiers in Psychiatry, 8,* 63.

Salami, T., Gordon, M., Coverdale, J., & Nguyen, P. T. (2018). What therapies are favored in the treatment of the psychological sequelae of trauma in human trafficking victims? *Journal of Psychiatric Practice, 24*(2), 87–96. https://doi.org/10.1097/PRA.0000000000000288

Schrader, E. M., & Wendland, J. M. (2012). Music therapy programming at an aftercare center in Cambodia for survivors of child sexual exploitation and rape and their caregivers. *Social Work & Christianity, 39*(4), 390–406.

Schultz, D. L. (2012). Translating intersectionality theory into practice: A tale of Romani-Gadûe feminist alliance. *Signs: Journal of Women in Culture and Society, 38*(1), 37–43. https://doi.org/10.1086/665802

Scott, J. T., Ingram, A. M., Nemer, S. L., & Crowley, D. M. (2019). Evidence-based human trafficking policy: Opportunities to invest in trauma-informed strategies. *American Journal of Community Psychology.* https://doi.org/10.1002/ajcp.12394

Shingal, A. (2015). The Devadasi system: Temple prostitution in India. *UCLA Women's Law Journal, 22*(1), 107–123.

Silverman, J. G., Decker, M. R., Gupta, J., Maheshwari, A., Willis, B. M., & Raj, A. (2007). HIV prevalence and predictors of infection in sex-trafficked Nepalese girls and women. *Journal of the American Medical Association, 298*(5), 536–542. https://doi.org/10.1001/jama.298.5.536

Spates, K., Evans, N. M., Watts, B. C., Abubakar, N., & James, T. (2019). Keeping ourselves sane: A qualitative exploration of Black women's coping strategies for gendered racism. *Sex Roles: A Journal of Research.* https://doi.org/10.1007/s11199-019-01077-1

Tesfay, N. (2015). *Impact of livelihood recovery initiatives on reducing vulnerability to human trafficking and illegal recruitment: Lessons from Typhoon Haiyan.* International Organization for Migration and International Labour Organization.

United Nations High Commissioner for Refugees. (2017, June 27). *2017 trafficking in persons report, India.* United States Department of State. https://www.refworld.org/docid/5959ecbba.html

United Nations Office on Drugs and Crime. (2004). *United Nations convention against transnational organized crime and the protocols thereto.* United Nations. https://www.unodc.org/documents/treaties/UNTOC/Publications/TOC%20Convention/TOCebook-e.pdf

United Nations Office on Drugs and Crimes. (2016). *Global report on trafficking in persons.* https://www.unodc.org/documents/data-and-analysis/glotip/2016_Global_Report_on_Trafficking_in_Persons.pdf

United Nations Office on Drugs and Crimes. (2018). *Global report on trafficking in persons.* https://www.unodc.org/documents/data-and-analysis/glotip/2018/GLOTiP_2018_BOOK_web_small.pdf

U.S. Department of Justice. (2020, June). *Human trafficking task force.* U.S. Attorney's Office, Middle District of Alabama. https://www.justice.gov/usao-mdal/human-trafficking-task-force

Walk Free Foundation. (2016, July 4). *Global slavery index.* https://reliefweb.int/report/world/global-slavery-index-2016

Williamson, E., Dutch, N., & Clawson, H. C. (2008). *National symposium on the health needs of human trafficking victims: Post-symposium brief.* Office of the Assistant Secretary for Planning and Evaluation, U.S. Department of Health and Human Services.

World Bank Group. (2016). *Poverty and shared prosperity 2016: Taking on inequality.*

Zimmerman, C., Hossain, M., & Watts, C. (2011). Human trafficking and health: A conceptual model to inform policy, intervention and research. *Social Science & Medicine, 73*(2), 327–335. https://doi.org/10.1016/j.socscimed.2011.05.028

10

The Rippling Effects of Unauthorized Status

Stress, Family Separations, and Deportation and Their Implications for Belonging and Development

Carola Suárez-Orozco, Guadalupe López Hernández, and Patricia Cabral

When Marieli was 4 years old, her father was assassinated in front of his wife and daughter.[1] Soon afterward, her mother reluctantly left Guatemala for the United States to support her family, leaving Marieli behind. Five years later, the grandmother who raised the children in the mother's absence died. The neighbor hired to take care of Marieli after the grandmother's death became increasingly abusive and neglectful. Though her mother had applied for asylum status, the processing of the request is still unresolved years later. Growing increasingly concerned for Marieli's well-being, the mother sent for her, on the cusp of adolescence, before documentation can be secured.

The reunification with the mother she barely remembers, as well as a new stepfather and stepsister, proves complicated and fraught with ambivalence. Further, the neighborhood where the family lives is one of the 10 most violent in the country. Marieli reports regularly overhearing gunshots, gang recruitment efforts as she travels from home to school, and frequent altercations involving other students in her school. She registers disdain expressed toward people who lack residency papers or whose English is marked by an accent and is deeply unsettled by that. Though she begins high school with straight A's and dreams of a soccer scholarship to college, as she begins to lose hope for finding a place in her new land, she disengages from school and becomes increasingly depressed.

---

[1] All case material has been altered to protect confidentiality.

https://doi.org/10.1037/0000214-011
Trauma and Racial Minority Immigrants: Turmoil, Uncertainty, and Resistance,
P. Tummala-Narra (Editor)

An estimated 5.1 million children under the age of 18 live with at least one unauthorized parent (Zong et al., 2019). Of these children over 4.5 million are U.S. citizens with at least one unauthorized parent, and about 959,000 children under the age of 18 do not have citizenship, permanent-resident status, refugee status, or any of the temporary statuses provided by the United States for long-term residence and work (Capps et al., 2016; Zong et al., 2019). In short, they are unauthorized migrants. As such, over a quarter (28%) of the 18.7 million first- and second-generation children and youth in the United States (Child Trends, 2013) are growing up directly affected by unauthorized status—either their own or their parents'. While they originate in multiple countries, those of Mexican and Central American origin represent the largest groups (Krogstad & Passel, 2015). Historically most crossed over the borders without inspection and the proper authorization. Indeed, recently, visa overstayers (immigrants who arrive with visas and become unauthorized as the visas expire) have surpassed those crossing the border without inspection (Warren & Kerwin, 2017).

A growing body of evidence has demonstrated that on average, relative to their authorized peers, children and youth with unauthorized status reveal less positive educational outcomes (Bean et al., 2011) as well as less positive mental health outcomes (Potochnick & Perreira, 2010) after adjusting for indicators of socioeconomic status. Moreover, the developmental issues associated with unauthorized status are not limited to youth who are unauthorized themselves. Research has indicated that having an unauthorized parent is associated with several concerning developmental and educational vulnerabilities in U.S.-born children and youth (Yoshikawa et al., 2017).

Like all immigrants, many children and youth with unauthorized status demonstrate an array of strengths including hope (Bahena, 2014), optimism (Kao & Tienda, 1995), motivation, and resilience (Perez et al., 2009). Nonetheless, the conferred societal disadvantage imposed upon these youths suggests clear increased risks (Yoshikawa et al., 2017). Children growing up in unauthorized families show higher levels of internalizing (e.g., depression, anxiety, withdrawal) as well as externalizing (aggression and acting out) behavioral problems relative to their counterparts with authorized or citizen status (Potochnick & Perreira, 2010; Yoshikawa et al., 2017). These domains of compromise include lower levels of cognitive development, academic achievement, and educational progress across early and middle childhood (Ortega et al., 2007) and into young adulthood (Yoshikawa et al., 2017). With the recent intensification of explicitly anti-immigrant federal policies (Kulish et al., 2017) as well as a postelection anti-immigration climate (Saldaña et al., 2018), these issues are of pressing concern (Rogers et al., 2019).

This chapter is grounded upon an application of stress theories (including traumatic, toxic, acculturative, and ethnocultural) as well as theories of social belonging and exclusion in the lives of unauthorized families and their children (Baumeister & Leary, 1995; Walton & Cohen, 2007). We consider a variety of stresses that accompany migration, with a particular eye to their implications for children and youth growing up in unauthorized homes. We also consider social exclusion and how it can compromise emotional and mental health as well as capacities for social belonging of immigrant children and youth.

MIGRATION, STRESS, AND TRAUMAS

By all accounts, immigration is a highly stressful process (Suárez-Orozco & Suárez-Orozco, 2001). Compounding classic acculturative stress, frequently pre- and postmigratory trauma may also have occurred, which has implications for the parents but also for their children through transgenerational pathways and toxic stress.

Trauma Prior to Migration and During the Voyage

Many immigrants choose to migrate because of traumatic experiences in their home country. Well-founded fears of persecution can include racial, ethnic, religious, and sexual orientation statuses. The migratory trauma can result from local conditions of sociopolitical violence (e.g., Central American or Middle Eastern individuals) or of personal violence (e.g., secondary to domestic violence). Natural disasters forcibly displacing many can also serve as a catalyst. Today, an estimated 80% of those seeking asylum have credible fear for their life and are at risk of persecution or death if they return home (U.S. Immigration and Customs Enforcement, 2018). Asylum seekers and refugees are particularly vulnerable to a heightened risk of mental health challenges (Fazel et al., 2012). Nonetheless, President Trump has made drastic changes to asylum policies by delaying and/or rejecting the paperwork asylum seekers need to enter the United States.

Today, a high rate of Central American asylum seekers, including women with children, are fleeing violence. By the time these immigrants reach the United States, many have already experienced assaults, abductions, and extortion from cartels, gang members, and police and immigration officials (Alberto & Chilton, 2019). As they attempt to seek asylum in the United States, many are subjected to detention under inhumane circumstances and concomitant family separations (e.g., Alberto & Chilton, 2019).

The adversity and risks many immigrants encounter before, during, and after immigration can complicate the adaptation process (Portes & Rumbaut, 2006; Suárez-Orozco & Suárez-Orozco, 2001). These "compound traumas" are rarely processed or entirely resolved before another trauma is experienced, which in turn affects "developmental and relational growth" (Cockersell, 2018, p. 27). In cases where children do not have direct exposure to trauma, caretaker exposure to physical and symbolic violence can lead to transgenerational transmission of trauma (Schwab, 2010). The rapid loss of familial social resources (Hobfoll, 1991), along with chronic exposure to stress, has been linked to post-traumatic stress disorder, depression, and somatic complaints and ailments

(Fazel et al., 2012; Vizek-Vidović et al., 2000) as well as to academic challenges essential for optimal functioning in the new land (American Psychological Association [APA] Presidential Task Force on Immigration, 2012; Bean et al., 2011; Suárez-Orozco, 2017; Suárez-Orozco et al., 2008).

Acculturative Stress

Acculturation is rooted in the immigration experience and is synonymous with undergoing the stressors associated with learning new cultural roles (Suárez-Orozco & Suárez-Orozco, 2001). Acculturative stress is most prevalent among newcomers but is also present in multigenerational families (those that include first-, second-, and third-generation members [Cervantes et al., 1991]). Acculturative dissonance typically emerges as immigrant family members learn how to negotiate and navigate the sociocultural norms of the dominant culture at different rates.

These new rules of cultural engagement are typically learned at different paces by children and their caregivers and depend on the context in which they interact with the host culture. Immigrant children are regularly immersed through their exposure in school (Suárez-Orozco & Suárez-Orozco, 2001). Immigrant caregivers, by contrast, who often work in ethnically homogeneous settings (e.g., ethnic enclaves) are more likely to experience lengthier routes to acculturation (Suárez-Orozco et al., 2015). Contrasting levels of acculturative stress across family members can contribute to observable generational tensions (Dinh & Nguyen, 2006), including those between traditional and more assimilated siblings (Pyke, 2005). Such disconnections are further amplified by family separations due to deportation or decisions to remigrate (Suárez-Orozco, Bang, & Kim, 2011).

Family Separations and Complicated Reunifications

Children in immigrant families are likely to experience periods of extended parent–child separation (Suárez-Orozco, Bang, & Kim, 2011). During the initial migration, parents often leave their children behind with caretakers with the intention of sending for them as soon as they are able to regularize their status; this often takes longer to arrange than anticipated (Dreby, 2012). Long backlogs, a byzantine bureaucracy, and high rates of denials are fomenting growing numbers of transnationally separated mixed-status families (Suárez-Orozco, Bang, & Kim, 2011).

Whereas citizen children can easily travel across borders, with the militarization of the southern border their unauthorized parents cannot reenter the United States without undergoing expensive, arduous, and clandestine crossings (Durand & Massey, 2004). Many families find themselves not only living apart from their extended families but also with parents and siblings, split between the United States and their country of origin (Suárez-Orozco, Bang, & Kim, 2011). Moreover, citizen children may be separated from their parents by deportation. Parent-child separation can harm children's learning and emotional development due to disruption in attachment, interruptions in schooling, as well as economic losses in the household (Suárez-Orozco, Yoshikawa, et al., 2011).

Although families typically expect to reunite quickly, they encounter ever-changing immigration policies that prolong separations (Menjívar & Abrego, 2009). Since 2012, the rate of unauthorized and unaccompanied children coming to the United States has increased (especially among those from Guatemala, Honduras, and El Salvador) in order to reunite family members (Menjívar & Perreira, 2019). These children often experience tensions as they rejoin their families (Suárez-Orozco, Bang, & Kim, 2011). Intergenerational conflict and detachment often occurs in life with immigrant parents in the new land and relationships do not align with children's expectations (Suárez-Orozco, Bang, & Kim, 2011). Reunited children and youth also frequently voice resentment toward their parent(s) for having left them behind or for having additional children (Abrego, 2014). Notably, while long-term separations are linked to higher levels of distress, children in families who arrive together are less likely to experience depression and anxiety than those who do not (Suárez-Orozco, Bang, & Kim, 2011).

Threats and Realities of Deportation

The most pervasive and immediately damaging family challenge associated with unauthorized status is the ever-present threat of deportation; this fear can center upon worries about the self as well as concerns about deportations of a loved one. Removal proceedings and removals themselves place extraordinary burdens on families and children (Rosenblum & Meissner, 2015). During President Obama's administration, there was a record high of about 2.5 million people deported. Between July 2010 and September 2012, over 22% of all removals were of parents with citizen children (Wessler, 2011). Upon inauguration, President Trump immediately targeted an estimated 2 million to 3 million people for deportation (Hirschfeld Davis & Preston, 2016). Indeed, apprehensions on the U.S.–Mexico border in the first 6 months of 2019 increased to about 361,087 (Pew Research Center, 2019), and during the 2018 fiscal year, there were about 256,086 deportations of unauthorized immigrants (U.S. Immigration and Customs Enforcement, 2018).

Further, new enforcement tactics are evident. News reports began to appear of immigrant women being swept up in court when requesting a restraining order after a domestic violence order, of a DACAmented youth being detained along with their unauthorized father, of ICE officers wearing police identification to gain entry to homes, of ICE sweeps in proximity to schools, and the like. Consequently, schools and day care centers reported drops in attendance after the election, intensifying a trend always present among precarious immigrant families living in the shadow of the law (National Public Radio, 2016).

The available research on the effects of parental removal is slim, as conducting studies of unauthorized families entails complex logistical and ethical issues (Hernández et al., 2013). Yet the evidence, not surprisingly, suggests that unexpected family separations precipitated by deportations have detrimental effects on family dynamics and separations (Brabeck et al., 2014). Many deportees have a family they leave behind; indeed, a quarter of them have a U.S.-citizen child (Koball et al., 2015). A majority of deportees are male (Mexican American Legal Defense and Educational Fund, 2014); as such, female partners are most often left to deal with the familial aftermath (Menjívar et al., 2018). These women are not only left to provide emotional support for their deported spouse and children left behind in the United States but often also have for the first time to deal with the finances of the home (Baker & Marchevsky, 2019). Many report struggling to pay their mortgage and car payment and working multiple jobs to make ends meet (Baker & Marchevsky, 2019). These circumstances often come at the expense of the children and youth contending with their loss.

The legal status of parents weighs heavily on children and youth (Dreby, 2012). A survey of 3,600 educators across the United States found that the majority (85%) had explicitly observed "overt expressions of fear" of immigration enforcement in their (or a loved one's) lives among their immigrant-origin students (Ee & Gándara, 2019). Multiple negative psychological outcomes have been linked to such forced separations (Lovato et al., 2018). Following a detention or deportation, children have been documented to experience short-term psychological effects including loss of appetite, nightmares, episodes of crying, and feeling afraid (Chaudry et al., 2010). These psychological effects can persist to become chronic and lead to severe episodes of anxiety and fear (Brabeck et al., 2014). Significant stress levels increase when children are placed under the care of extended family they are not familiar with, or, even worse, when they are placed in the foster system (Dreby, 2012; Wessler, 2011).

Further, many parents fear losing custody of their children as they undergo deportation proceedings (Dreby, 2012). Fear of parental removal can affect children regardless of whether the parent is actually detained; children in these unauthorized homes report living in constant fear that parents or other family members will vanish and never be seen again (Urban Institute for the National Council of La Raza, 2007). The fear of removal can be transmitted to children either directly or through more general parental stress, affecting the child's well-being (Enriquez, 2015). Children express a variety of fears, including fears of the family being split up, of both parents leaving the United States while the child stays behind, and generalized fear of the police (Dreby, 2012). At the core are high levels of anxiety and worry about a loved one being detained and deported (Enriquez, 2015).

In the face of such events, families must make difficult decisions about the fate of their children should the dreaded apprehension and deportation unfold. Often parents discuss contingency plans with their children in case they are detained or deported. A study of Latinx families found that among unauthorized parents, more than half (58%) had a plan in place for their children's care in case they were detained, and 40% had discussed the plan with their children (Brabeck & Xu, 2010). As Chavez (2013) documented, while the main concern of many unauthorized parents is to provide their children with stable futures, in this climate of deportation their ability to do so is heavily compromised.

Psychological Sequelae

In short, the adversity and risks many immigrants encounter before, during, and after immigration can complicate the adaptation process and activate "toxic stress" (Shonkoff et al., 2012). Perhaps not surprisingly, the large-scale survey of 3,600 educators noted earlier found that the majority of its respondents (79%) reported emotional or behavioral problems among their immigrant students that interfered with learning (Ee & Gándara, 2019). A growing body of research on trauma has demonstrated both the long-term health implications of exposure to trauma (Delva et al., 2013; Shonkoff et al., 2012) as well as its short-term implications for social-emotional functioning, learning, cognition, motivation, and learning (Navid & Nicholson, 2019; van der Kolk, 2015).

Simply put, traumatized children cannot learn optimally. For example, traumatic exposures can negatively affect children's learning at school by decreasing their ability to focus attention, regulate emotions and behavior, as well as to develop positive relationships with adults and peers (Navid & Nicholson, 2019). Students who have been exposed to trauma often "view the world as a perilous place" (Navid & Nicholson, 2019, p. 1). Day-to-day events can easily trigger fight, flight, or freeze survival responses that are not under the student's control, resulting in less ability to engage in problem-solving and rational thought (Navid & Nicholson, 2019). Traumatized students may appear anxious, are prone to perceiving intent of harm when criticized, and may engage in avoidance behaviors, placing them at risk for less than optimal learning experiences (van der Kolk, 2015).

SOCIAL BELONGING AND EXCLUSION

Deportation—and its perennial threat to the self as well as to loved ones— is the ultimate form of social exclusion. In the condition of actual deportation or its imminent threat, there is no ambiguity about whether one is being exiled from society. Yet for unauthorized individuals, the shadow of this status compromises belongingness in myriad other ways as well (Gonzales et al., 2013).

"The need to belong is a powerful, fundamental, and extremely pervasive" social motivation (Baumeister & Leary, 1995, p. 497) and human need (Maslow, 1943). Humans are a social species who long to belong across a variety of domains. These include kinship groups, schools, places of work, places of worship, mutual aid societies, voluntary associations, clubs, as well as in political groupings and social movements, and, of course, in the nation state (Crisp, 2010).

The converse of social belonging is the well-theorized concept of social exclusion (Crisp, 2010; Fangen, 2010; Lamont, 2018). However, for members of stigmatized groups—for example, people with disabilities, people of color, immigrants, and members of the LGBTQ community—a sense of social belonging is routinely compromised and at risk (Walton & Cohen, 2007) across a range of domains, including the sociopolitical, spatial, labor market, educational, and relational (Fangen, 2010).

Liminality

Liminality—belonging neither to the society left behind nor the society entered—also compromises the sense of social belonging (Menjívar, 2006). This is especially true in the midst of a contentious political landscape. Increasingly, children and youth live in households whose family members have liminal status. For example, many families with temporary protective status (TPS), which grants temporary conditions to reside in the United States, are currently in danger of losing this status and are under threat of deportation. The Trump administration has not renewed TPS for an array of communities, including those from Nepal, Nicaragua, Honduras, El Salvador, and Liberia among others (U.S. Citizenship and Immigration Services, 2019). Hundreds of thousands who have been living in the United States for decades—many of whom have citizen children—will no longer have legal protections to stay in the country. Deferred Action for Childhood Arrivals (DACA) provided an opportunity for its recipients to hold a temporary driver's license and work permit—in exchange for trusting the federal government and providing sensitive family information. Receiving these benefits transformed the outlook of life of DACA recipients, with many reported being more optimistic and hopeful, and having increased motivation about their future goals (Gonzales et al., 2018). Institutional trust was misplaced, as the program was rescinded by the Trump administration; while the U.S. Supreme Court ruled that his administration cannot immediately move forward with its plans to dismantle DACA, the program remains under attack (Liptak & Shear, 2020). As such, many unauthorized youths now face uncertain futures, extracting a heavy toll on the socioemotional development of children of unauthorized parents (Yoshikawa et al., 2017).

Structural Exclusion

The nation state can contribute to the sense of social exclusion in active ways, as in the case of deportation as well as by structuring access to resources (Fagan & MacDonald, 2013). These resources can include (quality of) jobs, housing, health care, and education, among others. Despite having working parents, children growing up in families in unauthorized homes face high levels of poverty (Tienda & Mitchell, 2006). Many families face declines in their economic well-being as they endure economic hardships due to the apprehension of a parent in an ICE raid, including costly efforts to contest deportation and job loss—with concurrent steep declines in income—as a result of workplace raids (Chaudry et al., 2010). Further, unauthorized individuals often work at below minimum wage in physically demanding conditions, with no benefits and little stability and no recourse in situations of labor law violations (Bernhardt et al., 2009). Parental work conditions such as these have been documented to have an array of negative consequences for academic, cognitive, and behavioral development of children and youth (Yoshikawa et al., 2006).

These economic hardships often result in food and housing instabilities (Chaudry et al., 2010). Many unauthorized families live in crowded conditions, as they often must "double up" with relatives to afford rent. Further, these families are prone to frequent moving either by being asked to leave by landlords who fear ICE raids, continually moving to avoid such encounters with ICE officials, or by unauthorized family members voluntarily moving to protect their loved ones (Chaudry et al., 2010). The economic constraints of unauthorized status, particularly in the wake of a parent's detainment, create difficulties affording food, with rates of hunger for unauthorized families far above the national norms (Chaudry et al., 2010).

Further, parents' legal status blocks access to such necessities of everyday life as valid social security numbers, driver's licenses, and bank accounts (Yoshikawa et al., 2017). Currently, unauthorized parents and children are ineligible for government health care benefits, with the exception of perinatal and emergency room care. Unauthorized Latinx immigrants in the United States visit doctors less frequently than immigrants who have legal status (Ortega et al., 2007). Citizen children of unauthorized parents are eligible for these benefits; however, their parents are fearful of revealing their own legal status and thus avoid applying for their children (Bernstein et al., 2019). Further, proposed legislation would block the acquisition of permanent status if families accessed public resources, including medical services, housing, and food stamps (Bernstein et al., 2019); evidence suggests that this proposed legislation has led to decreased use of services, including for citizen children (Bernstein et al., 2019).

Citizen children living in mixed-status families are less likely to be enrolled in programs such as preschool that help to foster their early learning, with negative longitudinal implications (Yoshikawa, 2011). Compromised access to learning resources in early life place children at a disadvantage for school readiness when compared to children of the authorized (Crosnoe, 2007). The schools where many unauthorized families typically enroll their children are often characterized by high dropout rates, inadequate postsecondary educational preparation, and low rates of matriculation into college (Ralph J. Bunche Center for African American Studies, 2004). For the small percentage who make it to college, most begin in community colleges that often have abysmal graduation rates (Osei-Twumasi & López-Hernández, 2019). Thus, unauthorized status can have educational ramifications that last a lifetime.

Symbolic Violence

While structural impediments such as those noted earlier have clear implications for social belonging, so do a variety of forms of symbolic violence (Bourdieu & Passeron, 1977). To legitimize the status quo, the dominant class imposes upon marginalized groups messages of subordination. These messages of "marginalizing, silencing, rejecting, isolating, segregating and disenfranchising [are] the machinery of exclusion" (Taket et al., 2009, p. 3). The messages of subordination are rendered all the more powerful when they are internalized by those who are disparaged (Bourdieu & Passeron, 1977). These social messages are transmitted to those who do (not) belong (Chavez, 2013) and can linger for years to create isolation that has a negative impact on well-being and academic self-efficacy (Walton & Cohen, 2007).

Whereas negative rhetoric about immigration has historically been a part of the United States' "ambivalent welcome" (Simon & Alexander, 1993), these relentless disparagements have increased significantly in recent years (Chavez et al., 2019). Under the current administration, those of immigrant origin have been particularly targeted as potential terrorists and criminals, and threats are repeatedly under way to withdraw automatic citizenship to children born to immigrants (Hagan et al., 2008). This polarizing social discourse around immigration has made unauthorized immigrants an especially frequent target of vitriol by politicians and anti-immigrant groups and is persistently played out in mainstream and social media (Chavez, 2013). Further, these narratives reinforce negative stereotypes legitimizing unabashed acts of covert and overt discrimination (Chavez, 2013). This type of rhetoric is linked to increased acts of violence against immigrants (e.g., Arikan, 2009), as well as to everyday stigmatizing encounters that "overscrutinize or underestimate" them (Lamont et al., 2016, p. 4).

Xenophobia and racism function to make the public imagine as "Other" those who are foreign-born (or perceived as such) and determine who is "us," who is "them," and who belongs. These biases serve to normalize stereotypes of criminality, sloth, and an unwillingness to learn the dominant language or the ways of the new land (Chavez-Dueñas et al., 2019). Further, they pit newcomers against long-standing residents regarding perceptions of competition over scarce resources as it delineates "who has the right to be cared for by the state and society" (Wimmer, 1997, p. 17). While immigrants have long been racialized (e.g., "Black" Irish), this pattern of response has been intensified in the last half-century as immigrants from Latin America, Asia, the Caribbean, and Africa are increasingly people of color (Sáenz & Manges Douglas, 2015). Immigrant-origin persons of color (across generations) may be more likely to experience discrimination associated with "perpetual foreigner" status (Lee et al., 2009), whereby becoming a full member of a White dominant society is thwarted. Resulting "ethno-racial trauma" (Chavez-Dueñas et al., 2019, p. 49)—experienced either directly or vicariously—has significant negative implications for both physical and psychological health (Comas-Díaz et al., 2019).

Hostile Learning Environments

The current xenophobic sociopolitical context has a clear "trickle-down effect" on the academic lives and learning contexts of immigrant-origin students. In a national survey of more than 500 school principals across the United States, Rogers et al. (2019) found a widespread increase in incivility across schools—with "an overwhelming majority of principals report[ing] problems such as contentious classroom environments, hostile exchanges outside of class, and demeaning and hateful remarks over political views" (p. v). In particular, 60% of participating principals reported that they had encountered issues around "derogatory comments about immigrants" (often drawing upon President Trump's "Build the Wall" rhetoric). A survey of 3,600 educators in the United States that considered school climate in regard to immigrant-origin students found a particularly high number of incidents of bullying toward such students in schools with higher percentages of White students (Ee & Gándara, 2019). Whereas in recent years bullying has been directed at students of Latinx origin, in the context of the COVID-19 pandemic such behavior has been targeted at the Asian community (Tarvernise & Oppel, 2020).

The problematic school climates that these studies point to should give us pause. Developmental scientists (Immordino-Yang et al., 2019) and educators (Cohen et al., 2009) have brought together ample evidence demonstrating that school and class climate have important implications for social-emotional functioning, motivation, and learning. Social scientists are demonstrating what students, parents, principals, and good teachers have always known: a healthy classroom climate is essential for optimal learning. Yet educational settings are at the frontlines of toxic (un)civil conversations (Rogers et al., 2019) that compromise the opportunity to develop an optimal sense of belonging in the new land.

RECOMMENDATIONS FOR PRACTICE AND RESEARCH

As we strive to serve immigrant families and their children, we should be ready to effectively reach out as our code of ethics and common humanity demands (Chavez-Dueñas et al., 2019; Suárez-Orozco, 2018). Appropriate and effective treatment begins with an awareness of the specific needs of families and of children growing up in unauthorized households, and the multiple levels of stress and social exclusion to which they are exposed. Clearly, many of the issues faced by immigrant-origin families and their children are structurally imposed by current policies of the sociopolitical land-scape. Given these constraints, how should we help families and children best cope?

Service begins with understanding. At a minimum, a mental health prac-titioner should be well-versed in the issues these children and families are facing. We encourage practitioners to take stock of pre- and postmigration stressors as part of assessment. It should be recognized that it takes time to build trust. Service providers ought to be aware of the various forms of trauma immigrant-origin families frequently encounter as they have significant impli-cations for mental health (Potochnick & Perreira, 2010). A trauma-informed lens should be incorporated; cognitive-behavioral therapy (Kataoka et al., 2003), narrative exposure therapy (Schauer et al., 2005), as well as creative expression techniques (Rousseau et al., 2005) have all been documented to decrease trauma-related symptoms in immigrants.

Mental health practitioners should address not only individual and familial trauma but also the historical and structural systems of oppression impeding the healing process. By grounding treatment in the HEART (Healing Ethno and Racial Trauma) framework (Chavez-Dueñas et al., 2019), practitioners can build trust, increase safety, and foster healing by providing immigrant-origin families a "sanctuary space" to "acknowledge and reprocess" (Chavez-Dueñas et al., 2019, p. 56) trauma within a historical context. Such practices can allow these individuals and their families to reframe their struggles through a collective lens (Chavez et al., 2019).

Isolation is yet another toll paid by immigrants entering a hostile social milieu; as such, finding ways to recognize and nurture sources of social support is essential (APA Presidential Task Force on Immigration, 2012). The community cultural wealth (Yosso, 2005) of immigrant-origin families should be recognized by incorporating familial and community (including faith-based) support systems into treatment and service (APA Presidential Task Force on Immigration, 2012; Goodman et al., 2017). It is important to include culturally relevant elements to treatment and intervention including, for example, integrating storytelling, community ceremonies, and indigenous healing practices (Brabeck et al., 2015).

To disrupt symbolic exclusion and increase a sense of belonging among these children and youth, practitioners and educators should signal allyship. Much in the way the rainbow symbolizes allyship to the LGBTQ+ community, small acts like displaying a butterfly can signal solidarity. When planning to take action, it is important to center advocacy on the specific needs of those who are served (NILC, 2017).

While our field has made strides in shedding light on the experiences of children and youth growing up in unauthorized households, it remains unclear which interventions have the greatest potential to disrupt the negative psychological effects of growing up in a "deportation nation" (Kanstroom, 2007). Future research should aim to address the impacts of liminality, structural exclusion, and symbolic violence on psychological well-being.

Research should be designed not simply to document but also to move toward developing context-specific interventions centered on trauma-informed care (Chavez et al., 2019).

Conducting culturally competent research requires bicultural and bilingual proficiencies, as well as the inclusion of immigrant communities, at all stages (APA Presidential Task Force on Immigration, 2012; Rivas-Drake et al., 2016). Children and youth residing in undocumented families are a hard-to-reach population; community involvement is essential to develop—and sustain—trust for participation (Parrado et al., 2005). Moreover, research should be carried out with, and not simply about, participants of immigrant origins (Hernández et al., 2013). Unless the specific benefits or tangible outcomes of the research endeavor can be delineated, the indirect benefits claimed may be perceived as exaggerated at the least and as a form of benevolent racism at the worst (Hernández et al., 2013).

While this field calls for more research, the dangers of participating are quite naturally of concern to participants who are part of undocumented families. As such, our first duty as researchers is to "do no harm" (Hernández et al., 2013, p. 43). Conducting studies with participants (or their parents) at risk of detention and deportation requires protections well beyond those regularly in place, for an ethical stance must be implemented. Protecting the identities of vulnerable participants must include minimizing identifying information, implementing multiple data encryption strategies, and storing separate portions of data in secured sites (see Hernández et al., 2013). Researchers should employ a waiver of signed consent to limit links to personal information. Moreover, Certificates of Confidentiality administered by the National Institutes of Health (NIH) can protect the privacy of research subjects by shielding investigators and institutions from being compelled to release information that could be used to identify subjects (NIH, 2019). This strategy supports investigators who have access to research records to refuse to disclose identifying information in any civil, criminal, administrative, legislative, or other proceeding at the federal, state, or local level.

CONCLUSION

In short, these are deeply unsettling times for immigrant families. Many of our most vulnerable families and children are being conferred heightened stress and profound disadvantage by a series of exclusionary policies and practices. Exposure to traumatic, cumulative, acculturative, and transgenerational stress are all too often part of the immigrant experiences. Further, multiple forms of social exclusion, ranging from its most extreme form—deportation—to restriction of access to resources, toxic media messages, and everyday hostile racial and ethnic social encounters have troubling implications for social belonging. In this chapter, we provided insights into these issues and suggested steps for practice and research to address these needs.

REFERENCES

Abrego, L. J. (2014). *Sacrificing families: Navigating laws, labor, and love across borders.* Stanford University Press.

Alberto, C., & Chilton, M. (2019). Transnational violence against asylum-seeking women and children: Honduras and the United States-Mexico border. *Human Rights Review, 20*(2), 205–227. https://doi.org/10.1007/s12142-019-0547-5

American Psychological Association Presidential Task Force on Immigration. (2012). *Crossroads: The psychology of immigration in the new century.* https://www.apa.org/topics/immigration/immigration-report.pdf

Arikan, H. (2009). Racist violence attacks on foreigners, mass-media and fear of crime. In M. Guggisberg & D. Weir (Eds.), *Understanding violence: Context and portrayals* (pp. 45–61). Interdisciplinary Press.

Bahena, S. (2014). *Examining immigrant optimism among Latino youth using the Children's Hope Scale* [Unpublished doctoral dissertation]. Harvard Graduate School of Education.

Baker, B., & Marchevsky, A. (2019). Gendering deportation, policy violence, and Latino/a family precarity. *Latino Studies, 17*(2), 207–224. https://doi.org/10.1057/s41276-019-00176-0

Baumeister, R. F., & Leary, M. R. (1995). The need to belong: Desire for interpersonal attachments as a fundamental human motivation. *Psychological Bulletin, 117*(3), 497–529. https://doi.org/10.1037/0033-2909.117.3.497

Bean, F. D., Leach, M. A., Brown, S. K., Bachmeier, J. D., & Hipp, J. R. (2011). The educational legacy of unauthorized migration: Comparisons across U.S.-immigrant groups in how parents' status affects their offspring. *International Migration Review, 45*(2), 348–385. https://doi.org/10.1111/j.1747-7379.2011.00851.x

Bernhardt, A., Milkman, R., Theodore, N., Heckathorn, D., Auer, M., & DeFilipppi, J. (2009). *Broken laws, unprotected workers: Violations of employment and labor laws in America's cities.* National Employment Law Project.

Bernstein, H., Gonzalez, D., Karpman, M., & Zuckerman, S. (2019). *One in seven adults in immigrant families reported avoiding public benefit programs in 2018.* https://www.urban.org/research/publication/one-seven-adults-immigrant-families-reported-avoiding-public-benefit-programs-2018

Bourdieu, P., & Passeron, J.-C. (1977). *Reproduction in education, society, and culture* (2nd ed.). SAGE.

Brabeck, K., & Xu, Q. (2010). The impact of detention and deportation on Latino immigrant children and families: A quantitative exploration. *Hispanic Journal of Behavioral Sciences, 32*(3), 341–361. https://doi.org/10.1177/0739986310374053

Brabeck, K. M., Lykes, M. B., & Hunter, C. (2014). The psychosocial impact of detention and deportation on U.S. migrant children and families. *American Journal of Orthopsychiatry, 84*(5), 496–505. https://doi.org/10.1037/ort0000011

Brabeck, K. M., Porterfield, K., & Loughry, M. (2015). Psychosocial and mental health issues assessment and intervention for individual and families. In D. Kanstroom & M. B. Lykes (Eds.), *The new deportation delirium* (pp. 167–192). New York University Press.

Capps, R., Fix, M., & Zong, J. (2016). *A profile of US children with unauthorized immigrant parents.* Migration Policy Institute.

Cervantes, R. C., Padilla, A. M., & Salgado de Snyder, N. (1991). The Hispanic Stress Inventory: A culturally relevant approach to psychosocial assessment. *Psychological Assessment, 3*(3), 438–447. https://doi.org/10.1037/1040-3590.3.3.438

Chaudry, A., Capps, R., Pedroza, J. M., Castañeda, R. M., Santos, R., & Scott, M. M. (2010). *Facing our future: Children in the aftermath of immigration enforcement.* Urban Institute.

Chavez, L. R. (2013). *The Latino threat: Constructing immigrants, citizens, and the nation.* Stanford University Press.

Chavez, L. R., Campos, B., Corona, K., Sanchez, D., & Ruiz, C. B. (2019). Words hurt: Political rhetoric, emotions/affect, and psychological well-being among Mexican-origin youth. *Social Science & Medicine, 228,* 240–251. https://doi.org/10.1016/j.socscimed.2019.03.008

Chavez-Dueñas, N. Y., Adames, H. Y., Perez-Chavez, J. G., & Salas, S. P. (2019). Healing ethno-racial trauma in Latinx immigrant communities: Cultivating hope, resistance, and action. *American Psychologist, 74*(1), 49–62. https://doi.org/10.1037/amp0000289

Child Trends. (2013). *Immigrant children: Indicators on children and youth.* https://www.childtrends.org/?indicators=immigrant-children

Cockersell, P. (2018). Compound trauma and complex needs. In P. Cockersell (Ed.), *Social exclusion, Compound trauma and recovery* (pp. 27–36). Jessica Kingsley.

Cohen, J., McCabe, L., Michelli, N. M., & Pickeral, T. (2009). School climate: Research, policy, practice, and teacher education. *Teachers College Record, 111*(1), 180–213.

Comas-Díaz, L., Hall, G. N., & Neville, H. A. (2019). Racial trauma: Theory, research, and healing: Introduction to the special issue. *American Psychologist, 74*(1), 1–5. https://doi.org/10.1037/amp0000442

Crisp, B. R. (2010). Belonging, connectedness and social exclusion. *Journal of Social Inclusion, 1*(2), 123–132. https://doi.org/10.36251/josi.14

Crosnoe, R. (2007). Early child care and the school readiness of children from Mexican immigrant families. *International Migration Review, 41*(1), 152–181. https://doi.org/10.1111/j.1747-7379.2007.00060.x

Delva, J., Horner, P., Martinez, R., Sanders, L., Lopez, W. D., & Doering-White, J. (2013). Mental health problems of children of undocumented parents in the United States: A hidden crisis. *Journal of Community Positive Practices, 13*(3), 25–35.

Dinh, K. T., & Nguyen, H. H. (2006). The effects of acculturative variables on Asian American parent–child relationships. *Journal of Social and Personal Relationships, 23*(3), 407–426. https://doi.org/10.1177/0265407506064207

Dreby, J. (2012). The burden of deportation on children in Mexican immigrant families. *Journal of Marriage and the Family, 74*(4), 829–845. https://doi.org/10.1111/j.1741-3737.2012.00989.x

Durand, J., & Massey, D. S. (Eds.). (2004). *Crossing the border: Research from the Mexican migration project.* Russell Sage Foundation.

Ee, J., & Gándara, P. (2019). The impact of immigration enforcement on the nation's schools. *American Educational Research Journal, 57*(2), 840–871. https://doi.org/10.3102/0002831219862998

Enriquez, L. E. (2015). Multigenerational punishment: Shared experiences of undocumented immigration status within mixed-status families. *Journal of Marriage and the Family, 77*(4), 939–953. https://doi.org/10.1111/jomf.12196

Fagan, J., & MacDonald, J. (2013). Policing, crime, and legitimacy in New York and Los Angeles: The social and political contexts of two historic crime declines. In D. Halle & A. A. Beveridge (Eds.), *New York and Los Angeles: The uncertain future.* Oxford University Press.

Fangen, K. (2010). Social exclusion and inclusion of young immigrants: Presentation of an analytical framework. *Young, 18*(2), 133–156. https://doi.org/10.1177/110330881001800202

Fazel, M., Reed, R. V., Panter-Brick, C., & Stein, A. (2012). Mental health of displaced and refugee children resettled in high-income countries: Risk and protective factors. *The Lancet, 379*(9812), 266–282. https://doi.org/10.1016/S0140-6736(11)60051-2

Gonzales, R., Suárez-Orozco, C., & Dedios-Sanguineti, M. C. (2013). No place to belong: Contextualizing concepts of mental health among undocumented immigrant youth in the United States. *American Behavioral Scientist, 57*(8), 1174–1199. https://doi.org/10.1177/0002764213487349

200 Suárez-Orozco, López Hernández, and Cabral

Gonzales, R. G., Ellis, B., Rendón-García, S. A., & Brant, K. (2018). (Un)authorized transitions: Illegality, DACA, and the life course. *Research in Human Development, 15*(3–4), 345–359. https://doi.org/10.1080/15427609.2018.1502543

Goodman, R. D., Vesely, C. K., Letiecq, B., & Cleaveland, C. L. (2017). Trauma and resilience among refugee and undocumented immigrant women. *Journal of Counseling and Development, 95*(3), 309–321. https://doi.org/10.1002/jcad.12145

Hagan, J., Levi, R., & Dinovitzer, R. (2008). The symbolic violence of the crime-immigration nexus: Migrant mythologies in the Americas. *Criminology & Public Policy, 7*(1), 95–112. https://doi.org/10.1111/j.1745-9133.2008.00493.x

Hernández, M. G., Nguyen, J., Casanova, S., Suárez-Orozco, C., & Saetermoe, C. L. (2013). Doing no harm and getting it right: Guidelines for ethical research with immigrant communities. *New Directions for Child and Adolescent Development, 2013*(141), 43–60. https://doi.org/10.1002/cad.20042

Hirschfeld Davis, J., & Preston, J. (2016). *What Donald Trump's vow to deport up to 3 million immigrants would mean.* https://www.nytimes.com/2016/11/15/us/politics/donald-trump-deport-immigrants.html

Hobfoll, S. E. (1991). Traumatic stress: A theory based on rapid loss of resources. *Anxiety Research, 4*(3), 187–197. https://doi.org/10.1080/08917779108248773

Immordino-Yang, M. H., Darling-Hammond, L., & Krone, C. R. (2019). Nurturing nature: How brain development is inherently social and emotional, and what this means for education. *Educational Psychologist, 54*(3), 185–204. https://doi.org/10.1080/00461520.2019.1633924

Kanstroom, D. (2007). *Deportation nation: Outsiders in American history.* Harvard University Press.

Kao, G., & Tienda, M. (1995). Optimism and achievement: The educational performance of immigrant youth. *Social Science Quarterly, 76*(1), 1–19.

Kataoka, S. H., Stein, B. D., Jaycox, L. H., Wong, M., Escudero, P., Tu, W., Zaragoza, C., & Fink, A. (2003). A school-based mental health program for traumatized Latino immigrant children. *Journal of the American Academy of Child & Adolescent Psychiatry, 42*(3), 311–318. https://doi.org/10.1097/00004583-200303000-00011

Koball, H., Capps, R., Perreira, K., Campetella, A., Hooker, S., Pedroza, J. M., Monson, W., & Huerta, S. (2015). *Health and social service needs of US-citizen children with detained or deported immigrant parents.* Urban Institute.

Krogstad, J. M., & Passel, J. (2015). *Five facts about illegal immigration in the United States.* Pew Research Center. http://www.pewresearch.org/facttank/2015/11/19/5-facts-about-illegal-immigration-inthe-u-s/

Kulish, N., Yee, V., Dickerson, C., Robbins, L., Santos, F., & Medinca, J. (2017, February 21). Trump's immigration policies explained. *The New York Times.* https://www.nytimes.com/2017/02/21/us/trump-immigration-policies-deportation.html?_r=0

Lamont, M. (2018). Addressing recognition gaps: Destigmatization and the reduction of inequality. *American Sociological Review, 83*(3), 419–444. https://doi.org/10.1177/0003122418773775

Lamont, M., Silva, G. M., Welburn, J., Guetzkow, J., Mizrachi, N., Herzog, H., & Reis, E. (2016). *Getting respect: Responding to stigma and discrimination in the United States, Brazil, and Israel.* Princeton University Press. https://doi.org/10.2307/j.ctv346qr9

Lee, S. J., Wong, N.-W. A., & Alvarez, A. N. (2009). The model minority and the perpetual foreigner: Stereotypes of Asian Americans. In N. Tewari & A. N. Alvarez (Eds.), *Asian American psychology: Current perspectives* (pp. 69–84). Routledge/Taylor & Francis Group.

Liptak, A., & Shear, M. D. (2020, June 18). Trump can't immediately end DACA, Supreme Court rules. *The New York Times.* https://www.nytimes.com/2020/06/18/us/trump-daca-supreme-court.html

Lovato, K., Lopez, C., Karimli, L., & Abrams, L. S. (2018, December). The impact of deportation-related family separations on the well-being of Latinx children and youth: A review of the literature. *Children and Youth Services Review, 95,* 109–116. https://doi.org/10.1016/j.childyouth.2018.10.011

Maslow, A. H. (1943). A theory of human motivation. *Psychological Review, 50*(4), 370–396. https://doi.org/10.1037/h0054346

Menjívar, C. (2006). Liminal legality: Salvadoran and Guatemalan immigrants' lives in the United States. *American Journal of Sociology, 111*(4), 999–1037. https://doi.org/10.1086/499509

Menjívar, C., & Abrego, D. (2009). Parents and children across borders. In N. Foner (Ed.), *Across generations: Immigrant families in America* (pp. 160–189). NYU Press.

Menjívar, C., Gómez Cervantes, A., & Alvord, D. (2018). The expansion of "crimmigration," mass detention, and deportation. *Sociology Compass, 12*(4), 1–15. https://doi.org/10.1111/soc4.12573

Menjívar, C., & Perreira, K. M. (2019). Undocumented and unaccompanied: Children of migration in the European Union and the United States. *Journal of Ethnic and Migration Studies, 45*(2), 197–217. https://doi.org/10.1080/1369183X.2017.1404255

Mexican American Legal Defense and Educational Fund. (2014). *Detention, deportation, and devastation: The disproportionate effect of deportations of the Latino community.* https://www.maldef.org/assets/pdf/DDD_050614.pdf

National Immigration Law Center (NILC). (2017). *Tips on how to be a better ally for the immigrants' rights cause.* https://www.nilc.org/news/the-torch/12-8-17/

National Institutes of Health (NIH). (2019). *Certificates of confidentiality (CoC): Human subjects.* https://grants.nih.gov/policy/humansubjects/coc.htm

National Public Radio. (2016). *Attendance drops at Maryland high school, as deportation fears rise.* https://www.npr.org/2016/01/17/463405722/attendance-drops-at-maryland-high-school-as-deportation-fears-rise

Navid, S., & Nicholson, J. (2019). *Creating trauma informed learning environments.* Mid-Atlantic Comprehensive Center at WestEd. https://www.wested.org/resources/trauma-informed-learning-environments/

Ortega, A. N., Fang, H., Perez, V. H., Rizzo, J. A., Carter-Pokras, O., Wallace, S. P., & Gelberg, L. (2007). Health care access, use of services, and experiences among undocumented Mexicans and other Latinos. *Archives of Internal Medicine, 167*(21), 2354–2360. https://doi.org/10.1001/archinte.167.21.2354

Osei-Twumasi, O., & López-Hernández, G. (2019). Resilience in the face of adversity: Undocumented students in community colleges. In C. Suárez-Orozco & O. Osei-Twumasi (Eds.), *Immigrant-origin students in community college: Navigating risk and reward in higher education.* Teacher's College Press.

Parrado, E. A., Flippen, C. A., & McQuiston, C. (2005). Migration and relationship power among Mexican women. *Demography, 42*(2), 347–372. https://doi.org/10.1353/dem.2005.0016

Perez, W., Espinoza, R., Ramos, K., Coronado, H. M., & Cortes, R. (2009). Academic resilience among undocumented Latino students. *Hispanic Journal of Behavioral Sciences, 31*(2), 149–181. https://doi.org/10.1177/0739986309333020

Pew Research Center. (2019). *What's happening at the U.S.-Mexico border in 6 charts.* https://www.pewresearch.org/fact-tank/2019/04/10/whats-happening-at-the-u-s-mexico-border-in-6-charts/

Portes, A., & Rumbaut, R. G. (2006). *Immigrant America: A portrait.* University of California Press.

Potochnick, S. R., & Perreira, K. M. (2010). Depression and anxiety among first-generation immigrant Latino youth: Key correlates and implications for future research. *Journal of Nervous and Mental Disease, 198*(7), 470–477. https://doi.org/10.1097/NMD.0b013e3181e4ce24

Pyke, K. (2005). "Generational deserters" and "black sheep": Acculturative differences among siblings in Asian immigrant families. *Journal of Family Issues, 26*(4), 491–517.

Ralph J. Bunche Center for African American Studies. (2004). Separate but certainly not equal: 2003 CAPAA findings. *Bunche Research Report.* https://bunchecenterdev. pre.ss.ucla.edu/wp-content/uploads/sites/97/2011/09/UCLA-Bunche-Research-Report-2004.pdf

Rivas-Drake, D., Camacho, T. C., & Guillaume, C. (2016). Just good developmental science: Trust, identity, and responsibility in ethnic minority recruitment and retention. *Advances in Child Development and Behavior, 50,* 161–188. https://doi.org/10.1016/bs.acdb.2015.11.002

Rogers, J., Ishimoto, M., Kwako, A., Berryman, A., & Diera, C. (2019). *School and society in the age of Trump.* UCLA's Institute for Democracy, Education, and Access. https://idea.gseis.ucla.edu/publications/school-and-society-in-age-of-trump/

Rosenblum, M. R., & Meissner, D. (2015). *The deportation dilemma: Reconciling tough and humane enforcement.* Migration Policy Institute.

Rousseau, C., Drapeau, A., Lacroix, L., Bagilishya, D., & Heusch, N. (2005). Evaluation of a classroom program of creative expression workshops for refugee and immigrant children. *Journal of Child Psychology and Psychiatry, and Allied Disciplines, 46*(2), 180–185. https://doi.org/10.1111/j.1469-7610.2004.00344.x

Sáenz, R., & Manges Douglas, K. (2015). A call for the racialization of immigration studies: On the transition of ethnic immigrants to racialized immigrants. *Sociology of Race and Ethnicity, 1*(1), 166–180. https://doi.org/10.1177/2332649214559287

Saldaña, M., Cueva Chacón, L. M., & García-Perdomo, V. (2018). When gaps become *huuuuge*: Donald Trump and beliefs about immigration. *Mass Communication and Society, 21*(6), 785–813. https://doi.org/10.1080/15205436.2018.1504304

Schauer, M., Neuner, F., & Elbert, T. (2005). *Narrative exposure therapy: A short-term intervention for traumatic stress disorders after war, terror, or torture.* Hogrefe & Huber.

Schwab, G. (2010). *Haunting legacies: Violent histories and transgenerational trauma.* Columbia University Press.

Shonkoff, J. P., Garner, A. S., The Committee on Psychosocial Aspects of Child and Family Health, The Committee on Early Childhood, Adoption, and Dependent Care, The Section on Developmental and Behavioral Pediatrics, Siegel, B. S., Dobbins, M. I., Earls, M. F., McGuinn, L., Pascoe, J., & Wood, D. (2012). The lifelong effects of early childhood adversity and toxic stress. *Pediatrics, 129*(1), e232–e246.

Simon, R. J., & Alexander, S. H. (1993). *The ambivalent welcome: Print media, public opinion, and immigration.* Praeger.

Suárez-Orozco, C. (2017). Conferring disadvantage: Behavioral and developmental implications for children growing up in the shadow of undocumented immigration status. *Journal of Developmental & Behavioral Pediatrics, 38*(6), 424–428. https://doi.org/10.1097/DBP.0000000000000462

Suárez-Orozco, C. (2018). Ecologies of care: Addressing the needs of immigrant origin children and youth. *Journal of Global Ethics, 14*(1), 47–53. https://doi.org/10.1080/17449626.2018.1496348

Suárez-Orozco, C., Abo-Zena, M. M., & Marks, A. K. (Eds.). (2015). *Transitions: The development of children of immigrants.* NYU Press.

Suárez-Orozco, C., Bang, H. J., & Kim, H. Y. (2011). I felt like my heart was staying behind: Psychological implications of family separations and reunifications for immigrant youth. *Journal of Adolescent Research, 26*(2), 222–257. https://doi.org/10.1177/0743558410376830

Suárez-Orozco, C., & Suárez-Orozco, M. M. (2001). *Children of immigration.* Harvard University Press. https://doi.org/10.2307/j.ctvjz82j9

Suárez-Orozco, C., Suárez-Orozco, M. M., & Todorova, I. (2008). *Learning a new land: Educational pathways of immigrant youth.* Harvard University Press.

Suárez-Orozco, C., Yoshikawa, H., Teranishi, T., & Suárez-Orozco, M. (2011). Growing up in the shadows: The developmental implications of unauthorized status. *Harvard Educational Review, 81*(3), 438–472. https://doi.org/10.17763/haer.81.3.g23x203763783m75

Taket, A., Crisp, B. R., Nevill, A., Lamaro, G., Graham, M., & Barter-Godfrey, S. (Eds.). (2009). *Theorising social exclusion*. Routledge. https://doi.org/10.4324/9780203874646

Tarvernise, S., & Oppel, R. A. (2020, March 23). Spit on, yelled at, attacked: Chinese Americans fear for their safety. *The New York Times*. https://www.nytimes.com/2020/03/23/us/chinese-coronavirus-racist-attacks.html

Tienda, M., & Mitchell, F. (2006). E Pluribus Plures or E Pluribus Unum? In M. Tienda & F. Mitchell (Eds.), *Hispanics and the future of America* (p. 1). National Academies Press.

Urban Institute for the National Council of La Raza (NCLR). (2007). *Paying the price: The impact of immigration raids on America's children*. https://www.urban.org/sites/default/files/publication/46811/411566-Paying-the-Price-The-Impact-of-Immigration-Raids-on-America-s-Children.PDF

U.S. Citizenship and Immigration Services. (2019). *Temporary protected status*. https://www.uscis.gov/humanitarian/temporary-protected-status

U.S. Immigration and Customs Enforcement. (2018). *Fiscal year 2018 ICE enforcement and removal operations report*. https://www.ice.gov/doclib/about/offices/ero/pdf/eroFY2018Report.pdf

van der Kolk, B. A. (2015). *The body keeps the score: Brain, mind, and body in the healing of trauma*. Penguin Books.

Vizek-Vidović, V., Kuterovac-Jagodić, G., & Arambasić, L. (2000). Posttraumatic symptomatology in children exposed to war. *Scandinavian Journal of Psychology*, *41*(4), 297–306. https://doi.org/10.1111/1467-9450.00202

Walton, G. M., & Cohen, G. L. (2007). A question of belonging: Race, social fit, and achievement. *Journal of Personality and Social Psychology*, *92*(1), 82–96. https://doi.org/10.1037/0022-3514.92.1.82

Warren, R., & Kerwin, D. (2017). The 2,000 mile wall in search of a purpose: Since 2007 visa overstays have outnumbered undocumented border crossers by a half million. *Journal on Migration and Human Security*, *5*(1), 124–136. https://doi.org/10.1177/233150241700500107

Wessler, S. (2011). *Shattered families: The perilous intersection of the immigration enforcement and child welfare system*. Applied Research Center.

Wimmer, A. (1997). Explaining xenophobia and racism: A critical review of current research approaches. *Ethnic and Racial Studies*, *20*(1), 17–41. https://doi.org/10.1080/01419870.1997.9993946

Yoshikawa, H. (2011). *Immigrants raising citizens: Undocumented parents and their children*. Russell Sage Foundation.

Yoshikawa, H., Suárez-Orozco, C., & Gonzales, R. G. (2017). Unauthorized status and youth development in the United States: Consensus statement of the Society for Research on Adolescence. *Journal of Research on Adolescence*, *27*(1), 4–19. https://doi.org/10.1111/jora.12272

Yoshikawa, H., Weisner, T. S., & Lowe, E. (Eds.). (2006). *Making it work: Low-wage employment, family life and child development*. Russell Sage.

Yosso, T. J. (2005). Whose culture has capital? A critical race theory discussion of community cultural wealth. *Race, Ethnicity and Education*, *8*(1), 69–91. https://doi.org/10.1080/1361332052000341006

Zong, J., Batalova, J., & Burrows, M. (2019). *Frequently requested statistics on immigrants and immigration in the United States*. Migration Policy Institute.

11

Interpersonal Violence and the Immigrant Context

Pratyusha Tummala-Narra

Alicia is a 48-year-old Bolivian American heterosexual, cisgender woman who emigrated from Bolivia to the United States as an adolescent, along with her older sister.[1] She was sexually assaulted twice, once by a relative in Bolivia and once by a stranger a few months before seeking help from a physician to cope with headaches. She did not disclose her sexual violations to her parents or sister. She confided in her adult daughter about being raped by a stranger, and her daughter encouraged her to meet with a physician, who then referred her to work with me in psychotherapy. When I met Alicia, she stated, "There is no way that I could have told my parents and no way for me to speak. I'm alive but I don't always feel like it. I just survive for my daughter. She needs me." Alicia's daughter attends college near their home and worries about her mother's deteriorating physical health and sadness. In her sessions, Alicia began to share her anxiety and sadness about her trauma, and her sense of fear and hopelessness about the dangerous environment in which her daughter lives. She stated, "I came here with my sister so that we don't have to live in an unsafe place, but now everything here is unsafe," referring to the rise in explicit xenophobia and misogyny in the United States. Sadly, Alicia is among many others whose traumatic stress based in interpersonal violence has been exacerbated in the current sociopolitical climate.

Interpersonal violence, such as childhood physical and sexual abuse, rape, and intimate partner violence (IPV), is a global crisis. Among racial minority

---

[1]All case material has been altered to protect confidentiality.

https://doi.org/10.1037/0000214-012
Trauma and Racial Minority Immigrants: Turmoil, Uncertainty, and Resistance,
P. Tummala-Narra (Editor)

immigrants in the United States, little attention has been directed to specific types of interpersonal violence, such as sexual abuse and assault, and how these experiences interact with other types of oppression, among them xenophobia, racism, homophobia, and poverty. Further, there is virtually no literature that addresses subgroups of immigrant survivors, for example, male survivors and LGBTQ survivors. Nevertheless, racial minority immigrant-origin survivors of interpersonal violence face unique challenges, as they navigate stress within multiple sociocultural contexts.

This chapter focuses on experiences of interpersonal violence that many immigrants face within their communities and in broader U.S. society, from the lens of socioecological and multicultural perspectives (American Psychological Association, 2012; Clauss-Ehlers et al., 2019; Comas-Díaz, 2012; García Coll & Marks, 2012). The socioecological framework, recently extended to the integrative contextual framework of minority youth development, emphasizes the importance of social position factors such as race, gender, immigration status, and social class as instrumental to either promoting or inhibiting individual growth and psychological well-being (García Coll & Marks, 2012). Multicultural psychologists have drawn attention to the role of culture, social location, and racial and ethnopolitical trauma in the experiences of immigrants and racial minorities. In this chapter, I provide an overview of (a) the prevalence of interpersonal violence, (b) factors pertaining to the conceptualization of interpersonal violence, (c) multiple marginalization occurring in families, (d) ethnic and/or religious communities and in the mainstream U.S. context, (e) the psychological impact of violence, and (f) the process of securing help in the aftermath of trauma. The chapter also includes a brief case vignette and recommendations for research and practice, with an emphasis on the coexistence of traumatic stress and resilience among survivors who face marginalization in multiple contexts, and a recognition of the heterogeneity of experience within and across different cultural groups. It is important to note that while this chapter focuses on the experiences of racial minority immigrant-origin survivors in the United States, it does so with a conscious effort to avoid any assumptions of interpersonal violence as a "cultural problem" specific to particular cultural groups. Rather, the global pervasiveness of interpersonal violence is the backdrop to a closer inquiry into the unique experiences of racial minority immigrant-origin survivors.

PREVALENCE AND CONTEXT OF INTERPERSONAL VIOLENCE

Amidst the COVID-19 outbreak, recent reports have noted that there has been a national and global rise in interpersonal violence, such as IPV and child abuse, which has been linked to various sources of stress These include loss of employment, financial hardship, school closures, confinement to physical spaces with perpetrators, limited social support and loss of social networks, and increased mental health and substance abuse problems (American

Psychological Association, 2020). There have also been increasing reports of interpersonal violence to crisis hotlines and in some cases, survivors of IPV have been reporting abuse using code words to staff in their local pharmacies. Further, there are fewer supports accessible to the most vulnerable survivors of interpersonal violence, such as undocumented immigrants who fear seeking help. Many racial minority immigrant survivors, families, and loved ones are also coping with illness, as hospitalizations and fatalities due to COVID-19 are disproportionately high among racial minorities (Centers for Disease Control and Prevention, 2020). As such, the COVID-19 outbreak has exacerbated the existing crisis levels of interpersonal trauma within a national and global context rife with economic, social, and health/health care disparities.

Before the COVID-19 outbreak, few studies examined the prevalence of sexual violence among various racial and ethnic minority communities in the United States. However, some research does indicate a high degree of interpersonal violence experienced by racial minority immigrant-origin women who are first generation (i.e., those arriving as adults) and second generation (i.e., those born and raised in the country). For example, estimates of IPV faced by immigrant women in Latina/x, Filipina/o, South Asian, and Korean communities have ranged from 30% to 50%, compared with 22.1% in the general U.S. population (Ammar et al., 2014; Choi, 2015). The prevalence of IPV reported by women of South Asian origin (Indian, Pakistani, Bangladeshi, Bhutanese, Nepalese, Sri Lankan) in the United States has ranged from 21% to more than 40% (Yoshihama et al., 2012). Despite higher educational levels and household incomes among many South Asians, particularly Indian Americans and Pakistani Americans, there are relatively high levels of interpersonal violence within these communities (Nagaraj et al., 2018). In one study of 368 South Asians in the United States, 25.2% of the sample reported experiencing childhood sexual abuse, 41.2% witnessed parental violence, 24% reported relationship violence, and participants who reported any relationship violence were more likely to have been victimized by sexual abuse in childhood (Robertson et al., 2016).

Research on interpersonal violence experienced by Latinas has also been emerging. According to some studies, over half of Latina women reported experiencing some form of victimization, such as physical violence, sexual assault, and stalking at some point in their lives (Cuevas et al., 2012), and Latinas are reported to experience IPV at higher rates than White women (Kyriakakis et al., 2012). Differences may also exist in the prevalence of victimization across immigrant generation. Some research suggests that Latina immigrant women report lower rates of being victimized by interpersonal violence when compared with U.S.-born Latina women. However, barriers related to language fluency, lack of economic resources, and documentation status may influence whether immigrant women report interpersonal violence (Zadnik et al., 2016).

It is important to note that racial minority immigrant-origin women (first and later generations) have been found to be less likely to report experiences of sexual violence when compared with White American women, contributing to the challenge of gathering accurate data on the prevalence of sexual violence. Further, limited literature exists concerning certain types of interpersonal violence such as sexual violence, and virtually no literature concerning interpersonal violence experienced by racial minority immigrant men and LGBTQ immigrants. No formal studies are yet available regarding the impact of COVID-19 on reports of sexual violence among racial minority immigrants, although reports of interpersonal violence have been on the rise among the general U.S. population. An additional gap in the literature concerns interpersonal violence that occurs in the premigration context and how immigrants experience, conceptualize, and respond to violence in both pre- and postmigration contexts. The impact of such violence can be pervasive, affecting mental and physical health across generations. As such, in the remainder of the chapter, I explore how various factors interplay in the experience of interpersonal violence among racial minority immigrants, including conceptualizations of violence, marginalization associated with violence, and the psychological impact of violence.

CONCEPTUALIZATIONS OF INTERPERSONAL VIOLENCE

Most of the literature in psychology concerning interpersonal violence, such as sexual abuse, rape, and IPV, reflects the perspectives of White, middle-class women. Therefore, the ways in which interpersonal violence is defined and conceptualized in psychology is largely embedded in White, Euro-American cultural values and norms. Both socioecological and multicultural perspectives (Bronfenbrenner, 1994; Comas-Díaz, 2012; García Coll & Marks, 2012) underscore the interplay of sociocultural context and individual histories in the experience of interpersonal violence. Specifically, García Coll and Marks (2012) described the role of social position factors, such as race, gender, and ethnicity, and how they interact with different contexts to shape development and mental health in ways that promote or inhibit this growth. Among many immigrants and subsequent generations, these social position factors shape conceptualizations of what constitutes abuse and violence, their decisions to disclose their experiences to others and seek help, and the ways in which they engage in healing. As there are no monolithic groups or communities of immigrants, it is critical to explore differences in conceptualizations of sexual violence within specific subgroups, such as those based on national origin, gender, and immigrant generation (e.g., first generation, second generation).

A few recent studies have examined the influence of cultural norms on how women from different cultural backgrounds understand IPV. For example, Asian American and South Asian American women have been found to be less likely than White women to categorize certain interpersonal interactions as constituting domestic violence or abuse. In one recent study of South Asian Americans, women conceptualized physical abuse as a type of sexual abuse, even though men and women had similar perceptions of what defines other aspects of sexual abuse (Ahmad et al., 2017). Scholars have noted that gender ideology rooted in a particular cultural context shapes how survivors conceptualize, experience, and respond to violence (Kallivayalil, 2010; Tummala-Narra et al., 2019). For example, a belief in karma, or the idea that suffering results from one's own past actions, may shape a survivor's understanding of who is responsible for the victimization, the survivor, or the perpetrator (Kallivayalil, 2010).

In a qualitative study of nineteen 1.5- and second-generation Indian American women (Tummala-Narra et al., 2019), contextual factors such as socialization within family and ethnic and religious communities, and acculturative stress, influenced participants' perspectives and experiences of sexual violence, as well as their responses to violence. In particular, these women described the importance of adhering to family and community-based expectations regarding gender roles and sexual behavior, including the expectation that women should uphold family unity, even when victimized by sexual violence. They also indicated a lack of discussion about violence within families and communities, and the challenge of identifying sexual violence in the context of silence and stigma associated with it. Further, cultural values and norms that shape conceptualizations of sexual violence in the premigration context continue to have intergenerational impact across subsequent generations of survivors of interpersonal violence. This stems from families' socializing their children with beliefs about violence rooted in the heritage culture and context. For example, in Tummala-Narra et al.'s (2019) study, parents' silence on sexual violence reflected a broader cultural stigma regarding open discussions about sex and violence in the Indian context. Yet, 1.5- and second-generation participants indicated that their conceptualizations of sexual violence were shaped through interactions both within and outside of their families (e.g., school, friends). The study also highlighted how women within the same family and the same immigrant generation can have distinct conceptualizations of sexual violence. Specifically, one participant described her experience of genital cutting as mutilation and violence, whereas her sister and other women in her family defined genital cutting as an accepted cultural and religious practice. This is an example of how individuals may define sexual violence in unique ways and of the complexity of developing a uniform definition of violence and abuse within any particular immigrant cultural group.

Cultural values and norms concerning gender, sexuality, and violence can also be used by perpetrators to exploit and abuse others within a given ethnic and/or religious community (Kyriakakis et al., 2012). As immigration often entails a sense of loss of a familiar cultural background along with a negative or hostile reception within the mainstream context, the need to adhere to cultural norms may intensify. This may place individuals in vulnerable positions in which upholding cultural norms rooted in the country of origin may become more prominent. In a qualitative study of Mexican immigrant survivors of IPV (Kyriakakis et al., 2012), cultural values and norms guided how women made meaning of their experiences of IPV. The findings revealed how women may come to view sexual abuse as a common or normal (although not acceptable) part of marriage, even while they recognized the negative emotional impact of the abuse.

The findings are not unique to Mexican immigrant women, but rather speak to the experiences of many racial minority immigrant survivors who face isolation within and outside of their families and communities. Survivors with disabilities can be especially vulnerable, as they may cope with stigma and isolation related to disability status and interpersonal violence. It is also important to note that the literature has historically associated interpersonal violence with a particular culture, cultural group, or cultural values, and therefore constructed violence within racial minority communities as a "cultural problem." However, interpersonal violence is a global problem, and violence contradicts values core to cultural and/or religious identity such as the value placed on respecting women or of caring for the most vulnerable. Rather than isolating violence as "cultural," emerging research suggests that it is critical to consider the unique ways in which immigrant and mainstream contexts shape the ways survivors experience and cope with trauma. There are also notable variations in how survivors deal with this trauma within broader cultural groups, for example, Latinx, Asian, Middle Eastern/North African, and Black immigrants (Tummala-Narra et al., 2019).

In addition to exploring variations in experiences of interpersonal violence within specific immigrant cultural groups, it is also important to consider differences across gender. Existing research indicates that one in four girls and one in six boys are sexually abused before the age of 18. On college campuses, one in five women and one in 16 men report being sexually assaulted, and over 90% of sexual assault cases are not reported (National Sexual Violence Resource Center, 2018). The experiences of men and gender nonconforming immigrants are largely invisible within psychology and other mental health disciplines. There is a paucity of research concerning IPV experienced by men and almost all of the research with male survivors of sexual abuse has been conducted primarily with White cisgender men. However, a recent study (French et al., 2019) examining sexual victimization among a racially diverse sample of 284 high school boys and college men found no differences in the prevalence of sexual victimization among White adolescents/men and adolescents/men of color. A total of 83% of adolescent boys/men reporting sexual victimization indicated that women were perpetrators in at least one incident. These findings call for a closer examination of socialization and sociocultural expectations that may interfere with inquiry and an accurate understanding of interpersonal violence.

Traditional masculine norms—for instance, a focus on competition and winning, self-reliance, and emotional control—interact with factors such as family dynamics, traumatic events, immigration, racial identity, and socioeconomic status to shape the extent to which a person conforms to gender role norms (Easton et al., 2016). In the case of sexual violence, many male survivors feel that is it not masculine to be seen as a victim, and struggle with issues of shame, stigma, and homophobia. For some men, a hypermasculine exterior defends against feelings of inadequacy. These sociocultural expectations of men are mirrored and reinforced in the broader U.S. context, and are even evident in clinical practice. In fact, studies indicate that male and female practitioners often dismiss the significance of gender role socialization and stereotypes in their work with male clients who are perceived as aggressive or abusive by nature, or shamed for having dependency needs (Mahalik et al., 2012). In a study concerning helpful and harmful practices with boys and men among practitioners, Mahalik and colleagues (2012) noted the problem of gender bias among some clinicians who refused to inquire about histories of trauma among male clients, as these clinicians assumed that men were really not victimized. The researchers highlighted the problem of assessing men's psychological distress in a standard clinical language that neglected the ways in which many men communicate their emotions (e.g., metaphor, humor). This research is consistent with men's experiences of calling suicide prevention hotlines and rape crisis hotlines and not being taken seriously, as clinicians may dismiss or minimize their victimization. As mentioned previously, the problem of silence about male victimization is largely unexplored among immigrant and racial minority men in the United States, contributing to unrecognized traumatic stress.

MULTIPLE MARGINALIZATIONS

Many immigrants and their children face multiple forms of trauma and marginalization that interact with and compound the negative effects of interpersonal violence. From a socioecological perspective (García Coll & Marks, 2012; Harvey, 2007), it is critical to examine the various contexts in which violence occurs, and how these contexts bear mutual influence on the well-being of survivors. The premigration context is important to consider, as immigrants may have experienced trauma, such as childhood abuse, IPV, or political violence, before leaving their countries of origin. For instance, studies indicate that approximately half of children in India experience sexual abuse, and that approximately 69% of Indian children are victimized by physical, mental, or emotional abuse, with more boys facing physical abuse compared with girls (Kanukollu & Mahalingam, 2011). With regard to sexual orientation and gender identity, Morales (2013) noted that a majority of murders of LGBT people in the world have been occurring in Latin American countries, with the vast majority of violent acts directed against gay men and transgender people. In the case of political trauma, exposure to premigration political violence among nonrefugee immigrants ranges from 11% to 69% (Gupta et al., 2009). Further, immigrant men who have experienced political violence in their countries of origin have been found to be more likely than men with no such exposure to perpetrate violence against a female partner (Gupta et al., 2009).

Relatedly, exposure to natural disasters such as earthquakes can contribute to higher rates of violence against women in both pre- and postmigration contexts (Campbell et al., 2016).

It is well documented that some immigrants experience physical and sexual violence on the journey to their destination country (American Psychological Association, 2012). Violence that occurs in transit is often connected with how immigrants travel and the length of their voyages (Kaltman et al., 2011). The trauma that occurs in the course of one's journey can play a critical role in how individuals adjust to living in the United States. In some cases, violence experienced in the premigration context or in transit is reproduced in the postmigration context. For example, LGBTQ immigrants may be targeted for violence within any of these different contexts (Cerezo et al., 2014). It is also important to note that trauma that occurs across multiple contexts can result in complex traumatic stress (Herman, 1992), affecting subsequent generations (i.e., children of immigrants).

In the postmigration context, racial minority immigrants and their children face discrimination based on race, ethnicity, gender, authorization/documentation status, religion, social class, sexual orientation, and dis/ability status. In a recent study (Garcini et al., 2018), undocumented Mexican immigrants' experiences of interpersonal discrimination (e.g., that occurring in everyday interpersonal interactions) based on their undocumented status was the strongest predictor of clinically significant emotional distress. The findings also indicated that men were more likely than women to experience interpersonal discrimination due to undocumented status, and that undocumented immigrants who lived in the United States for more than a decade and experienced interpersonal discrimination due to undocumented status were significantly more likely to have clinically significant psychological distress. Additionally, undocumented immigrants with histories of trauma perceived interpersonal discrimination as more stressful and were more likely to have clinically significant psychological distress. These findings (Garcini et al., 2018) underscore that the compounding effects of interpersonal violence and discrimination are profound for many immigrants, dispelling the notion that living in the United States for longer periods of time ensures healthier adjustment. In fact, ongoing experiences of discrimination have detrimental effects on various mental health outcomes for the first, 1.5, second, and later generations (García Coll & Marks, 2012; Tummala-Narra, 2016).

Since the election of Donald Trump in 2016, there has been a dramatic increase in explicit xenophobia, racist ideology, and harassment and violence based on race, gender, ethnicity, religion, sexual orientation, national origin, documentation status, and dis/ability status. The Trump administration's policies have intensified the profiling of racial minorities and have initiated traumatizing practices such as separating undocumented/unauthorized children from Mexico and Central America from their parents and other family members. Policies banning the entry of refugees from Syria and people from predominantly Muslim countries, and threats to end DACA, have further signaled the anti-immigrant sentiment in the United States. Most recent surges in such sentiment have centered on Chinese Americans and others perceived to be of Chinese origin (e.g., East Asian Americans, Southeast Asian Americans, Pacific Islander Americans) who have been targeted during the spread of COVID-19. With respect to children, scholars (Zimbardo & Sword, 2017) have coined the term "Trump effect" to describe the sharp rise in bullying of children in schools based on racism, xenophobia, misogyny, homophobia, and transphobia since Trump's presidential campaign. These sociopolitical conditions instill fear and uncertainty in immigrant families and communities and can exacerbate the effects of trauma resulting from interpersonal violence.

Other, subtle forms of discrimination, such as stereotyping and microaggressions, can also contribute to interpersonal violence. In particular, the internalization of racialized and sexualized stereotypes such as those applied to Latinx men as seductive, hypermasculine, and sexually aggressive, to East Asian women as sexually submissive and exotic, or to Black women as sexually promiscuous are associated with sexual behavior and victimization in the U.S. mainstream context (French et al., 2019). Additionally, even stereotypes considered to be positive can exacerbate the negative effects of interpersonal violence. For example, the model minority stereotype associated with Asian Americans poses an impossible dilemma of reconciling positive attributes such as academic and financial success with persistent notions of Asian Americans as foreigners, even when they are born and raised in the United States (Eng & Han, 2000). The model minority stereotype carries with it the notion that Asian Americans are a monolithic group and that, due to securing "success" and "not making waves," they do not face significant traumatic stress despite clear evidence for both historical and ongoing discrimination and violence. Moreover, violence experienced by Asian Americans is perceived to be located within individual and family contexts rather than as products of multiple traumatic contexts, such as stressful or traumatic home environments and racial trauma in mainstream society.

These stereotyped views further contribute to the notion that all Asian Americans share the same experience, which minimizes the impact of trauma among individuals and subgroups that are especially vulnerable to interpersonal violence. For example, Southeast Asian Americans have a higher prevalence of posttraumatic stress disorder and other mental health problems rooted in trauma experienced in pre- and postmigration contexts and have higher poverty rates compared with other Asian Americans (Pew Research Center, 2017). The circumstances of migration are highly varied across Southeast Asian, South Asian, and East Asian populations in the United States, with many Southeast Asian Americans being refugees (e.g., Cambodian refugees who survived the Pol Pot era's persecution) or children of refugees. As such, there are variations regarding access to resources such as finances, education, and family and other social supports, before, during, and after migration that protect against the negative effects of interpersonal and collective violence.

In examining the intersections of social location related to sexual violence, Kanukollu and Mahalingam (2011) underscored gender differences within the context of the model minority stereotype among South Asian Americans. Specifically, they noted that women's bodies are typically the "sites for maintaining the values that honor the group" (Kanukollu & Mahalingam, 2011, p. 219). As such, marginalization of women within an immigrant context (e.g., the South Asian American community) can contribute to the idealization of South Asian cultural identities, where women are praised for their self-sacrifice and devotion to the family. These processes of idealization can then influence disclosure of sexual violence and help seeking among South Asian American survivors. Further, consistent with recent studies of Latinx survivors, Sabina et al. (2015) observed that a greater degree of acculturation facilitates help-seeking outside of one's family or community. Yet, at the same time, the internalization of the model minority stereotype can inhibit help-seeking. The internalization of the model minority stereotype can also exacerbate the burden associated with traditional gender role expectations, as women tend to carry responsibility for passing on cultural traditions and maintaining family honor. For example, a South Asian American survivor of sexual assault may be less likely to report her assault and seek help from others if she internalizes the belief that her concerns are not as important as those of her perpetrator, family, or broader community, or that disclosing violence would disrupt a sense of family unity and reputation.

Among South Asian Americans, similar to other immigrant communities, many survivors of interpersonal violence struggle with disclosing violence to family and friends within their ethnic and religious communities. Often, doing so poses additional risk to one's safety and sense of isolation within different contexts. It is also notable that a stronger sense of affiliation and connection with one's ethnic group (e.g., ethnic identity) and foreign-born status have been found to be associated with more traditional gender role attitudes, which may make it more challenging to disclose gender-based violence to people within one's own ethnic community (Tummala-Narra et al., 2017). Given the lack of discussion on and stigma directed against talking openly about sexual and physical violence within many immigrant families, many survivors are reluctant to disclose violence to others within their families and communities. Male survivors may face unique barriers as they may not be viewed by others as potential victims due to their gender, or they may view the violence they endured as being less consequential despite suffering traumatic stress (French et al., 2019; Von Hohendorff et al., 2017; Sabina et al., 2014). The problem of disclosure to someone within or affiliated with one's ethnic or religious community can also manifest in counseling and psychotherapy, as survivors may have concerns about confidentiality and privacy in working with a therapist of a similar ethnic and/or religious background (Kanukollu & Mahalingam, 2011; Tummala-Narra, 2016).

In some cases, a survivor may create distance from people of a similar cultural, religious, or racial background if the traumatic event is associated with the heritage culture or community. Yi (2014) described the phenomenon of *cultural dissociation* where a person experiences a merging of traumatic suffering and a heritage culture. Yet, this type of dissociation can be problematic as traumatic stress affects survivors' relationships and sense of intrapsychic stability. As such, it is likely that a survivor at some later point copes with a sense of loss incurred in creating distance from the heritage culture or community, especially when faced with discrimination in the broader U.S. context. This tension lies at the core of an impossible dilemma faced by many racial minority immigrant-origin survivors of interpersonal violence.

In addition to complications regarding disclosure within one's ethnic and/or religious community, it is important to consider that disclosing interpersonal violence to others outside of one's community can also be precarious. In fact, many first- and later-generation immigrant-origin people have serious concerns about potential threats to connections with their families and communities, and about the responses to the violence they may face outside of their familiar networks (Kanukollu & Mahalingam, 2011; Tummala-Narra et al., 2019). For example, a survivor may fear that the perpetrator who is a family member, family friend, or a member of an ethnic or religious community will be imprisoned or deported due to interpersonal and/or systemic discrimination. Survivors may also hesitate to disclose violence to therapists who are mandated reporters of violence and abuse. Therapists, in turn, face the dilemma of securing and maintaining a strong working alliance with their clients while taking measures to protect clients and other vulnerable individuals (e.g., minors, older adults) from further victimization, including reporting violence to the appropriate authorities. Existing policies concerning mandated reporting typically do not consider these complexities of disclosure and reporting experienced by racial minority immigrant survivors and their therapists. The issue of reporting can be further complicated when what constitutes violence and abuse from the perspective of the client differs from that of the therapist.

It is important to note that the survivor's goals for establishing safety typically do not include reporting traumatic events to authorities, such as law enforcement agents. Rather, survivors may secure other ways to protect loved ones (e.g., children) from being harmed by the perpetrator. They tend to seek help from informal sources of support (e.g., friends, mentors, clergy) both within and outside of their ethnic and religious communities (American Psychological Association, 2012; Choi, 2015). In fact, authority figures within one's community can make a strong impact regarding responses to interpersonal violence. For example, Choi (2015) noted that clergy have the greatest degree of influence on individuals and families within Korean American churches, and therefore often play a critical role in responding to survivors even when the clergy may not be prepared to provide adequate assistance.

IMPACT OF INTERPERSONAL VIOLENCE

Interpersonal violence has a profound impact on survivors' physical and psychological well-being, relational life, and identity (Herman, 1992; Robertson et al., 2016). Exposure to specific types of victimization such as sexual violence has been found to increase the risk of HIV and sexually risky behaviors, placing survivors at further risk for violence (Draughon et al., 2015; French et al., 2019). There is also ample literature regarding the impact of physical and sexual trauma on substance abuse (Herman, 1992). Traumatic stress rooted in interpersonal violence is often unrecognized by the survivor and/or by others, and in some cases, manifests in physical symptomology, for example, headaches and gastrointestinal pain (Tummala-Narra, 2016). The negative, compounding effects of interpersonal violence and other forms of oppression, such as racial trauma, on mental health and relational life have been well documented (Sabina et al., 2015; Tummala-Narra, 2016). For example, in a recent study with 1.5- and second-generation Indian American women (Tummala-Narra et al., 2019), survivors of sexual violence reported post-traumatic stress such as anxiety, depressed mood, nightmares, flashbacks, suicidal ideation, guilt, self-blame, shame, and difficulty trusting and developing emotional and sexual intimacy with others. In addition to the complex traumatic stress (Herman, 1992) that these survivors may share with non-Indian American and nonimmigrant survivors, they experienced marginalization and isolation within their families and communities in both the United States and India, thereby accessing little support in coping with sexual trauma.

Other studies, such as those examining the IPV experiences of Iraqi and Muslim immigrants, highlight the compounded effects of interpersonal violence within the mainstream U.S. context where racism and sexism are pervasive. These studies note how the experience of IPV can be qualitatively distinct from that of other IPV survivors, as racism and discrimination disrupt social and economic opportunities and mobility, and contribute to survivors' vulnerability (Ammar et al., 2014; Barkho et al., 2011). Another important way in which interpersonal violence may be uniquely experienced by immigrant-origin survivors entails the experience of bilingualism and multilingualism. Specifically, traumatic memories may be encoded in and expressed in a specific language that may not be fully accessible to survivors across different contexts, for instance, the immigrant community and mainstream context (Tummala-Narra, 2014). As such, disclosing the details of traumatic events in a new language may affect a survivor's help-seeking decisions. Overall, racial minority immigrant survivors of interpersonal violence share some commonalities with other immigrant and nonimmigrant survivors. At the same time, these survivors have distinct experiences of trauma and complex trauma that are closely tied to specific cultural norms and expectations; social position factors such as race, gender, language, ethnicity, social class, dis/ability, sexual orientation, and documentation status; and ecological conditions such as sociopolitical climate and threat of deportation (García Coll & Marks, 2012; Kallivayalil, 2010).

It is also important to note that the psychological effects of interpersonal violence may vary across gender. For example, Easton and colleagues (2016) conducted a qualitative analysis of responses from 205 male survivors of sexual abuse by clergy, which focused specifically on the impact of the abuse on the men's sense of self. These researchers noted the impact of abuse on multiple layers of the self, such as relational self and spiritual self. One of the most significant findings was that many survivors described their self-identity as underdeveloped or nonexistent. One participant described his experience of sexual abuse as "a psychological castration," and another stated, "I don't have an identity. I am just a shell" (Easton et al., 2016) The sense of isolation, loneliness, and aloneness described by these participants was profound, as was a loss of sense of hope for the future. These findings highlight a social context that silences men and women from engaging with men's trauma and emotional needs. Notably, existing research and clinical theory concerning the experiences of male survivors of sexual violence and other forms of interpersonal violence has focused almost exclusively on the experiences of White men.

For immigrant survivors, interpersonal violence can have significant consequences for identity development. Specifically, ethnic and racial identity are negotiated across multiple contexts that foster resilience and recovery in some ways and that contribute to stress in other ways. For example, a survivor may feel a strong sense of connection and belonging to a heritage culture or community, and yet at the same time feel as though he/she/they cannot disclose traumatic experiences to people within this community due to the stigma associated with interpersonal violence. A survivor may also feel as though disclosing traumatic experiences to someone outside of the heritage community is more acceptable, but at the same time feel as though people outside of the community may not understand or accept other aspects of their identity. Additionally, many survivors cope with conflicting cultural identifications and loyalties to different sociocultural groups, which can foster a sense of disavowal of one or more aspects of identity and a sense of isolation (Tummala-Narra, 2014).

These conflicts underscore the role that communities play in healing from trauma. Recently, Herman (2019), through an analysis of accounts of survivors of complex trauma, emphasized the importance of the "moral community" in securing recovery and justice. The moral community refers to specific communities as well as broader society, which consist of bystanders (all of us). Specifically, when communities fail to hold perpetrators accountable and recognize the traumatic experiences of survivors, there is a profound break in trust (London, 2011). Herman (2019) proposed that when a survivor is isolated from the moral community, the survivor experiences "shame, defilement, and a disgraced identity," which are linked with posttraumatic stress, dissociation, and suicidality (p. 7). Justice for survivors involves recognizing trauma and placing responsibility for violence with those who perpetrate it rather than those who are victimized; survivors heal with recognition and support from multiple sources, including family, friends, partners, and the larger moral community (Herman, 2019). The emphasis on the role of communities cannot be overstated in the case of racial minority immigrant survivors, as they often contend with isolation, lack of recognition of trauma, structural inequalities, discrimination, and/or marginalization within their ethnic and religious communities and within broader mainstream U.S. society.

SECURING HELP

Securing help in coping with interpersonal violence can be challenging due to structural barriers, such as (a) unauthorized/undocumented status, (b) threats of deportations by perpetrator(s), (c) lack of English-language proficiency, (d) a dearth of financial resources and health insurance, (e) discrimination, (f) unfamiliarity with a new cultural environment and immigration policies, (g) misconceptions of policies such as the Violence Against Women Act of 1994, and (h) lack of familiarity with and access to culturally informed resources and services (American Psychological Association, 2012; Sabina et al., 2014). Additionally, broader public health concerns, such as the COVID-19 crisis, can impede securing help due to fears of contracting illness, being racially profiled by authorities, or being separated from family and/or deported. Other barriers to seeking help are both structural and interpersonal in nature (American Psychological Association, 2012; Clauss-Ehlers et al., 2019). For example, among some immigrant older adults, dependence on their children and partners can contribute to increased vulnerability to interpersonal violence (Souto et al., 2019).

Disclosure of interpersonal violence to formal supports such as school counselors, social services, police, physicians, and counselors is less likely among immigrant survivors; rather, there is a higher likelihood of disclosing to friends (Sabina et al., 2014). It is also less likely that survivors disclose violence, such as sexual violence, or discuss effects of trauma with parents and other members of their families (Tummala-Narra et al., 2019). Yet, families and ethnic and religious communities can play a critical role in supporting survivors to seek informal and formal supports.

In addition to structural and interpersonal barriers, culturally rooted barriers can pose challenges to survivors securing help. Survivors' experiences of shame in disclosing violence may be situated in a cultural stigma against openly sharing information about interpersonal violence or the belief that the survivor should tolerate violence to maintain family unity and honor. For survivors who have children, a primary goal may be to secure the family structure for their benefit, even if this requires bearing suffering. In a study examining the experiences of Muslim and non-Muslim immigrant battered women with police in the United States, Ammar and colleagues (2014) found that more Muslim women than non-Muslim women indicated that cultural and religious beliefs directed them away from leaving their abusive partners. They were fearful of negative reactions from their respective communities if they did so, and because their immigration documentation process was controlled by their spouses. These participants were also less likely to contact the police as they feared responses from the perpetrator and their families, or that police response would be irrelevant or ineffective (Ammar et al., 2014). As such, there are multiple layers of concerns (structural, interpersonal, and cultural) within families, ethnic and religious communities, and the broader mainstream context that can potentially obstruct access to help.

These barriers, unfortunately, contribute to ongoing stigma and silence concerning interpersonal violence, a reduced ability to recognize violence and its impact on survivors, and a lack of access to support (Tummala-Narra et al., 2019). However, survivors cope with interpersonal violence in creative and adaptive ways. For example, some survivors do, in fact, seek help from trusted friends and mental health professionals. They also make efforts to engage pro-actively in resisting violence for others, including their children. For example, in a previously mentioned study with Indian American women who experi-enced sexual violence (Tummala-Narra et al., 2019), participants indicated that they benefitted from disclosing their abuse to friends and therapists, and initiated conversations regarding sexual violence with their children in order to counter the lack of discussion on this issue with their families while growing up.

Recovery from interpersonal violence and trauma, for many immigrant survivors, can also entail social action. For example, some survivors advocate for legislation that protects vulnerable populations (e.g., survivors of IPV or trafficking, survivors with disabilities). Others try to raise awareness of the effects of interpersonal violence within their ethnic and religious communities through in-person and online discussion forums and artistic creation (e.g., theater, visual arts). Women's collectives and groups, such as Saheli (South Asian women's group in the Boston area), advocate for immigrant survivors of IPV. Here again, the significance of the moral community is underscored as critical to healing from trauma (Herman, 2019).

It is important to consider that resilience is a multidimensional and cultur-ally embedded construct. Survivors of interpersonal violence negotiate their recovery in ways that are sometimes congruent with the cultural beliefs of their families and communities, and other times correspond to another set of cultural beliefs in the broader U.S. society (Harvey, 2007; Singh et al., 2010; Tummala-Narra, 2016). The ways in which survivors experience and approach interpersonal violence are diverse and heterogeneous, and are multiply deter-mined through their social locations and interactions across sociocultural contexts. Next, I present a brief case vignette to illustrate the complex ways in which an immigrant-origin survivor may cope with trauma and negotiate the recovery process across different sociocultural contexts, and I then offer recommendations for research and practice.

CASE VIGNETTE: MITA

Mita is a 36-year-old Nepali American heterosexual, cisgender woman who sought help in coping with severe headaches and nightmares connected with being physically assaulted by her former husband. Mita was born and raised in the United States and her parents, both of whom work in a relative's restaurant business, emigrated from Nepal in their early adulthood to escape poverty. Mita is an only child who was often left alone in her home while growing up, as her parents worked long hours. She had a few friends in her neighborhood with whom she stays connected. However, while in middle school and high school, she was bullied by some White students who called her racial slurs and teased her for her dark skin color. I met Mita shortly after the election of Donald Trump, and in our first session, she stated, "I am so scared for my future in this country. It brings me back to when I was a kid, you know, a brown kid being bullied. I'm always anxious."

While in college, Mita met Larry, a White man in his late 40s, whom she would later marry. She described him as "intelligent and witty" and as someone she admired since he, like her, grew up in a working-class family and was the first in his family to attend college. As Mita became more independent, including earning a higher income than Larry, she noticed that his attitude toward her became belligerent. Over the course of a year, Larry became physically abusive to her, and called her racially offensive names (e.g., "dirty brown girl") as he beat her. Mita was reluctant to talk with her parents and relatives about the abuse, as she had chosen to marry someone outside of her ethnic community, which had triggered a rift between herself and her family. She decided to leave Larry after an incident when he beat her so severely that she had to call an ambulance. She did not press charges against him and ended the relationship shortly after this incident. She did not believe that the police would be helpful to her and was concerned that they would not protect a South Asian woman. However, Mita did not talk with her parents or anyone about the abuse for several years after the marriage dissolved.

When I asked Mita about how she coped with her trauma, she stated that she focused her energy on her work so that no one would ever have power over her again. Yet, over time, she suffered from growing isolation, depressed mood, anxiety, and headaches, and decided to seek the help of a therapist upon the suggestion of her primary care physician. In psychotherapy, she gradually shared in more detail her experience of victimization and began to recognize some helpful ways in which she had coped with her trauma in the past. For example, she drew on her artistic interests from childhood, and started taking a ceramics class in the evenings after work. She also joined a local South Asian women's collective where she met other women survivors of interpersonal violence. Her therapeutic work focused on both connecting with others and exploring her own wishes and needs as both distinct and overlapping with her family and friends.

Mita's case underscores the role of multiple contextual factors that contributed to both her experience of trauma and her decisions concerning disclosure and seeking help. Her long-standing stress of being bullied in school based on her race and ethnicity, and of being physically and psychologically abused by her former husband, was compounded by her concerns about people within and outside of her family responding sensitively and effectively to her. She often wondered in psychotherapy if there was anyone who could truly understand what it was like for her to be a Nepali American woman who both suffered and survived her violent relationship. In our work, it was important that we approached her dilemma by exploring traumatic experience in each context and how these contexts intersected or remained isolated from each other. In either case, living in multiple sociocultural contexts provided Mita with a sense of choice in terms of to whom she would disclose the violence, and yet at the same time contributed to a sense of being without a home. The growing anti-immigrant and misogynistic sentiment in the broader political climate in the United States triggered long-standing fears about deportation and having to leave the only physical home that she has known. In fact, she stated in one session, "I feel like we (Brown and Black people) will be rounded up and sent off somewhere away from the U.S.," referring to the Trump administration's immigration policies. There was a loss of a moral community to whom she could turn in the aftermath of being victimized and targeted. It has been critical for me to validate her experiences of the current political climate in the United States, and at the same time work toward securing reasonably safe spaces and social networks that Mita could access.

RECOMMENDATIONS FOR RESEARCH AND PRACTICE

Research concerning racial minority immigrant survivors of interpersonal violence is emerging. However, there are substantial gaps concerning the experiences of specific types of interpersonal violence, such as sexual violence, and the experiences of specific subgroups, such as male survivors, LGBTQ survivors, and undocumented/unauthorized survivors. There is also a need for closer inquiry into the experiences of survivors within specific ethnic and religious communities and immigrant generations (e.g., first generation, second generation). Quantitative and qualitative research should examine the multiple contexts within which survivors experience interpersonal violence, and how multiple forms of trauma and marginalization impact survivors. Further, empirical studies should pay closer attention to the contextual barriers (e.g., discrimination, poverty, undocumented status, COVID-19) to accessing appropriate help in coping with violence.

Relatedly, clinical interventions, including psychotherapy, advocacy, and community-based interventions, should attend to the ways in which survivors experience these various contextual factors intrapsychically and interpersonally. Practitioners should be aware that conceptualizations of interpersonal violence, responses to violence, and approaches to recovery and resilience are culturally embedded; therefore, they should listen closely to the survivor's cultural or indigenous narrative. At the same time, practitioners should examine their own assumptions about the survivor's sociocultural context as it relates to trauma (Tummala-Narra, 2016). In particular, it is important to recognize the heterogeneity and diversity of experience within immigrant communities as it intersects with traumatic experience. It is also critical that practitioners be informed about how policies and law enforcement potentially impact immigrant-origin survivors and be prepared to assist survivors in connecting to relevant legal resources. The risks of disclosing violence may also be exacerbated amidst shifting immigration policies and the COVID-19 crisis. Therefore, practitioners should be especially attuned to increased isolation and potential for harm faced by survivors.

Further, as interpersonal violence is most often stigmatized within immigrant communities, it would be important to implement outreach and community-based interventions (both in person and online) that engage individuals and families in dialogue and education concerning interpersonal violence and potential ways to support survivors (Garcini et al., 2018). These can be challenging due to concerns related to stigma or cultural beliefs prohibiting open discussions about interpersonal violence. As such, collaborating with communities in determining salient concerns and developing appropriate, culturally informed interventions to address these concerns is critical (Yoshihama et al., 2012). As community leaders, such as spiritual authorities, hold a significant place for many immigrant communities, it would be especially helpful to engage these leaders in discussion about interpersonal violence and invite them to connect survivors with appropriate resources both within and outside of their communities (Choi, 2015). Relatedly, it would be beneficial for practitioners to collaborate with law enforcement officials to develop culturally informed responses to survivors (Ammar et al., 2014).

CONCLUSION

The experiences of racial minority immigrant-origin survivors of interpersonal violence reflect a complex interplay of traumatic events, social position factors, and interpersonal interactions across different sociocultural contexts. Socio-ecological and multicultural perspectives inform how these various contexts influence traumatic experience, responses to violence, and the healing process. This chapter emphasized the importance of attending to how survivors conceptualize interpersonal violence, experience multiple types of oppression and marginalization, and cope with traumatic stress, all of which are linked to sociocultural context. I have also underscored approaching survivors with an appreciation for the heterogeneity of experiences and a culturally informed understanding of traumatic stress and resilience. Finally, it is important to situate the experience of interpersonal violence in the broader political climate where explicit racism, misogyny, homophobia, and other forms of discrimination have become heightened.

REFERENCES

Ahmad, F., Smylie, J., Omand, M., Cyriac, A., & O'Campo, P. (2017). South Asian immigrant men and women and conceptions of partner violence. *Journal of Immigrant and Minority Health, 19*(1), 57–66. https://doi.org/10.1007/s10903-015-0301-2
American Psychological Association. (2012). *Crossroads: The psychology of immigration in the new century.* Report of the APA Presidential Task Force on Immigration. https://www.apa.org/topics/immigration/executive-summary.pdf

American Psychological Association. (2020). *How COVID-19 may increase domestic violence and child abuse*. https://www.apa.org/topics/covid-19/domestic-violence-child-abuse

Ammar, N., Couture-Carron, A., Alvi, S., & San Antonio, J. (2014). Experiences of Muslim and non-Muslim battered immigrant women with the police in the United States: A closer understanding of commonalities and differences. *Violence Against Women, 19*(12), 1449–1471. https://doi.org/10.1177/1077801213517565

Barkho, E., Fakhouri, M., & Arnetz, J. E. (2011). Intimate partner violence among Iraqi immigrant women in Metro Detroit: A pilot study. *Journal of Immigrant and Minority Health, 13*(4), 725–731. https://doi.org/10.1007/s10903-010-9399-4

Bronfenbrenner, U. (1994). Ecological models of human development. In M. Gauvain & M. Cole (Eds.), *International encyclopedia of education* (2nd ed., Vol. 3, pp. 1643–1647). Elsevier.

Campbell, D. W., Campbell, J. C., Yarandi, H. N., O'Connor, A. L., Dollar, E., Killion, C., Sloand, E., Callwood, G. B., Cesar, N. M., Hassan, M., & Gary, F. (2016). Violence and abuse of internally displaced women survivors of the 2010 Haiti earthquake. *International Journal of Public Health, 61*(8), 981–992. https://doi.org/10.1007/s00038-016-0895-8

Centers for Disease Control and Prevention (CDC). (2020). *COVID-19 in racial and ethnic minority groups*. https://www.cdc.gov/coronavirus/2019-ncov/need-extra-precautions/racial-ethnic-minorities.html

Cerezo, A., Morales, A., Quintero, D., & Rothman, S. (2014). Trans migrations: Exploring life at the intersection of transgender identity and immigration. *Psychology of Sexual Orientation and Gender Diversity, 1*(2), 170–180. https://doi.org/10.1037/sgd0000031

Choi, Y. J. (2015). Korean American clergy practices regarding intimate partner violence: Roadblock or support for battered women? *Journal of Family Violence, 30*(3), 293–302. https://doi.org/10.1007/s10896-015-9675-0

Clauss-Ehlers, C. S., Chiriboga, D. A., Hunter, S. J., Roysircar, G., & Tummala-Narra, P. (2019). APA Multicultural Guidelines executive summary: Ecological approach to context, identity, and intersectionality. *American Psychologist, 74*(2), 232–244. https://doi.org/10.1037/amp0000382

Comas-Díaz, L. (2012). *Multicultural care: A clinician's guide to cultural competence*. American Psychological Association. https://doi.org/10.1037/13491-000

Cuevas, C. A., Sabina, C., & Milloshi, R. (2012). Interpersonal victimization among a national sample of Latino women. *Violence Against Women, 18*(4), 377–403.

Draughon, J. E., Lucea, M. B., Campbell, J. C., Paterno, M. T., Bertrand, D. R., Sharps, P. W., Campbell, D. W., & Stockman, J. K. (2015). Impact of intimate partner forced sex on HIV risk factors in physically abused African American and African Caribbean women. *Journal of Immigrant and Minority Health, 17*(5), 1313–1321. https://doi.org/10.1007/s10903-014-0112-x

Easton, S. D., Leone-Sheehan, D. M., & O'Leary, P. J. (2016). "I will never know the person who I could have become": Perceived changes in self-identity among adult survivors of clergy-perpetrated sexual abuse. *Journal of Interpersonal Violence, 34*(6), 1139–1162. https://doi.org/10.1177/0886260516650966

Eng, D. L., & Han, S. (2000). A dialogue on racial melancholia. *Psychoanalytic Dialogues, 10*(4), 667–700. https://doi.org/10.1080/10481881009348576

French, B. H., Teti, M., Suh, H. N., & Serafin, M. R. (2019). A path analysis of racially diverse men's sexual victimization, risk-taking, and attitudes. *Psychology of Men & Masculinity, 20*(1), 1–11. https://doi.org/10.1037/men0000159

García Coll, C., & Marks, A. K. (2012). *The immigrant paradox in children and adolescents: Is becoming American a developmental risk?* American Psychological Association. https://doi.org/10.1037/13094-000

Garcini, L. M., Chen, M. A., Brown, R. L., Galvan, T., Saucedo, L., Cardoso, J. A. B., & Fagundes, C. P. (2018). Kicks hurt less: Discrimination predicts distress beyond trauma among undocumented Mexican immigrants. *Psychology of Violence, 8*(6), 692–701. https://doi.org/10.1037/vio0000205

Gupta, J., Acevedo-Garcia, D., Hemenway, D., Decker, M. R., Raj, A., & Silverman, J. G. (2009). Premigration exposure to political violence and perpetration of intimate partner violence among immigrant men in Boston. *American Journal of Public Health, 99*(3), 462–469. https://doi.org/10.2105/AJPH.2007.120634

Harvey, M. R. (2007). Towards an ecological understanding of resilience in trauma survivors. *Journal of Aggression, Maltreatment & Trauma, 14*(1–2), 9–32. https://doi.org/10.1300/J146v14n01_02

Herman, J. L. (1992). *Trauma and recovery*. Basic Books.

Herman, J. L. (2019, November 14). *Truth and reconciliation: Envisioning justice from the victim's perspective* [Keynote address]. 35th Annual Meeting of the International Society for Traumatic Stress Studies, Boston, MA.

Kallivayalil, D. (2010). Narratives of suffering of South Asian immigrant survivors of domestic violence. *Violence Against Women, 16*(7), 789–811. https://doi.org/10.1177/1077801210374209

Kaltman, S., Hurtado de Mendoza, A., Gonzales, F. A., Serrano, A., & Guarnaccia, P. J. (2011). Contextualizing the trauma experience of women immigrants from Central America, South America, and Mexico. *Journal of Traumatic Stress, 24*(6), 635–642. https://doi.org/10.1002/jts.20698

Kanukollu, S. N., & Mahalingam, R. (2011). The idealized cultural identities model on help-seeking and child sexual abuse: A conceptual model for contextualizing perceptions and experiences of South Asian Americans. *Journal of Child Sexual Abuse, 20*(2), 218–243. https://doi.org/10.1080/10538712.2011.556571

Kyriakakis, S., Dawson, B. A., & Edmond, T. (2012). Mexican immigrant survivors of intimate partner violence: Conceptualization and descriptions of abuse. *Violence and Victims, 27*(4), 548–562.

London, R. (2011). *Crime, punishment and restorative justice: From the margins to the mainstream*. Boulder First Forum Press.

Mahalik, J. R., Good, G. E., Tager, D., Levant, R. F., & Mackowiak, C. (2012). Developing a taxonomy of helpful and harmful practices for clinical work with boys and men. *Journal of Counseling Psychology, 59*(4), 591–603. https://doi.org/10.1037/a0030130

Morales, E. (2013). Latino lesbian, gay, bisexual, and transgender immigrants in the United States. *Journal of LGBT Issues in Counseling, 7*(2), 172–184. https://doi.org/10.1080/15538605.2013.785467

Nagaraj, N. C., Vyas, A. N., McDonnell, K. A., & DiPietro, L. (2018). Understanding health, violence, and acculturation among South Asian women in the U.S. *Journal of Community Health, 43*(3), 543–551. https://doi.org/10.1007/s10900-017-0450-4

National Sexual Violence Resource Center. (2018). *NISVS 2015 data brief—Sexual violence by any perpetrator*. https://www.nsvrc.org/statistics

Pew Research Center. (2017). *Key facts about Asian Americans, a diverse and growing population*. https://www.pewresearch.org/fact-tank/2017/09/08/key-facts-about-asian-americans/

Robertson, H. A., Chaudhary Nagaraj, N., & Vyas, A. N. (2016). Family violence and child sexual abuse among South Asians in the U.S. *Journal of Immigrant and Minority Health, 18*(4), 921–927. https://doi.org/10.1007/s10903-015-0227-8

Sabina, C., Cuevas, C. A., & Rodriguez, R. M. (2014). Who to turn to? Help-seeking in response to teen dating violence among Latinos. *Psychology of Violence, 4*(3), 348–362. https://doi.org/10.1037/a0035037

Sabina, C., Cuevas, C. A., & Schally, J. L. (2015). The influence of ethnic group variation on victimization and help seeking among Latino women. *Cultural Diversity & Ethnic Minority Psychology, 21*(1), 19–30. https://doi.org/10.1037/a0036526

Singh, A. A., Hays, D. G., Chung, Y. B., & Watson, L. (2010). South Asian immigrant women who have survived child sexual abuse: Resilience and healing. *Violence Against Women, 16*(4), 444–458. https://doi.org/10.1177/1077801210363976

Souto, R. Q., Guruge, S., Merighi, M. A. B., & de Jesus, M. C. P. (2019). Intimate partner violence among older Portuguese immigrant women in Canada. *Journal of Interpersonal Violence, 34*(5), 961–979. https://doi.org/10.1177/0886260516646101

Tummala-Narra, P. (2014). Cultural identity in the context of trauma and immigration from a psychoanalytic perspective. *Psychoanalytic Psychology, 31*(3), 396–409. https://doi.org/10.1037/a0036539

Tummala-Narra, P. (2016). *Psychoanalytic theory and cultural competence in psychotherapy.* American Psychological Association. https://doi.org/10.1037/14800-000

Tummala-Narra, P., Gordon, J., Gonzalez, L. D., de Mello Barreto, L., Meerkins, T., Nguyen, M., Medzhitova, J., & Perazzo, P. (2019). Breaking the silence: Perspectives on sexual violence among Indian American women. *Asian American Journal of Psychology, 10*(4), 293–306. https://doi.org/10.1037/aap0000159

Tummala-Narra, P., Houston-Kolnik, J., Sathasivam-Rueckert, N., & Greeson, M. (2017). An examination of attitudes toward gender and sexual violence among Asian Indians in the United States. *Asian American Journal of Psychology, 8*(2), 156–166. https://doi.org/10.1037/aap0000078

Von Hohendorff, J. V., Habigzang, L. F., & Koller, S. H. (2017). "A boy, being a victim, nobody really buys that, you know?": Dynamics of sexual violence against boys. *Child Abuse & Neglect, 70*, 53–64. https://doi.org/10.1016/j.chiabu.2017.05.008

Yi, K. (2014). From no name to birth of integrated identity: Trauma-based cultural dissociation in immigrant women and creative integration. *Psychoanalytic Dialogues, 24*(1), 37–45. https://doi.org/10.1080/10481885.2014.870830

Yoshihama, M., Ramakrishnan, A., Hammock, A. C., & Khaliq, M. (2012). Intimate partner violence prevention program in an Asian immigrant community: Integrating theories, data, and community. *Violence Against Women, 18*(7), 763–783. https://doi.org/10.1177/1077801212455163

Zadnik, E., Sabina, C., & Cuevas, C. A. (2016). Violence against Latinas: The effects of undocumented status on rates of victimization and help-seeking. *Journal of Interpersonal Violence, 31*(6), 1141–1153. https://doi.org/10.1177/0886260514564062

Zimbardo, P., & Sword, R. (2017). Unbridled and extreme present hedonism. In B. X. Lee (Ed.), *The dangerous case of Donald Trump* (pp. 25–50). St. Martin's Press.

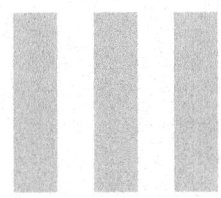

RESILIENCE AND IDENTITY

12

Coping With Trauma

Resilience Among Immigrants of Color in the United States

Germine H. Awad, Flor Castellanos, Jendayi B. Dillard, and Taylor Payne

People immigrate for many reasons (e.g., economics and work, family reunification, refuge) that vary in their level of exposure to trauma. In addition to typical stressors of immigration, immigrants of color may face additional challenges given their ethnic minority status (Suárez-Orozco et al., 2012). Various conditions precede immigration for those who come to the United States. This chapter utilizes the model of cumulative racial/ethnic trauma for Americans of Middle Eastern and North African (MENA) descent to frame a discussion of resilience among MENA Americans and other immigrants of color (Awad et al., 2019). We focus on the macro- and microlevel aspects of their immigration experiences. Specifically, macrolevel aspects related to historical trauma, national context, and institution discrimination are discussed. Further microlevel aspects such as interpersonal discrimination and identity are presented. The chapter concludes by discussing protective and resilience factors used to cope with the aforementioned factors and providing a brief case vignette that illustrates immigrants' navigation of stress and resilience.

MACROLEVEL FACTORS RELATED TO IMMIGRANT TRAUMA

Historical Trauma and the National Context

According to Awad et al. (2019), there are three macrolevel factors related to cumulative racial and ethnic trauma—historical trauma, national context, and institutional discrimination—that may also generally apply to immigrants

https://doi.org/10.1037/0000214-013
Trauma and Racial Minority Immigrants: Turmoil, Uncertainty, and Resistance,
P. Tummala-Narra (Editor)

of color. Many factors related to trauma often precede the event causing a person to immigrate to the United States (Birman & Tran, 2008; Heptinstall et al., 2004). War, politics, gender and religious oppression, and natural disasters are only a few of the reasons that lead a person to leave their own country in search of a new home (Suárez-Orozco et al., 2012). More recently, despite the spread of COVID-19 and various restrictions related to the pandemic, many people continue to flee their countries to secure safety. Leading up to this decision, immigrants may have experienced threats, malnutrition, loss of livelihood, separation from family members, and loss of family members or property. For example, recent immigrants from the Middle East and North Africa report fleeing persecution or violence based on gender, religion, or ethnic minority status and may have witnessed or experienced torture or political oppression (Kia-Keating et al., 2016; Kira & Wrobel, 2016). Immigrants, especially refugees and asylum seekers entering the United States, rarely experience a single traumatic event by the time they have reached postmigration status (Kira & Wrobel, 2016). In addition to experiences before arrival in the United States, recent immigrants may experience additional psychological distress due to fears for family that are still in situations where they are exposed to danger. These immigrants may also have to cope with cultural bereavement (Eisenbruch, 1990), or the grief associated with the loss of social structure and culture. This type of bereavement may manifest in continuing to focus on the past and feeling guilty for abandoning one's ancestral homeland (Eisenbruch, 1990).

Further, immigrants to the United States are not immune to the turbulent racist history of their new home. For example, until 1952, being "White" was a prerequisite for acquiring citizenship (Lopez, 1996). There was never any agreement on what was considered racially "White." Race as a product of national law has not only legal implications for people of color and immigrants but also mental health implications for these individuals working to navigate the U.S. legal system (Martinez et al., 2013). Shifting immigration flows have resulted from our nation's decisions about who is and who is not welcome to enter the country. The terms *chain migration* and *family reunification* have long been used to shift that flow on Capitol Hill (Garfing, 2018). The Immigration and Naturalization Act of 1924 set a quota for how many people would be allowed into the United States from each country. This national-origins system strongly favored immigration from Western and Northern Europe until 1952, when it established a quota for Asian countries (Hipsman et al., 2017). In 1965, as individuals continued to immigrate for occupational-related reasons, a shift began to include more migration for family reunification via sponsored visas (Khadria, 1991). This occurred after the civil rights movement encouraged a change from the national-origins to a seven-category system that prioritized family reunification (Chin, 1996). The Trump administration uses the term *chain migration* in place of *family reunification* to encourage anti-immigration sentiments and limit the number of immigrants allowed to enter the United States. Recently, Trump has used even worse tactics, such as travel bans on

Muslim immigrants and a parent–child separation policy for South and Central American immigrants (Syria Travel Advisory, n.d.).

National policies have the power to influence attitudes toward immigrants, which often result in discrimination (Awad & Amayreh, 2016). Trump's rhetoric in recent years has encouraged feelings of group status threats among White Americans by reminding them of shifting racial demographics (Major et al., 2018). The concern for status and security has been shown to have a relationship with pragmatic voting in favor of an anti-immigrant party or candidate, driven by the use of words such as "terrorism" or "crime" (Wright & Esses, 2018). This rhetoric has heightened prejudice and hostility toward immigrants of color (Awad & Amayreh, 2016; Crandall et al., 2018). Given that acculturation and social support are postmigration stressors that influence distress and psychological adjustment, the impact of a hostile national environment can have a negative effect on immigrants' adaptation to the host country (Li et al., 2016).

Institutional Discrimination

Another macrolevel factor concerning racial and ethnic trauma in the United States is institutional and societal discrimination. Trauma at this level stems from systemic, large-scale discrimination enacted through the laws, policies, and norms of large institutions, as opposed to discrimination expressed by individuals because of personal beliefs or prejudices (Feagin & Feagin, 1986; Sampson, 2008). These institutions may be considered as localized as the business in which one is employed or as far-reaching as the country in which one lives. Feagin and Feagin (1986) theorized that institutional discrimination develops as a mechanism for groups to maintain power over subjugated or colonized others. Groups in power fashion negative stereotypes and prejudices against those colonized in order to justify the hierarchy of power, and then create laws and policies to maintain that hierarchy. Over time, these laws and policies maintain and perpetuate an environment in which one group is systematically provided privileges at the expense of others.

Discrimination of this sort directly harms racial and ethnic minorities by restricting access to resources such as housing, education, and employment. Additionally, institutional discrimination harms these groups by restricting access to basic psychological needs, fostering an atmosphere of restriction instead of freedom (Awad et al., 2019). One notable example of such discrimination is a set of executive orders first instituted by Donald Trump in 2017 known as the "Muslim Bans." These policies severely restricted entry into the United States of immigrants and refugees from seven countries, primarily in the Middle East and North Africa (Yuhas & Sidahmed, 2017). Though multiple iterations of these policies have been revoked by judicial actors or expired, Executive Order 13780 does remain in effect pending intervention by the Supreme Court of the United States. Additionally, policies such as extreme vetting of nationals from the targeted countries and reduction of annual refugee admissions have worked less officially to target MENA nationals (National Immigration Law Center, 2018).

Another example of institutional discrimination are policies and practices aimed at restricting immigrants from Mexico and Central America. Immigration enforcement in the United States has a long history of racial and ethnic bias and discrimination. Currently, most of that bias is targeted at Latinx immigrants, especially those from Mexico and Central America (Provine, 2013). Over the past 2 decades, federal funding and resources allocated for the deportation of unauthorized immigrants have increased steadily. This has culminated in the longest government shutdown in American history, precipitated by Donald Trump over funding for a wall along the Mexican border to prevent unauthorized border crossings (Paletta & Werner, 2019; Provine & Doty, 2011; Zaveri et al., 2019). Policies aimed at enforcing immigration laws are nominally race-blind. Yet investigations by Human Rights Watch have found evidence of heavy overrepresentation of Mexican-origin immigrants, who made of about 78% of deportees with criminal convictions but only about 28% of foreign-born individuals living in the United States (Parker & Root, 2009).

MICROLEVEL FACTORS RELATED TO IMMIGRANT TRAUMA: INTERPERSONAL DISCRIMINATION

Interpersonal discrimination occurs on the individual level when a person treats another individual unfairly due to that individual's identity or membership in a group. Interpersonal discrimination can sometimes include overt acts such as verbally attacking someone or making stereotypic remarks. But it usually refers to negative nonverbal communications—for example, staring at someone, ignoring them, or excluding them from activities—or microaggressions (Dovidio et al., 2002; Singletary & Hebl, 2009). Immigrants of color face prejudice due not only to being perceived as a threat to the in-group, but also because of their ethnicity and race. These immigrants' multiple outgroup status, which tends to increase the perception that they are outsiders, may lead to discrimination (Ashforth & Mael, 1989; Lee & Fiske, 2006; Tajfel & Turner, 1979).

One common predictor of prejudice toward immigrants is social dominance orientation (SDO). Individuals high in SDO are more likely to subscribe to the ideology that their own group is superior to others, and that a hierarchy of groups is natural. SDO has been shown to be positively related to nationalism, negatively related to concern for others, altruism, and tolerance, and is a strong predictor of discrimination and prejudice (Pratto et al., 1994). Since the 2016 election, there has been an increase in anti-immigration rhetoric; claims that immigrants are taking American jobs, don't pay taxes, or are a threat to national security abound. Much of the rhetoric has been directed at Mexican immigrants (the largest immigrant group) and immigrants from the

Middle East, although other groups are often subject to the same xenophobic rhetoric (Awad & Amayreh, 2016). Additionally, the language used to describe immigrants of color and immigration tends to be widely adopted and perpetuates prejudice toward targeted groups (Wei et al., 2019). For example, Mexican and Latinx immigrants have been called "rapists" and "criminals" while Arab and Muslim immigrants have been called "radical," "jihadists," and "terrorists" (Wei et al., 2019).

PROTECTIVE AND RESILIENCE FACTORS

The extent to which immigrants successfully cope with the stressors of the immigration process typically depends on protective and resilience factors. There are several definitions of resilience. For example, scholars in the field of human development define resilience as the capacity to endure or effectively cope with hardship (Ledesma, 2014; Werner & Smith, 2001). Other definitions focus on the extent to which an individual can recover from unfavorable life events and gain strength from experiencing adversity (Henderson & Milstein, 1996). The theoretical lens guiding our conceptualization of resilience in this chapter involves using an ecological system approach that focuses on the individual within a system and takes into consideration the family system as well as macrolevel factors such as the society and the institutional structures that interact with the individual (Vesely et al., 2017). In this section, we discuss resilience and protective factors such as understanding legal protections, cultural strengths, identity, religiosity, and social support especially as it relates to the experience of MENA immigrants.

Understanding Legal Protections

One major protective factor for coping with macrolevel stressors is understanding the legal system and resources available to immigrants. Under current immigration law, lawful permanent residents have constitutional rights that include the right to work legally in the United States and the eligibility for certain public benefits (USCIS, 2015). Lawful permanent residents also have the right to speak to a lawyer before signing any documents, and the right to request a search or arrest warrant before allowing an officer into their home. Furthermore, any stops or searches by law enforcement based on a person's religion, national origin, or ethnicity are illegal and discriminatory. It is important that immigrants become aware of these rights in order to feel that they can advocate for themselves and feel protected under U.S. law enforcement (Rhodes et al., 2015). Knowing how to advocate for yourself under these circumstances can foster a sense of empowerment and autonomy (Salas et al., 2013).

Having an awareness of the legal system and receiving guidance to navigate the many systems that provide access to health care and other social services is important for any member of a society. The ability to receive medical care and secure appropriate housing, for example, can have significant effects on a person's mental health (Rhodes et al., 2015). Access to resources can also provide the immigrant population a sense of safety and security and allows for easier integration into the new society (Strunk & Leitner, 2013). Immigrant families who are able to secure housing in a neighborhood populated by both immigrant and nonimmigrant families are more likely to have a positive adjustment and potentially a positive ethnic identity (Miller et al., 2009).

Cultural Strengths

Across the United States a wide range of cultures are frequently celebrated during festivals and in individual homes. Families celebrate various milestones of life in ways that reflect their values, religion, and culture. These cultural traditions and norms reflect sources of resilience for immigrants. Arab/MENA immigrants tend to have several protective factors that help increase resilience and ease stressors associated with immigration. These cultural strengths include valuing high educational attainment and close-knit family structures. One reason that Arab/MENA immigrants choose to immigrate is for better educational opportunities for themselves or their children. This is viewed as the main vehicle for upward mobility. Therefore, Arab/MENA Americans usually enjoy higher educational attainment than other ethnic groups residing in the United States (Haboush & Barakat, 2014).

Another cultural strength that is not typically discussed is an individual's approach to mourning loss. Loss is processed in unique ways across cultural contexts. Mourning rituals, for example, vary widely among different cultures (Stroebe & Schut, 1998). When loss disrupts life, mourning has a way of bringing healing and restoration to the disruption (Neimeyer, 2015). The opportunity to culturally appropriately mourn losses such as friend networks, familiar social structures, and access to cultural resources within the host country is a powerful tool for healing and helps promote positive mental health outcomes in immigrant populations (Betz & Thorngren, 2006; Bhugra & Becker, 2005).

Ethnic Identity

There is a link between cultural identity and emotional distress that is important to consider (Bhugra, 2005). A sense of pride among immigrants that involves valuing their cultural norms, beliefs, and values has been shown to be a protective factor against mental health problems (Mossakowski et al., 2019; Umaña-Taylor & Updegraff, 2007). For example, given that immigrants tend to be portrayed negatively in the media (Esses et al., 2013), a strong cultural or ethnic identity may serve to protect against these messages being internalized. Therefore, ethnic identity exploration may serve as a protective factor against discrimination for immigrants of color (Umaña-Taylor & Updegraff, 2007). Ethnic identity seems to serve as a buffer against the stress related to discrimination, particularly for foreign-born individuals. Conversely, for U.S.-born citizens a strong ethnic identity appears to exacerbate the effects of discrimination (Mossakowski et al., 2019). Therefore, a strong ethnic identity may be an especially important asset for immigrants.

Further, immigrants with a strong sense of identity have been shown to be resilient regarding the negative psychological outcomes associated with prejudice and discrimination (Cobb et al., 2019; Greenaway et al., 2015; Jetten et al., 2015; Smith & Silva, 2011). This phenomenon, also termed *identity centrality* or *identity salience*, describes the extent to which an individual sees oneself as a part of a particular group, in this case on the basis of ethnic, racial, or cultural affiliations (Phinney & Ong, 2007). Therefore, immigrants who strongly identify with their respective racial, ethnic, or cultural group are better able to cope with discrimination. Theorists hypothesize that this is because while prejudice and discrimination predict negative mental health outcomes, a strong ethnic identity may allow one to access feelings of belonging among group members due to their shared experiences of discrimination (Branscombe et al., 1999).

The association between ethnic identity and positive psychological outcomes is well documented. A meta-analysis of 184 studies found a significant, positive effect of ethnic identity and well-being among people of color in North America (Smith & Silva, 2011). Similarly, Cobb and colleagues (2019) examined the experiences of unauthorized Hispanic immigrants during the 2016 presidential campaign season (a period in which unauthorized immigrants, especially those of Hispanic origin, were especially susceptible to anti-immigration rhetoric). These researchers found that while discrimination had a significant, negative impact on immigrants' flourishing and life satisfaction, ethnic identity moderated both relationships such that the association was weakened in individuals high in ethnic identity.

Religiosity

Religiosity, or the degree to which a person adheres to and engages with a system of beliefs, rituals, and practices (Cervantes & Parham, 2005; Moreno & Cardemil, 2018), is another factor that may contribute to resilience among immigrant communities in the face of discrimination. Religiosity is an especially important resource for Arab/MENA immigrants (Kira & Wrobel, 2016). Research has shown that communities facing traumatic circumstances use religion and spirituality to cope with distress. This is also true of incarcerated individuals serving long sentences (Begovic-Juhant et al., 2014), and survivors of genocide (Fox, 2012). More generally, researchers have linked high religious involvement with decreased rates of depression and mood disorders (Kasen et al., 2012; Maselko et al., 2009).

Among immigrant populations, religiosity may help individuals to reestablish the community they were forced to leave behind when resettling in another country. Moreno and Cardemil (2018) found that 95% of first-generation Mexican immigrants interviewed identified social support gained through religious engagement as an important coping resource for managing their stress.

Similarly, Maliepaard and Schacht (2018) found that Muslim immigrants who attended mosque more frequently before resettling developed more social contacts than their less religious peers.

Additionally, religiosity may help individuals cope with discrimination and injustice by allowing them to reaffirm those values through spiritual beliefs. African immigrants experiencing intimate partner violence claimed that maintaining a personal relationship with God allowed them to have hope for their situation and future justice (Ting & Panchanadeswaran, 2016). Mexican-born immigrants expressed that shifting locus of control externally—relegating control to supernatural powers such as saints, God, and the Virgin Mary—positively impacted their well-being (Moreno & Cardemil, 2018).

Social Support

Upon arrival, immigrants must navigate a new society that typically involves new sociocultural systems. Therefore, a strong social support system is necessary to cope effectively with acculturative stress. Immigrants must learn to navigate new educational systems and workplaces, contend with language barriers, and may generally experience feelings of inadequacy due to a change in job or socioeconomic status (Davies et al., 2011; Martinez et al., 2013). Research indicates that having a network of social support and a sense of belonging with one's ethnic community is predictive of positive mental health outcomes (Schweitzer et al., 2006). In fact, an environment that is welcoming and supportive is critical to immigrants' well-being; this holds true regardless of their English language proficiency. In fact, even individuals with better language skills who typically have higher expectations for coping with acculturative stress may experience more posttraumatic stress disorder (PTSD) outcomes than those with less language fluency if they have poor social support systems (Chu et al., 2012).

Arab/MENA immigrants tend to have extended social support networks given that one of the cultural strengths of this group is that they often seek out social support and provide it to others (Kira & Wrobel, 2016). Social support networks provide a feeling of connectedness in which members can share cultural practices and knowledge and help other group members find ways to reduce acculturative stress. Social support becomes an integral part of new rerooting processes that take place after immigration (Kira & Wrobel, 2016). It is important to note that immigrants may face dilemmas of how and where to secure social support, especially if they have recently immigrated and/or are undocumented.

RECOMMENDATIONS FOR RESEARCH AND INTERVENTION

Although it is important to note the struggles of immigrants of color, much of the literature is presented in terms of pathology and risk as opposed to protective and resilience factors. There should be a more concerted effort to better understand cultural strengths and protective factors. Understanding specific cultural features of groups who immigrate to a new country may help in the development of effective interventions designed to lessen the negative effects of immigration. A concerted effort in implementation science is needed to understand which aspects of interventions are generalizable across immigrant groups and which should be culturally tailored for specific ethnic groups. Randomized control trials should be conducted when possible to ensure that interventions that target immigrant groups are truly effective in treating poor mental health.

Further, more research about the differences between immigrants of color and European-descended immigrants, and the impact of intersectionality on immigrants' resiliency, is needed. Additional studies of underrepresented immigrants of color are also important. For example, immigrants of MENA descent are often left out of the immigration literature unless it is focused on refugees of Middle Eastern wars. Generally, there is a lack of representation of Arab/MENA individuals in psychological research because most study demographics do not collect data in a separate Arab/MENA category. To develop interventions that are effective with all immigrants and refugees entering the United States, it is important to ensure that all groups are represented.

CASE EXAMPLE: THE HANNA FAMILY

Arab/MENA Americans are a marginalized ethnic minority group in U.S. society. In addition to the documented discrimination they face (Awad et al., 2019; Awad & Amayreh, 2016), this population is underrepresented in many aspects. Little representative data are available on this pan-ethnic group and, as a result, disparity statistics are often unavailable. Arab/MENA individuals hold the precarious position of being both hypervisible and invisible in U.S. society. They are hypervisible because of the constant "othering" and discrimination they face and invisible because their experiences as people of color tend to be undocumented or invalidated. These experiences contribute to cumulative ethnic/racial trauma among this population (Awad et al., 2019). The following case example presents the immigration experience of Ibrahim Hanna and his family.[1] This case study specifically addresses the notions of historical trauma, discrimination, and opportunity as discussed in the Model of Cumulative Racial-Ethnic Trauma for MENA Americans (Awad et al., 2019).

In 1979, Ibrahim Hanna immigrated to the United States from Egypt when he was 32 years old. He was joined by his new bride, Nora, age 25, and their 1-year-old child, Lamise. As a Coptic Egyptian, he was worried that economic opportunities would be limited given the ongoing discrimination against Coptic Egyptians (an ethnic and religious minority in Egypt). He was excited about the "American Dream" that he had heard so much about. People spoke

---

[1]All case material has been altered to protect confidentiality.

of the United States as if money grew on trees and everyone flourished. He had attended college for one semester in Egypt but realized that he could not afford to continue and therefore dropped out. Ibrahim was looking forward to providing for his family and giving his daughter the life that he never could have dreamt of in Egypt. They moved to Jersey City, New Jersey, as that is where his brothers and his sisters-in-law lived along with their children. His brother took him and his wife to the Coptic Orthodox Church to meet the Jersey City Egyptian community. His brother helped him and his wife find an affordable apartment, and other Egyptian immigrants provided used furniture. Ibrahim found a job as a dishwasher after looking for a few days and being denied other positions due to his limited English-speaking skills and accent. He also acquired a second job at a gas station. He left one job and went straight to the other, sometimes falling asleep at the bus station. About 3 months after they settled in Jersey City, Ibrahim reported sleep disturbances and experienced flashbacks to his time in the Egyptian Army when he fought in the 1967 Arab–Israeli War. Nora often had to wake him from his nightmares in which he was reliving losing his platoon members in an explosion. She witnessed that his undiagnosed PTSD symptoms had worsened recently and suggested that they start regularly attending church, hoping that would help ease his symptoms. At church, he met another veteran of the Arab–Israeli War, who told him about a doctor that helped him sleep better. The doctor, who was a psychiatrist, diagnosed Ibrahim with PTSD and prescribed an antianxiety medication to help with feelings of anxiousness and hypervigilance.

As time progressed, Ibrahim and Nora welcomed two more children, Mark and Dalia. Nora noted challenges with adjusting to the American school system and also trying to instill a strong Coptic Egyptian identity in their children so that they understood that they were not only "American." Nora especially felt pressure to make sure her kids excelled in the United States. She spent time with other Egyptian mothers to discuss child-rearing practices. She valued the social support she received from her network. Ibrahim spent time teaching his children about Egypt and its contribution to world civilization. He often claimed that Egyptians were the source of most major discoveries and often pointed out famous Egyptian contributions. He did an excellent job of instilling a strong Egyptian identity in his children such that his oldest daughter, Lamise, was convinced that she was good at math simply because she was Egyptian. Her Egyptian identity gave her a sense of confidence in her academic work. Because education was always described as "the way to make it," Lamise, Mark, and Dalia excelled in school. Ibrahim and Nora wanted to set a good example for their children, and so they studied for the citizenship test and became naturalized citizens, automatically granting U.S. citizenship to Lamise in the sixth grade. The children did experience prejudice and discrimination especially during the Iraq wars and after 9/11. The two younger children, Mark and Dalia, were in high school when 9/11 occurred and had to cope with being called racial epithets and being told to go back home by their classmates. They shared these experiences with other Egyptians at their church and usually found emotional support among their peers.

All three of Ibrahim and Nora's children graduated college and two earned postgraduate degrees. Ibrahim and Nora credit their success in the United States to the grit and resilience that they acquired while in Egypt. Both came from poor families that had to be resourceful. Therefore, when they immigrated, they believed they had the skills to survive in a harsh and hostile environment. The Hanna family's immigration journey reflected some of the tenets of the cumulative racial/ethnic trauma model (Awad et al., 2019), given that Ibrahim's PTSD from fighting in the Arab–Israeli War was a source of historical trauma and the family experienced discrimination pre- and post-9/11. Overall, the Hanna family's sources of resilience included social support from extended family and religious communities. Their strong familial bonds helped them persevere and thrive in a U.S. environment that has not always been welcoming to the Arab/MENA community.

CONCLUSION

This chapter examined common sources of cumulative ethnic/racial trauma faced by immigrants of color and the protective factors that mitigate the negative effects of acculturation stressors. Macrolevel factors such as historical trauma, national context, and institutional discrimination were discussed along with the microlevel factor of interpersonal discrimination and belonging. Experiences such as war, political strife (i.e., historical trauma), and national context (e.g., U.S. anti-immigration rhetoric) along with discrimination experiences contribute to acculturative stress experienced by immigrants of color. Protective factors such as cultural strengths, identity, religiosity, and social support were discussed as resilience factors that aid in coping with the negative aspects of immigration. Immigrants bring with them many strengths that are often unacknowledged in the research literature. A movement toward incorporating a resilience approach as opposed to a deficit approach is needed. The chapter ended with a case example of the Hanna family that illustrates many of these themes.

REFERENCES

Ashforth, B. E., & Mael, F. (1989). Social identity theory and the organization. *Academy of Management Review, 14*(1), 20–39. https://doi.org/10.5465/amr.1989.4278999

Awad, G. H., & Amayreh, W. (2016). Discrimination: Heightened prejudice post 9/11 and psychological outcomes. In M. M. Amer & G. H. Awad (Eds.), *Handbook of Arab American psychology* (pp. 63–75). Routledge.

Awad, G. H., Kia-Keating, M., & Amer, M. M. (2019). A model of cumulative racial-ethnic trauma among Americans of Middle Eastern and North African (MENA) descent. *American Psychologist, 74*(1), 76–87. https://doi.org/10.1037/amp0000344

Begovic-Juhant, A., Collins, E., Kopera-Frye, K., & Hughes, J. (2014). Spirituality and social support as coping mechanisms among older adult inmates. *International Journal of Aging & Society, 3*(4), 37–52. https://doi.org/10.18848/2160-1909/CGP/v03i04/35123

Betz, G., & Thorngren, J. M. (2006). Ambiguous loss and the family grieving process. *The Family Journal, 14*(4), 359–365. https://doi.org/10.1177/1066480706290052

Bhugra, D. (2005). Cultural identities and cultural congruency: A new model for evaluating mental distress in immigrants. *Acta Psychiatrica Scandinavica, 111*(2), 84–93. https://doi.org/10.1111/j.1600-0447.2004.00454.x

Bhugra, D., & Becker, M. A. (2005). Migration, cultural bereavement and cultural identity. *World Psychiatry, 4*(1), 18–24.

Birman, D., & Tran, N. (2008). Psychological distress and adjustment of Vietnamese refugees in the United States: Association with pre-and postmigration. *American Journal of Orthopsychiatry, 78*(1), 109–120.

Branscombe, N. R., Schmitt, M. T., & Harvey, R. D. (1999). Perceiving pervasive discrimination among African Americans: Implications for group identification and well-being. *Journal of Personality and Social Psychology, 77*(1), 135–149. https://doi.org/10.1037/0022-3514.77.1.135

Cervantes, J. M., & Parham, T. A. (2005). Toward a meaningful spirituality for people of color: Lessons for the counseling practitioner. *Cultural Diversity and Ethnic Minority Psychology, 11*(1), 69–81. https://doi.org/10.1037/1099-9809.11.1.69

Chin, G. J. (1996). The civil rights revolution comes to immigration law: A new look at the Immigration and Nationality Act of 1965. *North Carolina Law Review, 75*(1), 273–345.

Chu, T., Keller, A. S., & Rasmussen, A. (2012). Effects of post-migration factors on PTSD outcomes among immigrant survivors of political violence. *Journal of Immigrant and Minority Health, 15*(5), 890–897. https://doi.org/10.1007/s10903-012-9696-1

Cobb, C. L., Meca, A., Branscombe, N. R., Schwartz, S. J., Xie, D., Zea, M. C., Fernandez, C. A., & Sanders, G. L. (2019). Perceived discrimination and well-being among unauthorized Hispanic immigrants: The moderating role of ethnic/racial group identity centrality. *Cultural Diversity & Ethnic Minority Psychology, 25*(2), 280–287. https://doi.org/10.1037/cdp0000227

Crandall, C. S., Miller, J. M., & White, M. H., II. (2018). Changing norms following the 2016 U.S. presidential election: The Trump effect on prejudice. *Social Psychological & Personality Science, 9*(2), 186–192. https://doi.org/10.1177/1948550617750735

Davies, B., Larson, J., Contro, N., & Cabrera, A. P. (2011). Perceptions of discrimination among Mexican American families of seriously ill children. *Journal of Palliative Medicine, 14*(1), 71–76. https://doi.org/10.1089/jpm.2010.0315

Dovidio, J. F., Gaertner, S. L., Kawakami, K., & Hodson, G. (2002). Why can't we just get along? Interpersonal biases and interracial distrust. *Cultural Diversity & Ethnic Minority Psychology, 8*(2), 88–102. https://doi.org/10.1037/1099-9809.8.2.88

Eisenbruch, M. (1990). The cultural bereavement interview: A new clinical research approach for refugees. *Psychiatric Clinics of North America, 13*(4), 715–735. https://doi.org/10.1016/S0193-953X(18)30345-9

Esses, V. M., Medianu, S., & Lawson, A. S. (2013). Uncertainty, threat, and the role of the media in promoting the dehumanization of immigrants and refugees. *Journal of Social Issues, 69*(3), 518–536. https://doi.org/10.1111/josi.12027

Feagin, J. R., & Feagin, C. B. (1986). *Discrimination American style: Institutional racism and sexism* (2nd ed.). Robert E. Krieger.

Fox, N. (2012). "God must have been sleeping": Faith as an obstacle and a resource for Rwandan genocide survivors in the United States. *Journal for the Scientific Study of Religion, 51*(1), 65–78. https://doi.org/10.1111/j.1468-5906.2011.01624.x

Garfing, S. (2018). *A primer on family reunification/chain migration.* Retrieved from https://www.law.georgetown.edu/immigration-law-journal/online/a-primer-on-family-reunification-chain-migration/

Greenaway, K. H., Haslam, S. A., Cruwys, T., Branscombe, N. R., Ysseldyk, R., & Heldreth, C. (2015). From "we" to "me": Group identification enhances perceived personal control with consequences for health and well-being. *Journal of Personality and Social Psychology, 109*(1), 53–74. https://doi.org/10.1037/pspi0000019

Haboush, K. L., & Barakat, N. (2014). Education and employment among Arab Americans: Pathways to individual identity and community resilience. In S. C. Nassar-McMillan, K. J. Ajrouch, & J. Hakim-Larson (Eds.), *Biopsychosocial perspectives on Arab Americans: Culture, development, and health* (pp. 229–255). Springer. https://doi.org/10.1007/978-1-4614-8238-3_11

Henderson, N., & Milstein, M. M. (1996). *Management of organizational behavior: Utilizing human resources* (5th ed.). Corwin Press.

Heptinstall, E., Setha, V., & Taylor, E. (2004). PTSD and depression in refugee children: Associations with pre-migration trauma and post-migration stress. *European Child & Adolescent Psychiatry, 13*(6), 373–380.

Hipsman, F., Hipsman, D. M., & Meissner, D. (2017). *Immigration in the United States: New economic, social, political landscapes with legislative reform on the horizon.* Migration Policy Institute. https://www.migrationpolicy.org/article/immigration-united-states-new-economic-social-political-landscapes-legislative-reform

Jetten, J., Branscombe, N. R., Haslam, S. A., Haslam, C., Cruwys, T., Jones, J. M., Cui, L., Dingle, G., Liu, J., Murphy, S., Thai, A., Zoe, W., & Zhang, A. (2015). Having a lot of a good thing: Multiple important group memberships as a source of self-esteem. *PLOS ONE, 10*(5), e0124609. https://doi.org/10.1371/journal.pone.0124609

Kasen, S., Wickramaratne, P., Gameroff, M. J., & Weissman, M. M. (2012). Religiosity and resilience in persons at high risk for major depression. *Psychological Medicine, 42*(3), 509–519. https://doi.org/10.1017/S0033291711001516

Khadria, B. (1991). Contemporary Indian immigration to the United States—Is the brain drain over? *Revue Européenne des Migrations Internationales, 7*(1), 65–96. https://doi.org/10.3406/remi.1991.1278

Kia-Keating, M., Ahmed, S. R., & Modir, S. (2016). Refugees and forced migrants: Seeking asylum and acceptance. In M. Amer & G. Awad (Eds.), *Handbook of Arab American psychology* (pp. 160–172). Routledge.

Kira, I. A., & Wrobel, N. H. (2016). Trauma: Stress, coping, and emerging treatment models. In M. M. Amer & G. H. Awad (Eds.), *Handbook of Arab American psychology* (pp. 188–205). Routledge.

Ledesma, J. (2014). Conceptual frameworks and research models on resilience in leadership. *SAGE Open, 4*(3), 1–8. https://doi.org/10.1177/2158244014545464

Lee, T. L., & Fiske, S. T. (2006). Not an outgroup, not yet an ingroup: Immigrants in the stereotype content model. *International Journal of Intercultural Relations, 30*(6), 751–768.

Li, S. S. Y., Liddell, B. J., & Nickerson, A. (2016). The relationship between post-migration stress and psychological disorders in refugees and asylum seekers. *Current Psychiatry Reports, 18*(9), 82. https://doi.org/10.1007/s11920-016-0723-0

Lopez, I. H. (1996). *White by law.* NYU Press.

Major, B., Blodorn, A., & Blascovich, G. M. (2018). The threat of increasing diversity: Why many White Americans support Trump in the 2016 presidential election. *Group Processes & Intergroup Relations, 21*(6), 931–940. https://doi.org/10.1177/1368430216677304

Maliepaard, M., & Schacht, D. D. (2018). The relation between religiosity and Muslims' social integration: A two-wave study of recent immigrants in three European countries. *Ethnic and Racial Studies, 41*(5), 860–881. https://doi.org/10.1080/01419870.2017.1397280

Martinez, O., Wu, E., Sandfort, T., Dodge, B., Carballo-Dieguez, A., Pinto, R., & Chavez-Baray, S. (2013). Evaluating the impact of immigration policies on health status among undocumented immigrants: A systematic review. *Journal of Immigrant and Minority Health, 17*(3), 947–970. https://doi.org/10.1007/s10903-013-9968-4

Maselko, J., Gilman, S. E., & Buka, S. (2009). Religious service attendance and spiritual well-being are differentially associated with risk of major depression. *Psychological Medicine, 39*(6), 1009–1017. https://doi.org/10.1017/S0033291708004418

Miller, A. M., Birman, D., Zenk, S., Wang, E., Sorokin, O., & Connor, J. (2009). Neighborhood immigrant concentration, acculturation, and cultural alienation in former Soviet Immigrant women. *Journal of Community Psychology, 37*(1), 88–105. https://doi.org/10.1002/jcop.20272

Moreno, O., & Cardemil, E. (2018). Religiosity and well-being among Mexican-born and U.S.-born Mexicans: A qualitative investigation. *Journal of Latina/o Psychology, 6*(3), 235–247. https://doi.org/10.1037/lat0000099

Mossakowski, K. N., Wongkaren, T., Hill, T. D., & Johnson, R. (2019). Does ethnic identity buffer or intensify the stress of discrimination among the foreign born and U.S. born? Evidence from the Miami-Dade Health Survey. *Journal of Community Psychology, 47*(3), 445–461. https://doi-org.ezproxy.lib.utexas.edu/10.1002/jcop.22130. https://doi.org/10.1002/jcop.22130

National Immigration Law Center. (2018). *Understanding Trump's Muslim ban.* National Immigration Law Center.

Neimeyer, R. A. (2015). Reconstructing meaning in bereavement. In D. A. Winter & N. Reed (Eds.), *The Wiley handbook of personal construct psychology* (pp. 254–264). Wiley-Blackwell.

Paletta, D., & Werner, E. (2019, January 2). Trump falsely claims Mexico is paying for wall, demands taxpayer money for wall in meeting with Democrats. *The Washington Post.* Retrieved from https://www.washingtonpost.com/business/economy/trump-falsely-claims-mexico-is-paying-for-wall-demands-taxpayer-money-before-meeting-with-top-democrats/2019/01/02/408bf86e-0e97-11e9-8938-5898adc28fa2_story.html

Parker, A., & Root, B. (2009). *Forced apart (by the numbers): Non-citizens deported mostly for nonviolent offenses.* Human Rights Watch.

Phinney, J. S., & Ong, A. D. (2007). Conceptualization and measurement of ethnic identity: Current status and future directions. *Journal of Counseling Psychology, 54*(3), 271–281. https://doi.org/10.1037/0022-0167.54.3.271

Pratto, F., Sidanius, J., Stallworth, L. M., & Malle, B. F. (1994). Social dominance orientation: A personality variable predicting social and political attitudes. *Journal of Personality and Social Psychology, 67*(4), 741–763. https://doi.org/10.1037/0022-3514.67.4.741

Provine, D. M. (2013). Institutional racism in enforcing immigration law. *Norteamérica: Revista Académica Del CISAN-UNAM, 8*(3), 31–53. https://doi.org/10.20999/nam.2013.c002

Provine, D. M., & Doty, R. L. (2011). The criminalization of immigrants as a racial project. *Journal of Contemporary Criminal Justice, 27*(3), 261–277. https://doi.org/10.1177/1043986211412559

Rhodes, S. D., Mann, L., Simán, F. M., Song, E., Alonzo, J., Downs, M., Lawlor, E., Martinez, O., Sun, C. J., O'Brien, M. C., Reboussin, B. A., & Hall, M. A. (2015). The impact of local immigration enforcement policies on the health of immigrant Hispanics/Latinos in the United States. *American Journal of Public Health, 105*(2), 329–337. https://doi.org/10.2105/AJPH.2014.302218

Salas, L. M., Ayón, C., & Gurrola, M. (2013). Estamos Traumados: The effect of anti-immigrant sentiment and policies on the mental health of Mexican immigrant families. *Journal of Community Psychology, 41*(8), 1005–1020. https://doi.org/10.1002/jcop.21589

Sampson, W. A. (2008). Institutional discrimination. In R. Schaefer (Ed.), *Encyclopedia of race, ethnicity, and society* (pp. 727–729). https://doi.org/10.4135/9781412963879.n289

Schweitzer, R., Melville, F., Steel, Z., & Lacherez, P. (2006). Trauma, post-migration living difficulties, and social support as predictors of psychological adjustment in resettled Sudanese refugees. *The Australian and New Zealand Journal of Psychiatry, 40*(2), 179–187. https://doi.org/10.1080/j.1440-1614.2006.01766.x

Singletary, S. L., & Hebl, M. R. (2009). Compensatory strategies for reducing inter-personal discrimination: The effectiveness of acknowledgments, increased positivity, and individuating information. *Journal of Applied Psychology, 94*(3), 797–805. https://doi.org/10.1037/a0014185

Smith, T. B., & Silva, L. (2011). Ethnic identity and personal well-being of people of color: A meta-analysis. *Journal of Counseling Psychology, 58*(1), 42–60. https://doi.org/10.1037/a0021528

Stroebe, M., & Schut, H. (1998). Culture and grief. *Bereavement Care, 17*(1), 7–11. https://doi.org/10.1080/02682629808657425

Strunk, C., & Leitner, H. (2013). Resisting federal–local immigration enforcement partnerships: Redefining "secure communities" and public safety. *Territory, Politics. Governance: An International Journal of Policy, Administration and Institutions, 1*(1), 62–85.

Suárez-Orozco, C., Birman, D., Casas, J. M., Nakamura, N., Tummala-Narra, P., & Zárate, M. (2012). *Crossroads: The psychology of immigration in the new century. Report of the APA Presidential Task Force on Immigration.* American Psychological Association. http://www.apa.org/topics/immigration/report.aspx

Syria Travel Advisory. (n.d.). Retrieved from https://travel.state.gov/content/travel/en/traveladvisories/traveladvisories/syria-travel-advisory.html

Tajfel, H., & Turner, J. C. (1979). An integrative theory of intergroup conflict. In W. G. Austin & S. Worchel (Eds.), *The social psychology of intergroup relations* (pp. 33–47). Brooks-Cole.

Ting, L., & Panchanadeswaran, S. (2016). The interface between spirituality and violence in the lives of immigrant African women: Implications for help seeking and service provision. *Journal of Aggression, Maltreatment & Trauma, 25*(1), 33–49. https://doi.org/10.1080/10926771.2015.1081660

Umaña-Taylor, A. J., & Updegraff, K. A. (2007). Latino adolescents' mental health: Exploring the interrelations among discrimination, ethnic identity, cultural orientation, self-esteem, and depressive symptoms. *Journal of Adolescence, 30*(4), 549–567. https://doi.org/10.1016/j.adolescence.2006.08.002

USCIS. (2015). *Rights and responsibilities of a Green Card holder (permanent resident).* https://www.uscis.gov/green-card/after-green-card-granted/rights-and-responsibilities-permanent-resident/rights-and-responsibilities-a-green-card-holder-permanent-resident

Vesely, C. K., Letiecq, B. L., & Goodman, R. D. (2017). Immigrant family resilience in context: Using a community-based approach to build a new conceptual model. *Journal of Family Theory & Review, 9*(1), 93–110. https://doi.org/10.1111/jftr.12177

Wei, K., Jacobson López, D., & Wu, S. (2019). The role of language in anti-immigrant prejudice: What can we learn from immigrants' historical experiences? *Social Sciences, 8*(3), 93. https://doi.org/10.3390/socsci8030093

Werner, E. E., & Smith, R. S. (2001). *Journeys from childhood to midlife: Risk resilience and recovery.* Cornell University Press.

Wright, J. D., & Esses, V. M. (2018). It's security, stupid! Voters' perceptions of immigrants as a security risk predicted support for Donald Trump in the 2016 US presidential election. *Journal of Applied Social Psychology, 49*(1), 36–49. https://doi.org/10.1111/jasp.12563

Yuhas, A., & Sidahmed, M. (2017, January 31). Is this a Muslim ban? Trump's executive order explained. *The Guardian.* https://www.theguardian.com/us-news/2017/jan/28/trump-immigration-ban-syria-muslims-reaction-lawsuits

Zaveri, M., Gates, G., & Zraick, K. (2019, January 9). The government shutdown was the longest ever. Here's the history. *The New York Times.* https://www.nytimes.com/interactive/2019/01/09/us/politics/longest-government-shutdown.html

13

Resilience and Identity

Intersectional Migration Experiences of LGBTQ People of Color

Matthew D. Skinta and Nadine Nakamura

Lesbian, gay, bisexual, transgender, and queer (LGBTQ) immigrants share many similarities to other immigrants to the United States: Most were born in Latin America or Asia and become members of racial and ethnic minority groups within the United States; about the same number of these immigrants enter via documented versus undocumented routes (Gates, 2013). There are notable differences, however: LGBTQ immigrants are more likely to be younger than 30, more likely to be cisgender men, and less likely to be Latinx than non-LGBTQ immigrants. Immigration Equality (an LGBTQ immigrant rights organization that handles asylum cases) reports a record caseload due to the worldwide persecution of LGBTQ people resulting in increases in immigration from regions that have historically comprised a lower percentage of immigration to the United States, including Russia, the Middle East, and Sub-Saharan Africa. This chapter begins with an overview of the primary theoretical lenses that we use to explore LGBTQ intersectional identities, and how the global context of race, culture, and anti-LGBTQ persecution shapes identities and contributes to traumatic experiences among LGBTQ immigrants of color—before, during, and after the immigration process. Further, despite traumatic experiences frequently reported by LGBTQ racial minority immigrants and asylum seekers and the challenges that they face, many exhibit a great deal of resilience (Alessi, 2016; Hopkinson & Keatley, 2017; Nakamura & Morales, 2016). A vignette illustrating this complexity will tie together how a therapist may attend to an immigrant's experiences, shaped by

https://doi.org/10.1037/0000214-014
Trauma and Racial Minority Immigrants: Turmoil, Uncertainty, and Resistance,
P. Tummala-Narra (Editor)

minority stress, intersectional identities, and complex trauma. Finally, we make recommendations for research and intervention to better support and promote resilience among LGBTQ immigrants of color.

THEORETICAL FRAMEWORK

To understand the unique stressors that LGBTQ immigrants face related to their sexual orientation and/or gender identity, we use two theoretical frameworks. The first is minority stress theory, which Ilan Meyer (2003) developed to explain why sexual minorities are at an increased risk for psychiatric disorders compared with heterosexuals. Minority stress has several components, including *distal stress*, which refers to objective sources of stress such as experiencing discriminatory acts of violence, and *proximal stress*, which refers to subjective experiences of stress (Feinstein, 2016). Proximal stressors include the internalization of negative attitudes toward sexual minorities (e.g., internalized homophobia), vigilance for cues of potential negative consequences resulting in distrust and interpersonal guardedness, and concealing one's sexual identity to avoid potential harm or rejection. More recently, research has found that minority stress impacts not only the mental health of sexual minorities but also their physical health and relationships (e.g., Frost et al., 2015; Mohr & Daly, 2008). For instance, Frost et al. (2015) found that externally rated prejudice events were associated with greater odds of experiencing physical health conditions over the course a one year, even when participants did not self-rate stressors as resulting from prejudice. In addition, Hatzenbuehler (2009) extended the theory to recognize the role of structural stigma. Minority stress theory can also be applied to the experiences of transgender people, who are at an increased risk for mental and physical health disparities due to high rates of distal and proximal stressors and structural stigma (Hendricks & Testa, 2012; White Hughto et al., 2015). The gender minority stress model, which was tested on a large sample of transgender and nonbinary participants, found that minority stress factors developed with sexual minorities was a good fit for transgender and nonbinary individuals as well (Testa et al., 2015).

We also draw from intersectionality theory to conceptualize how immigrants' diverse social identities impact their experiences. Intersectionality theory was originally conceptualized to consider the experiences of Black women who faced oppression based on both race and gender (Crenshaw, 1989). Intersectionality recognizes "how multiple social identities such as race, gender, sexual orientation, SES, and disability intersect at the micro level of individual experience to reflect interlocking systems of privilege and oppression (i.e., racism, sexism, heterosexism, classism) at the macro social–structural level" (Bowleg, 2012, p. 1267). Intersectionality asserts that lives cannot be explained by taking into account single categories (e.g., gender, race, and socioeconomic status [SES]), that lived realities are shaped by different factors and social dynamics operating together, that people can experience privilege and oppression simultaneously, and that it depends on what situation or specific context they are in (Hankivsky, 2014). At the most basic level, this suggests that immigrants are not a monolithic group. In the case of LGBTQ immigrants, there is a great deal of diversity in terms of sexual orientation and gender identity in addition to the diversity of country of origin, as well as other factors such as race, SES, religion, and disability.

Bearing both of these theories in mind, we note that LGBTQ immigrants are likely to experience oppression based on their sexual orientation and/or gender identity and may also experience racism and xenophobia. They may be subjected to *heterosexism*, which promotes the notion that heterosexuality is the only "normal" sexual orientation, and laws and policies that privilege heterosexuality (Rumens, 2016). *Homonegativity* encompasses negative attitudes toward LGBTQ people, which can be expressed at both individual and institutional levels (Bolen & McGreehan, 2016). Bi+ individuals (an umbrella term including people who identify as bisexual, pansexual, etc.) are further subjected to *monosexism*, which presumes that people should only be attracted to one gender (Eisner, 2016). Transgender immigrants will likely face *transphobia*, also referred to as *cisgenderism*, defined as hatred and intolerance toward trans people or people who do not conform to narrow gender norms (Hill, 2016).

INTERSECTIONAL IDENTITIES IN CONTEXT: PEELING BACK THE LAYERS

The stressors that LGBTQ immigrants are subject to vary by the country of origin, before and during the migratory process and after arriving in a destination country. Relative minority or majority status based upon one's race, ethnicity, or religion change the context of safety and support that individuals experience at each stage.

Global Factors: Causes to Leave

LGBTQ people have a host of reasons for emigrating. Many of these are similar to the reasons of non-LGBTQ immigrants, such as a desire to reunite with family; for educational or occupational purposes; or for safety from war, conflict, or environmental catastrophes (American Psychological Association [APA], 2012). LGBTQ immigrants also have other reasons related to their sexual orientation or gender identity that might compel them to leave their countries of origin, such as the desire to be "out" as an LGBTQ person. Carrillo (2004) referred to this concept as *sexual migration*, whereby a person immigrates to a new country because of their sexual orientation. Bianchi and colleagues (2007) conducted qualitative interviews with Brazilian, Colombian, and Dominican immigrant men who have sex with men to understand their motivations for migration and their sexual behavior postmigration. Common reasons given were to improve their economic situation, further their education, join family members, escape political instability, escape homonegativity in their home country, and have more sexual freedom. Likewise, Nieves-Lugo and colleagues (2019) examined a sample of Brazilian, Colombian, and Dominican immigrant men who have sex with men to understand the relationship between sexual migration and HIV risk. The top five reasons that they endorsed as reasons to migrate to the United States were to improve their financial situation (49%), to affirm their sexual orientation (40%), to pursue education (37%), to join family members who decided to migrate (i.e., not participant's decision) (33%), and stayed after initially arriving as a tourist (20%). LGBTQ people may wish to leave their countries of origin if they are subjected to attempts to change their sexual orientation or gender identity. For example, Ojanen et al. (2019) wrote about a gay man whose family tried to change his sexual orientation, which led to him experience depression until he was able to move to the United States to study, and, in the process, was able to gain self-confidence as a gay man.

Although there is limited research on LGBTQ immigrants, a few studies have examined reasons that LGBTQ immigrants from Latin America come to the United States. For example, Morales et al. (2013) conducted a qualitative study to identify individual and contextual factors affecting the adaptation and transition of Latino immigrant gay men. The participants had a variety of reasons for immigrating, including coming as children with their families, to be with a romantic partner, or because they felt unsafe in their home country due to anti-LGBTQ violence or discrimination. Participants also experienced discrimination related to their sexual orientation and immigration status. Coping strategies included accessing social support, attending English as a Second Language classes, exercising, attending social gatherings, and recognizing their personal strengths as immigrants and gay men. In a qualitative study of Latinx transgender women, Cerezo et al. (2014) found that motivations to come to the United States included the freedom to express their gender identity more safely, greater acceptance of transgender individuals leading to an increased sense of safety, economic opportunities, and employment. Participants reported experiencing discrimination related to their gender identity both in their home country and in the United States, as well as xenophobia and racism in the United States. Further, the researchers found sub-themes related to a lack of socioemotional support, being targets of violence, and the impact of discrimination on symptoms of anxiety, trauma, or general distress. Another theme was difficulty finding employment, which was related to problems with legal documents, and led some to engage in survival work. Participants also expressed resilience, specifically connected to religious faith, social support, and a desire to help others.

In addition, there are LGBTQ people who flee their home countries to seek asylum from persecution. In many countries, including Jamaica, Iran, and Sudan, LGBTQ individuals are persecuted, imprisoned, and sometimes sentenced to death on the basis of their sexual orientation or gender identity (Itaborahy & Zhu, 2014). Horne and White (2019) noted that there has been an increased number of asylum applications by Russians to the United States, as well as ethnic Chechens to Germany, since specific persecution began in Chechnya in 2017. This demonstrates that anti-LGBTQ persecution in various regions of the world drives migration of LGBTQ people who are fleeing for their lives.

Domestic Factors: Challenges Upon Arrival

For those motivated to immigrate or seek asylum, a cost–benefit analysis of the challenges of relocation and the relative difference between anti-LGBTQ bias at home or abroad is likely considered. Such calculations may under-estimate other forms of bias, however, such as the relative level of racism or Islamophobia in one's new host nation. This may occur due to both a lack of available information on levels of bias in Western nations as well as limited time to prepare due to the necessity of fleeing a current threat. For these reasons, often the first decision an immigrant must make is whether to disclose their sexual orientation or gender identity to others. Of practical importance is that once asylum is granted, an individual cannot return to their country of origin without risk of losing their asylum status, potentially permanently severing ties with parents and siblings or forcing a disclosure about one's sexual orientation or gender. At the same time, attempting to immigrate under other grounds and, later in the process, disclosing one's identity and seeking asylum can jeopardize a person's standing in the application process (Burns et al., 2013). Relatedly, an individual may have already learned that the rate of successful asylum in the United States based upon one's sexual orientation or gender identity is about 30% lower than for other asylum-seeker types, and therefore, relocation may be perceived as a riskier option (Burns et al., 2013).

Additional challenges may arise as a result of stereotypes held by govern-ment employees and gatekeepers once the decision to seek asylum has been made. The United States and the European Union both recognize LGBTQ identity, as well as HIV status, as grounds for political asylum (Tiven & Neilson, 2016). A number of high profile cases, however, have illustrated that arbitrary stereotypes held by government agents may be barriers to consideration, such as rejections of application based upon gendered behavior (i.e., cisgender lesbians appearing stereotypically feminine or cisgender gay men appearing stereotypically masculine) or a corresponding perception that an individual can "pass" as heterosexual to avoid discrimination. In 2018, an Afghani asylum seeker was rejected by Austrian authorities after he failed to accurately describe what each color on the rainbow flag represents, despite this being a task unlikely to be easily reproduced by members of the LGBTQ communities within the United States or Europe (Schuetze & Hauser, 2018). In 2015, a Hungarian psychologist conducting an interview for an LGBTQ asylum seeker based his rejection on the use of a Rorschach test and the determination that the gay applicant's responses did not indicate the gender stereotypes the psychologist expected from a gay man (Koester, 2018).

In recent years, detention of asylum seekers has increased nearly threefold from 2010 (15,683; 45% of all asylum seekers in removal proceedings) to 2014 (44,228; 77% of all asylum seekers in court proceedings; Human Rights First, 2016). Transgender asylum seekers are especially vulnerable in detention, facing additional violence and abuse based on their gender identity (Bach, 2013; Gruberg, 2013; Nakamura & Morales, 2016), and are 13 times more likely to be sexually assaulted compared with other detainees. Abuses are perpetrated by both peer detainees and detention officers; according to the American Civil Liberties Union, 20% of confirmed sexual abuse cases of people in the custody of U.S. Immigration and Customs Enforcement involve a transgender detainee. Many transgender detainees are placed into "administrative segregation," which is essentially solitary confinement, in order to "protect" them from these abuses. However, placing LGBTQ people in solitary confinement to isolate them from others is considered a form of torture, according to the United Nations, and can exacerbate preexisting psychological problems (McCauley & Brinkley-Rubinstein, 2017; Tabak & Levitan, 2013). It is important to note that many transgender immigrants experience psychological problems, such as depression, anxiety, and posttraumatic stress disorder (PTSD), as a result of the trauma faced in their home countries and in detention centers (Chávez, 2011; Robjant et al., 2009; Shidlo & Ahola, 2013).

Finally, it is worth considering that barriers to integration do not disappear or ameliorate upon completing the immigration process. As noted earlier, the vast majority of LGBTQ immigrants are people of color and will face racism in addition to anti-LGBTQ bias (e.g., Adames et al., 2018). Further, while cisgender, heterosexual immigrants of color might have full access to the broader community of immigrants with shared identities, LGBTQ immigrants may experience exclusion or bias within those communities, as well as xenophobia or racism within LGBTQ communities (Bowleg, 2013). These various, ongoing sources of exclusion have led to the creation of community-centered spaces in some larger cities. For instance, community organizers have carved out spaces in bars and nightclubs specifically to foster inclusion and safety among LGBTQ immigrants of color, ranging from Paris's Black Blanc Beur parties, to the Middle East and North African emphasis of Gayhane in Berlin or ASHEq in San Francisco (Mack, 2017).

TRAUMA AND RESILIENCE

Many LGBTQ immigrants have experienced trauma in their countries of origin, which may have propelled them to immigrate in the first place. This is especially true for refugees and asylum seekers. Piwowarczyk et al. (2017) conducted a retrospective chart review of 50 patients self-identified as lesbian, gay, or bisexual who were asylum seekers or refugees seen through a program for survivors of torture between 2009 and 2014. The majority of the participants were from Uganda, and about three fourths had been in the United States for less than a year at the time of intake. Ninety-eight percent had experienced persecution due to their sexual orientation, and 84% were survivors of torture. All had symptoms of depression and anxiety, and 70% were diagnosed with PTSD. Persecution by the police, arrest or detention, and history of torture were all significantly associated with a PTSD diagnosis.

Persecution related to sexual orientation takes places at the hands of many perpetrators. Hopkinson et al. (2017) conducted a study with clients from a torture survivors' program ($n = 61$) who reported persecution due to LGBTQ identity. The study included clients from 29 countries in Eastern Europe, Africa, the Americas, Central Asia, and the Middle East. Of these participants, 66% had experienced sexual violence; 59% had experienced beatings; 30% had experienced threats; 23% had experienced slapping, kicking, and punching; and 20% had experienced blows with heavy objects. The most common perpetrators were government officials (65%), community members (60%), family members (46%), gangs or organized crime (19%), and religious groups (4%). Sixty-nine percent experienced persecution before the age of 18. Thirty-five clients who experienced persecution due to their LGBTQ identity were matched by sex and country of origin with clients who experienced persecution for other reasons. LGBTQ asylum seekers had higher incidences of sexual violence, persecution during childhood, persecution by family members, and suicidal ideation. However, despite their higher rates of sexual violence and persecution, they did not have higher PTSD symptom severity. The authors noted that the decision to seek asylum itself reflects asylum seekers' resilience. Asylum seekers, unlike refugees, do not have access to housing, health insurance, and employment. Therefore, they must largely rely on their own abilities to find resources and overcome barriers, which is an indication of their resilience.

While many LGBTQ asylum seekers attempt to escape violence in their home countries, they often experience further violence along the way, as well as after reaching their destinations. An example of this is described in a case study of "Scarlett," a Central American transgender woman who sought asylum in the United States after receiving death threats from gang members when she would not agree to sell drugs for them (Nakamura & Morales, 2016). Scarlett reported that there was daily violence directed at LGBTQ people and that murders went unpunished. She further reported being targeted by gang members and receiving death threats before fleeing the country. She described how the police could not be counted on for protection, and that they were often the perpetrators of violence against LGBTQ people, stating,

> We have a government where the police officers themselves are the delinquents. They are the ones that pursue us, they beat us, they force us to do immoral acts. They force us to do . . . sex at gunpoint. (Nakamura & Morales, 2016, p. 53)

Scarlett paid smugglers to help her cross the Mexican border into the United States and when she was injured on the journey, she was abandoned and wandered alone for 3 days and nights. When she found her way to the border, she turned herself over to Immigration and was detained. At first, she was housed with the general population, where she experienced assault. She was later put in solitary confinement for a month. Despite the trauma that Scarlett described premigration, during migration, and postmigration, she expressed hope for the future. She credited this to her desire to help others and her religious faith.

Although many LGBTQ immigrants experience trauma and could benefit from mental health services, various barriers prevent them from accessing these and other services. Chávez (2011) conducted a needs assessment of LGBTQ immigrants and refugees in Southern Arizona through interviews with service providers, LGBTQ migrants, and their allies. Results indicated a lack of formal support services for LGBTQ immigrants and refugees. Barriers to health care included cultural insensitivity, lack of discreet services, and fear of having their documentation status revealed. Participants also had concerns related to housing, including challenges with securing housing, particularly for those who are undocumented, and lack of adequate housing resources. Participants also identified concerns related to fear of deportation. The need for culturally sensitive services across the board was highlighted as a major one for this population. In a study of Mexican transgender asylum seekers, Gowin and colleagues (2017) found that participants reported little or no use of health or social services due to shame, fear of government entities, language, or transportation barriers. Some reported having experienced abuse, including harassment and physical or sexual assault, within programs by staff or other members. Those who accessed services often withheld information from providers or did not follow through with treatments.

Another barrier for many LGBTQ immigrants is the lack of a sense of belonging within the LGBTQ community and/or their ethnic community. For example, in a study concerning stress, challenges, and resilience of gay Latinx immigrants, participants described feelings of both connectedness and disconnectedness to the LGBTQ community (Gray et al., 2015). While they spoke of feeling welcomed by the LGBTQ community, many of the same participants spoke at length about the ways in which they felt disconnected from this community. Ethnic group differences, gender roles, and gender expression were mentioned as reasons for the disconnection. Participants expressed that the LGBTQ community was very White and privileged and that they had experienced racism and objectification. Another finding reflected feelings of (dis)connection to the Latinx community. In many cases, participants reported that they felt a strong connection to the Latinx community, but many also spoke of how they felt disconnected. Catholicism was frequently cited as a reason for this disconnection. In particular, they described institutional discrimination from the Catholic church and from individual Catholics who used their religious beliefs as a justification for their homophobia. Gender norms and expectations were another reason that participants stated for feeling disconnected from the Latinx community. Participants also identified intersectional challenges and opportunities, as they noted feeling as though they had to choose one identity over the other. Many felt that the LGBTQ community did not care about immigrant issues and that the Latinx community did not care about LGBTQ issues. Some strategies for dealing with this included avoidance or seeking out certain people for support, altering behavior to fit different social contexts, and keeping their social spheres separate. A final theme described by participants entailed well-being, strength, and resilience. Importantly, social support and psychotherapy were identified as contributing to resilience.

Similar themes of disconnection emerged in a qualitative study of Asian Canadian immigrants, which revealed two major themes of experiences in the LGBTQ community and experiences in the ethnic community (Nakamura et al., 2013). Participants' reports were mixed with regard to feelings about the LGBTQ community. About equal numbers reported that the LGBTQ was accepting as those who reported that it was rejecting. Disconnection from the LGBTQ community was attributed to challenges with social involvement and with discrimination and objectification. In an effort to gain access to the LGBTQ community, many participants reported volunteering at events and stated that meeting people and making friends was difficult. Similarly, equal numbers stated that the LGBTQ community was overtly racist as those who stated that it was not overtly racist. Regardless of whether they labeled it as racist, most participants said that they had seen the phrase "No Asians" when accessing online dating sites. Others described being pursued by White men who only wanted to date Asians. When it comes to the Asian community, only a small minority of participants said that they found their ethnic community to be accepting. Other findings in the study revealed sex as a taboo subject of discussion, stereotypes about being gay, and negative attitudes toward homosexuality being rooted in religion. Sex as a taboo subject in general in Asian communities exacerbates discomfort towards homosexuality and an avoidance of the topic. This avoidance seemed to intensify misunderstandings about being gay. Participants noted that when coming out to family members, there was often a conflation of HIV/AIDS and homosexuality, as well as the idea that homosexuality is a Western phenomenon. Further, religion was seen as a barrier to ethnic community acceptance, with some participants concealing their sexual orientation around religious ethnic community members and others experiencing excommunication from their churches.

LGBTQ immigrants of color experience many forms of oppression. Intersectionality theory suggests that people with multiple marginalized identities experience unique interlocking oppressions that must be understood in context. It is important to recognize the specific forms of discrimination that LGBTQ immigrants of color face and to be mindful of the gaps that form when we focus only on the dominant narratives of White LGBTQ individuals or heterosexual, cisgender immigrants of color. Minority stress theory suggests that animus directed toward LGBTQ individuals contributes to negative mental health outcomes. Therefore, it is imperative that psychologist conceptualize LGBTQ immigrants of color through the lenses of both minority stress theory and intersectionality in order to not pathologize their clinical presentations.

VIGNETTE: KAMAL'S EXPERIENCE

Kamal[1] came to therapy as a 26-year-old, gay-identified, cisgender asylum seeker from Egypt. His concerns centered around his struggles with his sexuality, acculturation challenges, and his relationship with his family. Though he had realized at an early age that he was attracted only to other men, he had been raised in a conservative Sunni family and immersed himself in religious observance in hopes that this might change his sexual orientation. As he approached young adulthood, he began to lose hope that his attraction would change. Taking advantage of his parents' offer to support him studying in the United States, he began researching therapists who advertised sexual orientation change efforts, so that he might clandestinely "fix" himself before returning home after graduation.

His therapy experience did not unfold as planned. While he committed himself deeply to the process, he never experienced any shift in his attractions, though in hindsight reported finding a great deal of value in meeting other men who struggled with and took their religious experiences seriously. Over the course of his undergraduate studies in computer sciences, he began the process of exploring the gay community and dating, and leapt at the opportunity for a job offer on the West Coast at a large company in a coastal city with a visible gay community. Kamal enjoyed his experiences and ability to live openly as a gay man in his new city, though he knew that this could end at any time as a result of his visa being linked to his job. He also began noticing more news out of Egypt shared on social media describing an environment of persecution (Aboulenein, 2017), and he began exploring the decision to seek asylum status. This was difficult, as he had maintained a close relationship with his family, particularly his mother, and knew that he would likely never see her again in his childhood home if he were to be granted asylum, since travel to a country one has been granted asylum from is prohibited. Also, as Kamal became more comfortable and less focused on his sexuality, he also began to notice daily microaggressions that he experienced both as a person of color and based upon the assumption that he practiced Islam.

The therapist began the assessment with the use of the ADDRESSING model (Hays, 1996, 2016). This framework orients the therapist to consider the following: age and generation, disability (developmental), disability (acquired), religion, ethnicity and race, SES, sexual orientation, Indigenous heritage, national origin and language, and gender/gender identity. The ADDRESSING model serves multiple purposes. First, it ensures that aspects of diversity that may be invisible are not ignored in the assessment process. Next, it undermines the risk that a clinician, unaware of their own biases, might make stereotypes about other aspects of diversity based upon limited information regarding a client's race and ethnicity.

---

[1] All case material has been altered to protect confidentiality.

As described above, Kamal is 26, and therefore unlikely to experience ageism, particularly within LGBTQ spaces. He left Egypt as a young adult. Many of his same-age peers may have been involved in the "Arab Spring" and may subsequently be more oriented toward political events than same-age peers within the United States. He identifies with Arab culture, and while his relationship to Islam has shifted, it is his primary lens of exposure to spiritual practice and was a source of support earlier in his life. In being under 30 years of age and a person of color, he is similar to the majority of LGBTQ people seeking to immigrate. As a person of Arab descent, he is still in a group that comprises a minority of immigrant groups; this may subject him to micro-aggressions related to misperceptions or inaccurate assumptions about his ethnicity and race. The following is an exchange illustrating the conflict Kamal feels in pursuing asylum status:

KAMAL: I met with my immigration attorney again. I'm so afraid of taking the next step.

THERAPIST: Tell me more about the fear?

KAMAL: Well, first, if they say no, then I'm back where I started from, only I know that it isn't an option to stay. It might be harder not to be out to other people from home, though. I'd been thinking of telling my mom soon, but it seems like too much to do it this way.

THERAPIST: I hear how important your relationship with your family is, and I also can hear that there are other considerations coming to mind that make this less simple?

KAMAL: Yes, I really want this! I hate the idea of being closeted again, but I am afraid to live openly and what the impact on me and my family would be back home if I were made to move back tomorrow. Before I got so overwhelmed thinking about this decision, I had been starting to think I might be married one day, and live happily with a partner.

THERAPIST: So there's a side of you that feels uncertain or unready about saying goodbye to home, and about feeling that the timing of coming out to your family might be forced, while on the other hand this situation feels very urgent and there's a sense of pressure to resolve it immediately?

KAMAL: Exactly!

In this opening of the vignette, the therapist explores the ambivalence the client is feeling using the basic motivational interviewing (MI) skills of Open questions, Affirmation, Reflective listening, and Summary reflections in order to explore discrepant desires in a nonconfrontational, nonargumentative way (OARS; Miller & Rollnick, 2013). Many clinical resources are available for the integration of MI with other approaches, such as cognitive behavior therapy (e.g., Naar & Safren, 2017), though in working with LGBTQ immigrant clients the stance of nondirective, empathic recognition of the dilemma of immigration may be an important stage in therapy.

KAMAL: I also struggle with this decision because I know it isn't like anywhere is perfect. Sometimes I'll try and sound more stereotypically gay while talking with friends on the bus if I notice people acting nervous to be close to me. I also still have a coworker who makes tasteless jokes about radical Islam every time he sees me wearing a backpack.

THERAPIST: How is this for you being with me doing this work? I am White, a nonimmigrant, with few of the barriers you've described. How does this affect you?

KAMAL: I thought about it a lot before I came in, but I needed support and wanted a gay therapist. I often have White coworkers express shock about the process of asylum seeking and visa status, and sometimes I do have the thought that instead of empathy, you'll get overwhelmed or treat me like I'm exaggerating. I haven't felt that yet.

THERAPIST: I'm glad to hear—though with permission, I'd like to check in regularly about this, to make sure that doesn't happen. How would that be for you?

KAMAL: I'd like that.

THERAPIST: I also want to support you in connecting with other LGBTQ people of color. I wondered if you'd had any success connecting with others in the community, such as at the queer North African dance parties, film festivals, or political organizations?

KAMAL: I had been nervous about going to those. I'm not sure where to begin?

People of color are much less well-represented within professional psychology than in the general population (Lin et al., 2015), and though desirable, it is unlikely that an LGBTQ immigrant of color might find a therapist who matches their race, ethnicity, sexual orientation, gender identity, and immigration status. For these reasons, it is imperative that a therapist be comfortable with labeling and discussing the majority identities they hold that differ from the client, to continually assess its impact on the therapy, and to refer out if a history of xenophobia, Islamophobia, or homophobia have resulted in the client's not being comfortable with some identity the therapist holds. For additional guidance, psychologists should be familiar with the range of relevant APA publications, including *Crossroads: The Psychology of Immigration in the New Century* (APA Presidential Task Force on Immigration, 2012); "Guidelines for Psychological Practice With Lesbian, Gay, and Bisexual Clients" (APA, 2012); "Guidelines for Psychological Practice With Transgender and Gender Non-conforming People" (APA, 2015); and *Multicultural Guidelines: An Ecological Approach to Context, Identity, and Intersectionality* (APA, 2017). Relatedly, therapists should seek their own education regarding immigrant community events and media, both for their own education and to provide resources to clients. The first author has written previously of using bibliotherapy with LGBTQ immigrants of color to normalize experiences and provide a reflection of common struggles that a White, nonimmigrant therapist cannot personally provide (Farhadi Langroudi & Skinta, 2019).

RECOMMENDATIONS

Growth is needed in a number of areas related to the experiences of LGBTQ immigrants. Of primary importance is the limited access to and availability of advanced training or mentorship programs. During the recent development of a fact sheet on LGBTQ asylum seekers on behalf of the APA Committee on Sexual Orientation and Gender Diversity (CSOGD; 2019), the authors of this chapter found that the few certification and training sites specific to the needs of LGBTQ immigrants listed on the APA website had been discontinued since their advertisement online. While there are resources and trainings available for working with asylum seekers, these typically do not include experiences of LGBTQ people. This may leave providers with having to assemble knowledge piecemeal about working with heterosexual immigrants with general knowledge about LGBTQ people in the United States. The lack of intersectional awareness and knowledge can lead to making erroneous assumptions and conclusions about LGBTQ immigrant clients. There is no single set of guidelines that would guide practice in this area, as effective work requires professional awareness and experience surrounding sexual orientation, gender diversity, race, ethnicity, and the challenges of the asylum process. The intersectional nature of these challenges highlights the need for a greater awareness of how the law treats same-sex couples and gender diverse applicants. Clients may arrive in greater distress as a result of minority stress if their immigration involved time spent in refugee centers or detention centers.

There is also a greater need for more centralized resources within APA and other professional organizations to increase provider knowledge and provision of treatment. LGBTQ immigrants are particularly vulnerable to the rapidly changing political nature of LGBTQ rights, in addition to immigration specific policies. For example, prior to the *United States v. Windsor* (2013) decision that overturned the Defense of Marriage Act, a lack of federal recognition meant that binational, same-sex couples with a legal marriage in either a U.S. state or abroad were unable to petition for citizenship or to seek relief from removal based upon their marriage (Geidner, 2011). The differential treatment of same-sex couples or gender diverse individuals of color by law enforcement and immigration poses challenges for those experiencing concerns such as intimate partner violence, where the provision of services may elicit fears of contact with law enforcement (Messinger, 2017). This lack of information among providers is compounded by a lack of clinical guidance. While some frameworks have been published for treatment integrating minority stress and complex trauma for LGBTQ immigrants (e.g., Alessi & Kahn, 2017), outcome data on the implementation of such guides are needed to determine how well psychological interventions are meeting the needs of those clients. This is an area where research could be of great benefit to providers. Either additional pilots, case studies, or randomized-controlled trials of interventions specific to the needs of LGBTQ immigrants would provide helpful, meaningful guidance. Further research priorities might include longitudinal studies that can provide insight into the course of community connection and integration for LGBTQ immigrants, as well as a better understanding of the alternate community structures being developed by LGBTQ asylum seekers of color.

CONCLUSION

LGBTQ immigrants, the majority of whom are people of color, often arrive in the United States with experiences of both trauma and resilience (Alessi, 2016; Hopkinson, Keatley, Glaeser, et al., 2017; Nakamura & Morales, 2016), and cultural identities and histories related to their sexual orientation and gender identity that may vary from other immigrants with similar cultural backgrounds. The intersectional identities of LGBTQ immigrants also require a greater familiarity with working with race, culture, sexual orientation, gender diversity, and an awareness of a rapidly changing legal landscape. The development of clinician resources, guidance, and training opportunities are all important to increase the usefulness that psychologists can have for LGBTQ immigrant clients. Clinicians should explore and be knowledgeable regarding not only the relevant treatment guidelines for informed care, but also of the increasingly rich and diverse resources developed by and for LGBTQ immigrants.

As we finish writing this chapter, the COVID-19 pandemic rages on, with more than 400,000 deaths and over 7 million cases worldwide (Washington Post Staff, 2020). It is important to highlight that there are disparities in infection rates and other impacts related to COVID-19. For example, in the United States, early data indicate that African Americans are disproportionately affected by COVID-19 (Garg et al., 2020). Without a vaccine available, COVID-19 prevention efforts include social distancing and stay-at-home orders. Some of these efforts have already worsened conditions for transgender people in some Latin American countries (Perez-Brumer & Silva-Santisteban, 2020). Social distancing measures also lessen access to supportive communities, which can lead to feelings of isolation (Brennan et al., 2020). Asylum seekers in Immigration and Customs Enforcement (ICE) detention centers are vulnerable as COVID-19 is present among inmates and staff, and conditions are crowded and unsanitary (Amon, 2020). Transgender asylum seekers are especially vulnerable because they are more likely to have underlying health conditions that put them at high risk for developing serious complications from COVID-19 (Castro, 2020). Unfortunately, this global pandemic further highlights how racist, xenophobic, heterosexist, and cissexist policies and practices harm LGBTQ immigrants of color. This serves as an important reminder that we must address the added burdens and barriers that LGBTQ immigrants of color experience.

REFERENCES

Aboulenein, A. (2017, October 6). *Rainbow raids: Egypt launches its widest anti-gay crackdown yet.* Reuters. https://www.reuters.com/article/us-egypt-rights/rainbow-raids-egypt-launches-its-widest-anti-gay-crackdown-yet-idUSKBN1CB1HE

Adames, H. Y., Chavez-Dueñas, N. Y., Sharma, S., & La Roche, M. J. (2018). Intersectionality in psychotherapy: The experiences of an AfroLatinx queer immigrant. *Psychotherapy, 55*(1), 73–79. https://doi.org/10.1037/pst0000152

Alessi, E. J. (2016). Resilience in sexual and gender minority forced migrants: A qualitative exploration. *Traumatology, 22*(3), 203–213. https://doi.org/10.1037/trm0000077

Alessi, E. J., & Kahn, S. (2017). A framework for clinical practice with sexual and gender minority asylum seekers. *Psychology of Sexual Orientation and Gender Diversity, 4*(4), 383–391. https://doi.org/10.1037/sgd0000244

American Psychological Association. (2012). Guidelines for psychological practice with lesbian, gay, and bisexual clients. *American Psychologist, 67*(1), 10–42. https://doi.org/10.1037/a0024659

American Psychological Association. (2015). Guidelines for psychological practice with transgender and gender nonconforming people. *American Psychologist, 70*(9), 832–864. https://doi.org/10.1037/a0039906

American Psychological Association. (2017). *Multicultural guidelines: An ecological approach to context, identity, and intersectionality.* http://www.apa.org/about/policy/multicultural-guidelines.pdf

American Psychological Association Presidential Task Force on Immigration. (2012). *Crossroads: The psychology of immigration in the new century.* https://www.apa.org/topics/immigration/executive-summary.pdf

Amon, J. J. (2020). COVID-19 and detention: Respecting human rights. *Health and Human Rights Journal, 23.* https://www.hhrjournal.org/2020/03/covid-19-and-detention-respecting-human-rights/

Bach, J. (2013). Assessing transgender asylum claims. *Forced Migration Review, 42,* 34–36. https://www.fmreview.org/sites/fmr/files/FMRdownloads/en/fmr42full.pdf

Bianchi, F. T., Reisen, C. A., Zea, M. C., Poppen, P. J., Shedlin, M. G., & Penha, M. M. (2007). The sexual experiences of Latino men who have sex with men who migrated to a gay epicentre in the USA. *Culture, Health & Sexuality, 9*(5), 505–518. https://doi.org/10.1080/13691050701243547

Bolen, D., & McGreehan, D. (2016). Homophobia. In A. Goldberg (Ed.), *The SAGE encyclopedia of LGBTQ studies* (pp. 545–547). SAGE. https://doi.org/10.4135/9781483371283.n198

Bowleg, L. (2012). The problem with the phrase women and minorities: Intersectionality—an important theoretical framework for public health. *American Journal of Public Health, 102*(7), 1267–1273. https://doi.org/10.2105/AJPH.2012.300750

Bowleg, L. (2013). "Once you've blended the cake, you can't take the parts back to the main ingredients": Black gay and bisexual men's descriptions and experiences of intersectionality. *Sex Roles, 68*(11–12), 754–767. https://doi.org/10.1007/s11199-012-0152-4

Brennan, D. J., Card, K. G., Collict, D., Jollimore, J., & Lachowsky, N. J. (2020). How might social distancing impact gay, bisexual, queer, trans and two-spirit men in Canada? *AIDS and Behavior, 24,* 2480–2482. https://doi.org/10.1007/s10461-020-02891-5

Burns, C., Garcia, A., & Wolgin, P. E. (2013). *Living in dual shadows: LGBT undocumented immigrants.* Center for American Progress. https://www.americanprogress.org/issues/immigration/reports/2013/03/08/55674/living-in-dual-shadows/

Carrillo, H. (2004). Sexual migration, cross-cultural sexual encounters, and sexual health. *Sexuality Research & Social Policy, 1*(3), 58–70. https://doi.org/10.1525/srsp.2004.1.3.58

Castro, A. (2020, April 23). *TLC, Ballard Spahr, & Rapid Defense Network announce class action lawsuit to free all transgender people in ICE custody.* https://transgenderlawcenter.org/archives/15791

Cerezo, A., Morales, A., Quintero, D., & Rothman, S. (2014). Trans migrations: Exploring life at the intersection of transgender identity and immigration. *Psychology of Sexual Orientation and Gender Diversity, 1*(2), 170–180. https://doi.org/10.1037/sgd0000031

Chávez, K. R. (2011). Identifying the needs of LGBTQ immigrants and refugees in Southern Arizona. *Journal of Homosexuality, 58*(2), 189–218. https://doi.org/10.1080/00918369.2011.540175

Committee on Sexual Orientation and Gender Diversity. (2019). *LGBTQ asylum seekers: How clinicians can help.* https://www.apa.org/pi/lgbt/resources/lgbtq-asylum-seekers.pdf

Crenshaw, K. (1989). *Demarginalizing the intersection of race and sex: A Black feminist critique of antidiscrimination doctrine, feminist theory and antiracist politics.* University of Chicago Legal Forum, 1989, 139–167. https://chicagounbound.uchicago.edu/cgi/viewcontent.cgi?article=1052&context=uclf

Eisner, S. (2016). Monosexism. In A. Goldberg (Ed.), *The SAGE encyclopedia of LGBTQ studies* (pp. 793–796). SAGE. https://doi.org/10.4135/9781483371283.n274

Farhadi Langroudi, K., & Skinta, M. (2019). Working with gender and sexual minorities in the context of Islamic culture: A queer Muslim behavioural approach. *The Cognitive Behaviour Therapist, 12,* E21. https://doi.org/10.1017/S1754470X19000096

Feinstein, B. (2016). Minority stress. In A. Goldberg (Ed.), *The SAGE encyclopedia of LGBTQ studies* (pp. 781–785). SAGE. https://doi.org/10.4135/9781483371283.n271

Frost, D. M., Lehavot, K., & Meyer, I. H. (2015). Minority stress and physical health among sexual minority individuals. *Journal of Behavioral Medicine, 38*(1), 1–8. https://doi.org/10.1007/s10865-013-9523-8

Garg, S., Kim, L., Whitaker, M., O'Halloran, A., Cummings, C., Holstein, R., Prill, M., Chai, S. J., Kirley, P. D., Alden, N. B., Kawasaki, B., Yousey-Hindes, K., Niccolai, L., Anderson, E. J., Openo, K. P., Weigel, A., Monroe, M. L., Ryan, P., Henderson, J., . . . Fry, A. (2020, April 17). Hospitalization rates and characteristics of patients hospitalized with laboratory-confirmed coronavirus disease 2019—COVID-NET, 14 States, March 1–30, 2020. *Morbidity and Mortality Weekly Report, 69*(15), 458–464. https://doi.org/10.15585/mmwr.mm6915e3

Gates, G. (2013). *LGBT adult immigrants in the United States.* The Williams Institute.

Geidner, C. (2011, March 30). Immigration official: "The hold is over." *Metro Weekly.* https://web.archive.org/web/20110401043538/http://metroweekly.com/poliglot/2011/03/immigration-official-the-hold.html

Gowin, M., Taylor, E. L., Dunnington, J., Alshuwaiyer, G., & Cheney, M. K. (2017). Needs of a silent minority: Mexican transgender asylum seekers. *Health Promotion Practice, 18*(3), 332–340. https://doi.org/10.1177/1524839917692750

Gray, N. N., Mendelsohn, D. M., & Omoto, A. M. (2015). Community connectedness, challenges, and resilience among gay Latino immigrants. *American Journal of Community Psychology, 55*(1–2), 202–214. https://doi.org/10.1007/s10464-014-9697-4

Gruberg, S. (2013). *Dignity denied: LGBT immigrants in U.S. immigration detention.* Center for American Progress. http://cdn.americanprogress.org/wp-content/uploads/2013/11/ImmigrationEnforcement-1.pdf

Hankivsky, O. (2014). Rethinking care ethics: On the promise and potential of an intersectional analysis. *The American Political Science Review, 108*(2), 252–264. https://doi.org/10.1017/S0003055414000094

Hatzenbuehler, M. L. (2009). How does sexual minority stigma "get under the skin"? A psychological mediation framework. *Psychological Bulletin, 135*(5), 707–730. https://doi.org/10.1037/a0016441

Hays, P. A. (1996). Addressing the complexities of culture and gender in counseling. *Journal of Counseling & Development, 74*(4), 332–338. https://doi.org/10.1002/j.1556-6676.1996.tb01876.x

Hays, P. A. (2016). *Addressing cultural complexities in practice: Assessment, diagnosis, and therapy* (3rd ed.). American Psychological Association.

Hendricks, M. L., & Testa, R. J. (2012). A conceptual framework for clinical work with transgender and gender nonconforming clients: An adaptation of the Minority Stress Model. *Professional Psychology: Research and Practice, 43*(5), 460–467. https://doi.org/10.1037/a0029597

Hill, D. (2016). Transphobia. In A. Goldberg (Ed.), *The SAGE encyclopedia of LGBTQ studies* (pp. 1272–1273). SAGE. https://doi.org/10.4135/9781483371283.n447

Hopkinson, R., & Keatley, E. S. (2017). LGBT Forced Migrants. In K. L. Eckstrand & J. Potter (Eds.), *Trauma, resilience, and health promotion in LGBT patients* (pp. 121–131). Springer. https://doi.org/10.1007/978-3-319-54509-7_11

Hopkinson, R. A., Keatley, E., Glaeser, E., Erickson-Schroth, L., Fattal, O., & Sullivan, M. N. (2017). Persecution experiences and mental health of LGBT asylum seekers. *Journal of Homosexuality, 64*(12) 1650–1666. https://doi.org/10.1080/00918369.2016.1253392

Horne, S. G., & White, L. (2019). The return of repression: Mental health concerns of lesbian, gay, bisexual, and transgender people in Russia. In N. Nakamura & C. H. Logie (Eds.), *LGBTQ mental health: International perspectives and experiences* (pp. 75–88). American Psychological Association. https://doi.org/10.1037/0000159-006

Human Rights First. (2016). *Lifeline on lockdown: Increased U.S. detention of asylum seekers.* https://www.humanrightsfirst.org/resource/lifeline-lockdown-increased-us-detention-asylum-seekers

Itaborahy, L. P., & Zhu, J. (2014). *State-sponsored homophobia—A world survey of laws: Criminalisation, protection and recognition of same-sex love.* https://ilga.org/downloads/ILGA_State_Sponsored_Homophobia_2014.pdf

Koester, S. (2018, January 25). *EU court bars "gay test" for asylum seekers.* Reuters. https://www.reuters.com/article/us-eu-lgbt-extradition/eu-court-bars-gay-test-for-asylum-seekers-idUSKBN1FE1G1

Lin, L., Nigrinis, A., Christidis, P., & Stamm, K. (2015). *Demographics of the US psychology workforce: Findings from the American Community Survey.* American Psychological Association Center for Workforce Studies.

Mack, M. A. (2017). *Sexagon: Muslims, France, and the sexualization of national culture.* Fordham University Press.

McCauley, E., & Brinkley-Rubinstein, L. (2017). Institutionalization and incarceration of LGBT individuals. In K. L. Eckstrand & J. Potter (Eds.), *Trauma, resilience, and health promotion in LGBT patients* (pp. 149–161). Springer. https://doi.org/10.1007/978-3-319-54509-7_13

Messinger, A. M. (2017). *LGBTQ intimate partner violence: Lessons for policy, practice, and research*. University of California Press. https://doi.org/10.1525/california/9780520286054.001.0001

Meyer, I. H. (2003). Prejudice, social stress, and mental health in lesbian, gay, and bisexual populations: Conceptual issues and research evidence. *Psychological Bulletin, 129*(5), 674–697. https://doi.org/10.1037/0033-2909.129.5.674

Miller, W. R., & Rollnick, S. (2013). *Motivational interviewing: Helping people change.* (3rd ed.). Guilford Press.

Mohr, J. J., & Daly, C. A. (2008). Sexual minority stress and changes in relationship quality in same-sex couples. *Journal of Social and Personal Relationships, 25*(6), 989–1007. https://doi.org/10.1177/0265407508100311

Morales, A., Corbin-Gutierrez, E., & Wang, S. C. (2013). Latino, immigrant, and gay: A qualitative study about their adaptation and transitions. *Journal of LGBT Issues in Counseling, 7*(2), 125–142. https://doi.org/10.1080/15538605.2013.785380

Naar, S., & Safren, S. A. (2017). *Motivational interviewing and CBT: Combining strategies for maximum effectiveness.* Guilford Press.

Nakamura, N., Chan, E., & Fischer, B. (2013). "Hard to crack": Experiences of community integration among first- and second-generation Asian MSM in Canada. *Cultural Diversity & Ethnic Minority Psychology, 19*(3), 248–256. https://doi.org/10.1037/a0032943

Nakamura, N., & Morales, A. (2016). Criminalization of transgender immigrants: The case of Scarlett. In R. Furman, G. Lamphear, & D. Epps (Eds.), *The immigrant other: Lived experiences in a transnational world* (pp. 48–61). Columbia University Press. https://doi.org/10.7312/furm17180-004

Nieves-Lugo, K., Barnett, A., Pinho, V., Reisen, C., Poppen, P., & Zea, M. C. (2019). Sexual migration and HIV risk in a sample of Brazilian, Colombian and Dominican immigrant MSM living in New York City. *Journal of Immigrant and Minority Health, 21*(1), 115–122. https://doi.org/10.1007/s10903-018-0716-7

Ojanen, T. T., Newman, P. A., Ratanashevorn, R., de Lind van Wijngaarden, J. W., & Suchon Tepjan, S. (2019). Whose paradise? An intersectional perspective on mental health and gender/sexual diversity in Thailand. In N. Nakamura & C. H. Logie (Eds.), *LGBTQ mental health: International perspectives and experiences* (pp. 137–151). American Psychological Association. https://doi.org/10.1037/0000159-010

Perez-Brumer, A., & Silva-Santisteban, A. (2020). Covid-19 policies can perpetuate violence against transgender communities: Insights from Peru. *AIDS and Behavior, 24*, 2477–2479. https://doi.org/10.1007/s10461-020-02889-z

Piwowarczyk, L., Fernandez, P., & Sharma, A. (2017). Seeking asylum: Challenges faced by the LGB community. *Journal of Immigrant and Minority Health, 19*(3), 723–732. https://doi.org/10.1007/s10903-016-0363-9

Robjant, K., Hassan, R., & Katona, C. (2009). Mental health implications of detaining asylum seekers: Systematic review. *The British Journal of Psychiatry, 194*(4), 306–312. https://doi.org/10.1192/bjp.bp.108.053223

Rumens, N. (2016). Heterosexism. In A. Goldberg (Ed.), *The SAGE encyclopedia of LGBTQ studies* (pp. 497–501). SAGE. https://doi.org/10.4135/9781483371283.n184

Schuetze, C. F., & Hauser, C. (2018, August 17). Gay Afghan boy denied asylum in Austria. *The New York Times*, p. A10.

Shidlo, A., & Ahola, J. (2013). Mental health challenges of LGBT forced migrants. *Forced Migration Review, 42*, 9–11. https://www.fmreview.org/sites/fmr/files/FMRdownloads/en/fmr42full.pdf

Tabak, S., & Levitan, R. (2013). LGBTI migrants in immigration detention. *Forced Migration Review, 42*, 47–49. https://www.fmreview.org/sites/fmr/files/FMRdownloads/en/fmr42full.pdf

Testa, R. J., Habarth, J., Peta, J., Balsam, K., & Bockting, W. (2015). Development of the Gender Minority Stress and Resilience measure. *Psychology of Sexual Orientation and Gender Diversity, 2*(1), 65–77. https://doi.org/10.1037/sgd0000081

Tiven, R. B., & Neilson, V. (2016). Working with lesbian, gay, bisexual, and transgender immigrants. In F. Chang-Muy & E. P. Congress (Eds.), *Social work with immigrants and refugees* (pp. 257–267). Springer.

United States v. Windsor, 570 U.S. 744 (2013).

Washington Post Staff. (2020, June 12). *Mapping the worldwide spread of the coronavirus.* https://www.washingtonpost.com/graphics/2020/world/mapping-spread-new-coronavirus/

White Hughto, J. M., Reisner, S. L., & Pachankis, J. E. (2015). Transgender stigma and health: A critical review of stigma determinants, mechanisms, and interventions. *Social Science & Medicine, 147,* 222–231. https://doi.org/10.1016/j.socscimed.2015.11.010

IV

KEY STRATEGIES FOR INTERVENTION

14

Bullying Prevention for Asian American Families

Collaborations With School Districts and Community Organizations

Cixin Wang, Jia Li Liu, Kavita Atwal, and Kieu Anh Do

A substantial proportion of American children and adolescents experience bullying with negative developmental consequences. *Bullying* refers to a "form of proactive or reactive aggressive behavior inflicted by one or more individuals with intent to cause harm or discomfort to another individual" (Maynard et al., 2016, p. 337) and occurs repeatedly and between individuals where a power imbalance exists (Olweus, 1999). Approximately 30% of American children are involved in bullying, including physical (e.g., assault, destruction of property), verbal (e.g., taunts, threats, name-calling), and/or psychological/relational (e.g., peer exclusion, gossiping, spreading rumors) behavior in schools either as bullies, victims, or both (Nansel et al., 2001). Victims of bullying are at greater risk of lowered academic performance, increased psychosocial distress, physical health complaints, and suicidal thoughts and behaviors (Crepeau-Hobson & Leech, 2016; Davis et al., 2018; Juvonen et al., 2011; Nishina, 2012; Vergara et al., 2019). Community-wide bullying prevention programs can help reduce the prevalence of bullying (and its insidious effects) and foster environments where optimal learning and development can occur. Our work is guided by the integrative risk and resilience model (Suárez-Orozco et al., 2018), which suggests individual (ethnic identity), microsystems (schools, families), political and social contexts (attitudes toward migrants), and global forces all contribute to the adaptation of immigrant-origin youth. In this chapter, we highlight bullying of immigrant youth, specifically focusing on the Asian American experience, and share our

https://doi.org/10.1037/0000214-015
Trauma and Racial Minority Immigrants: Turmoil, Uncertainty, and Resistance,
P. Tummala-Narra (Editor)

experiences of developing school and community partnerships in order to prevent bullying of Asian American families in general (not solely for East Asians or South Asians).

BULLYING OF IMMIGRANTS

According to Child Trends (2018), the population of immigrant children in the United States increased by 51% (19.6 million) between 1994 and 2017, accounting for one out of every four American children today. *Ethnic bullying* refers to bullying that targets another's ethnic background or cultural identity and may encompass direct forms of aggression (e.g., racial taunts and slurs, derogatory references to culturally specific customs, foods, costumes), as well as indirect forms of aggression, such as exclusion from a mainstream group of peers as a result of ethnic differences (McKenney et al., 2006). Relatedly, *immigrant bullying* involves "bullying that targets another's immigrant status or family history of immigration in the form of taunts and slurs, derogatory references to the immigration process, physical aggression, social manipulation, or exclusion because of immigration status" (Scherr & Larson, 2010, p. 225).

The research on whether immigrant youth experience higher rates of bullying compared with their native-born peers has yielded mixed findings. For example, Maynard et al. (2016) found that even after controlling for age, gender, race/ethnicity, grade level, and family affluence, immigrant youth between fifth and 10th grades were significantly more likely to experience one or more forms of bullying compared with their U.S.-born peers. In a similar vein, Sulkowski et al. (2014) found that American youth from immigrant families are more likely than their nonimmigrant peers to report being victimized by physical aggression and to be victimized because of race, religion, and family income issues.

However, other researchers have not found evidence for elevated bullying victimization rates among immigrant youth (e.g., Peguero, 2009), possibly due to different samples being used and other contextual factors, such as school climate, socioeconomic status, and the amount of ethnic and cultural diversity within schools. In terms of context, we do see that immigrant youth reported being exposed to pervasive anti-immigrant rhetoric through media, anti-immigrant comments, and insults from peers in the current sociopolitical climate. In 2016, the Southern Poverty Law Center administered a survey to approximately 2,000 kindergarten to 12th grade teachers. Over 67% of the teachers in the study reported that Muslim students, students of color, and children from immigrant backgrounds expressed concerns about what might happen to them and their families after the 2016 presidential election. An increase in racial slurs and negative comments directed at students of color and those of the Islamic faith and immigrant backgrounds have also been noted, such as being called "terrorist or ISIS or bomber" (Costello, 2016, p. 5) and "dirty Mexican" (Costello, 2016, p. 9).

The effects of peer victimization may be especially insidious for immigrant youth when combined with the unique stressors they already face (e.g., intergenerational conflict, acculturative stress, acculturative family distancing, poverty, language barriers, limited social networks). Yet these students often are at a loss for specific strategies for combatting discrimination (Romero et al., 2015). Given the sizeable (and growing) segment of this population and bullying's adverse effects, a more contextualized understanding of ethnic and immigrant bullying is essential. Unfortunately, immigrant youths reported that bystanders and authorities do not effectively respond to these victimization incidents (Sulkowski et al., 2014). Therefore, greater bullying prevention efforts are needed for this population.

Given that family, peer, and school factors are related to bullying victimization across racial/ethnic groups (Spriggs et al., 2007), maximizing the effectiveness of bullying interventions for immigrant children requires "joint efforts of parents, teachers/administrators to build safe and culturally sensitive school and home environments" (Shea et al., 2016, p. 92). It is important to address family interactions in future bullying prevention efforts given the negative association between family communication and bullying behaviors for ethnically diverse adolescents (Spriggs et al., 2007). For immigrant families, such endeavors must incorporate culture-responsive parent training that goes beyond the problems and deficits, and takes into consideration the family's worldviews and cultural assets (e.g., collectivist coping strategies and family connectedness; Shea et al., 2016). Immigrant parents (Latinx, Afro Caribbean, and Asian in particular) experience unique parenting challenges, including financial pressures, contextual pressures (e.g., language barriers, limited educational experience, limited time and energy), and acculturative stress that negatively impact parental efficacy when it comes to preventing and intervening in school bullying. These same parents express a dire need for help and intervention services in a bicultural context while simultaneously acknowledging their expectation for schools and teachers to be heavily involved in fostering positive child development and school experiences (Shea et al., 2016). In this next section, we discuss the research on bullying toward Asian Americans.

BULLYING TOWARD ASIAN AMERICANS

Asian Americans represent a diverse group of people from more than 20 countries in East and Southeast Asia and the Indian subcontinent (López et al., 2017). However, they face similar social and cultural experiences here in the United States, including prejudice, racism, discrimination, and xenophobia (Koo et al., 2012). Additionally, for Asian American youth, the insidious and pervasive "model minority" myth often places undue stress or pressure on many youth and prevents them from receiving the services and support they need in school settings. For example, one qualitative study found that 15% of Chinese American respondents ($n = 120$) reported that poor treatment and bullying was directly related to "getting good grades," "being too smart," "studying too much," and "not having fun" (Qin et al., 2008).

Prevalence of Bullying Victimization of Asian American Youth

Research shows that Asian American adolescents reported higher levels of victimization and discrimination at school than adolescents of other ethnic backgrounds (Greene et al., 2006; Hoglund & Hosan, 2013). For example, as many as 54% of Asian students reported being bullied in the classroom setting compared with 31% of White students (U.S. Department of Education, 2011). Fisher et al. (2000) found that although adolescents of all ethnic groups experienced racial name-calling, it was most frequently experienced by East Asian and South Asian youth. Asian American students also experienced more verbal harassment (e.g., racial slurs, teasing, mocking) and physical victimization than White peers (Hoglund & Hosan, 2013) and other ethnic groups (Rosenbloom & Way, 2004). Recently, during COVID-19, as President Trump has labeled it the "Chinese virus," there has been a surge of racism and xenophobia toward Chinese/Asian Americans (both adults and youth), ranging from name-calling and social exclusion to physical assault/violence, resulting in high levels of stress for Asian American families.

The experiences of harassment that first- and second-generation Chinese Americans face originate from assumptions about academic ability (i.e., the model minority stereotype), students' immigrant status and language barriers, within-group conflicts, and differences in physical appearance that set Asian American students apart from other ethnic minority or majority students (Qin et al., 2008). Additionally, Asian American youth who do not conform to commonly held stereotypes are at greater risk of being victimized. Compared with third- or later-generation students, first- and second-generation Asian American students are more likely to be victimized, and they report being more afraid at school than do their White peers (Peguero, 2009).

For Asian American students, racial discrimination and bullying are often related. For example, many students attribute the reasons for their victimization to cultural differences, including language, the model minority myth, physical appearance, and poor performance in sports compared with non–Asian American students. Interestingly, although interscholastic sports participation is a protective factor against bullying and victimization for White and Black/African American adolescents, it is a risk factor for Asian Americans, as well as Latinx students (Peguero & Williams, 2013).

Also, the school climate factor, respect for diversity, is a significant predictor for victimization for Asian American students in California, but not for non–Asian American students (Wang et al., 2016). Qualitative interviews with adult children of Korean and Vietnamese immigrants suggest that intra-ethnic bullying can also occur with recent immigrant youth being subjected to social exclusion by their more assimilated Asian peers (Pyke & Dang, 2003).

Bullying Against Sikh American Youth

Sikh Americans are a specific subgroup of Asian Americans who experience elevated rates of bullying. In the aftermath of 9/11, violence and discrimination of Sikhs in the United States rose exponentially. Prevalence rates of bullying victimization of Sikh American youth range from 47% to 56%, and increase to 69% when considering Sikh students who wear religious head coverings (Asian American Legal Defense and Education Fund, 2013; The Sikh Coalition, 2010, 2014; United Sikhs, 2010). Bajaj et al. (2016) identified five relevant forms of xenophobic bullying in South Asian American youth (including Sikh Americans). This includes (a) name-calling and verbal bullying in relation to one's assumed Muslim identity (e.g., "terrorist," "raghead"); (b) physical assaults and intimidation (e.g., cutting off hair, violently removing the hijab or turban); (c) religious-based verbal or physical bullying (e.g., taunts that non-Christians are going to hell, they cannot be American if they are not Christian); (d) attacks on families and communities (e.g., "Go back where you came from," physical damage of property such as homes and places of worship); and (e) ridicule and taunting based on food, appearance, dress, or smell. High prevalence rates of bullying victimization of Sikh Americans has been cited as one of the reasons for the formation of the Asian Americans and Pacific Islanders (AAPI) Bullying Prevention Task Force (Ahuja, 2014). This task force was formed by The White House Initiative on Asian Americans and Pacific Islanders (WHIAAPI), in partnership with the U.S. Department of Justice, the U.S. Department of Education, and the U.S. Department of Health and Human Services. To bring awareness to and address this issue, various Sikh organizations have conducted studies to examine the bullying victimization of Sikh American youth. Atwal and Wang (2019) found 76.4% Sikh American students experienced bullying, and wearing a religious head covering is related to being perceived as a foreigner, which relates to more victimization and adjustment difficulties.

Negative Outcomes of Bullying Victimization

Victimization confers negative consequences across multiple domains, including internalizing symptoms and lower academic achievement (Baker & Tanrikulu, 2010; Dempsey et al., 2009; Fredstrom et al., 2011; Nakamoto & Schwartz, 2010). Immigrant bullying victims disclose that they have poorer health; fewer close friends; greater dissatisfaction with family relationships; more frequent experiences of loneliness; greater levels of negative body image; somatic symptomatology; dissatisfaction with life; and greater tobacco, alcohol, and marijuana use within the past 30 days (Maynard et al., 2016). Korean

American adolescents who reported being bullied experienced high levels of depression. (Shin et al., 2011). In Goebert et al.'s (2011) predominantly Asian American and Pacific Islander sample, cyberbullying victimization significantly increased the likelihood of substance use (e.g., binge drinking, marijuana), depression, and suicide attempts. Across instances of peer discrimination, Asian American adolescents' distress scores were consistently high (Fisher et al., 2000). Because of these negative associations, it is imperative to identify and maximize resiliency factors.

COLLABORATION WITH ASIAN AMERICAN COMMUNITY ORGANIZATIONS AND SCHOOL DISTRICTS

The community, school, and family contexts serve important roles in combatting the negative psychosocial and academic consequences of bullying. In a systematic review of 18 meta-analyses, community factors (e.g., positive communities) and school factors (e.g., school safety, positive school climate) protected children against bullying and cyberbullying victimization (see Zych et al., 2019, for a full review). Family characteristics, such as a positive family environment, authoritative parenting, high parent–child interaction, parental involvement, support, parental communication, parental warmth, parental supervision, mediation, and monitoring of technology, were also related to lower victimization (Zych et al., 2019).

Involving families and schools is necessary to build safe and culturally sensitive bullying prevention programs (Shea et al., 2016). Most commonly, researchers and practitioners offer training (once or twice) to school staff through staff development training on bullying prevention. However, without ongoing coaching and support that includes parents and communities, it is difficult for the school district to implement the evidence-based bullying prevention efforts. To date, there is a paucity of research addressing how to build university and community partnerships with Asian American communities, and bridge the gap between research and practice to reduce bullying and discrimination and promote Asian American youth development.

Despite its benefits, community-based participatory research among Asian American communities is very rare (Ma et al., 2004). Guided by the participatory culture-specific consultation model (PCSC, Nastasi, 2017), we built a university–community partnership between a university research team and community organizations (a Chinese American Parent Organization, Chinese language schools, and a large school district on the East Coast). Together, these partners developed culturally informed interventions for Asian American students and parents to prevent bullying. PCSC offers a culture-sensitive framework for the development of interventions across different cultural settings. It encompasses a multistep process involving learning about the culture and relationship building, formative investigation of target problems, culture-informed adaptation of existing interventions, and evaluation (Nastasi, 2017). Next, we describe our process.

RELATIONSHIP BUILDING WITH THE COMMUNITY

Our initial step was to identify and get to know local community organizations that share our values, goals, priorities, and empirical decision-making methods. Our expertise in bullying prevention led to an invitation by a local nonprofit, nonpartisan organization called Communities United Against Hate, which hosted a series of countywide conferences with school staff and leaders, county council members, community organizations, parents, and youth to address hate crime and bullying toward minority students, and promote inclusiveness and diversity. The conference series was sponsored by more than 20 organizations (including schools). Some Asian American community groups also attended the workshop (e.g., The Chinese American Parent Association). An event like this was a prime opportunity for us to get to know other community organizations and find potential collaborators. We were invited to be part of the opening plenary panel to discuss the topic of school climate, particularly as it relates to bullying of Asian American children in the school system. In our presentation, we emphasized how the school system can respond effectively to bullying incidents and underscored how schools should make their reporting form and process more accessible to parents. To be culturally inclusive, special considerations should be given to translating the form and making it available in multiple languages.

Other speakers covered topics relating to other ethnic/racial minority groups such as Muslim Americans and African Americans. For example, one schoolteacher showed a video project that she and her fourth grade class created to address bias and promote understanding. A school staff member described her efforts to monitor different bus stops in a low-income neighborhood. Many negative peer-to-peer interactions, including bullying, often occur at these bus stops due to the lack of adult supervision. In her intervention, she brought activities for the children to do while they were waiting for the school bus. Her presence inspired parents to begin supervising their children at the bus stop. The panel also included a student and a teacher from a local high school, and a representative from an LGBTQ+ ally organization, PFLAG. They discussed the harassment and bullying experiences of sexual minority students in the schools. These initial contacts and interactions with community organizations reiterated the importance of collaborating with school districts and connecting with parents to prevent bullying.

In deciding which organizations to partner with, we prioritized community entities that have previous experience with research, are open to continuing participation in research, and share our goals and mission. Our partners included a Chinese American parent organization, a school district, a Pan Asian volunteer health clinic, and several Chinese language schools. Additionally, we sought out organizations with established infrastructure and community networks to make mobilization and the organization of community events more successful. The leaders from the parent organization and the school district were already using data to make decisions in their programming and were open to data collection. The university team and community leaders spent time together during meetings, meals, and community events to build rapport before establishing the formal partnership. Relationship building is an ongoing process that occurs throughout our collaboration.

PROBLEM IDENTIFICATION

The Chinese American Parent Association of Montgomery County (CAPA-MC) invited us to share our expertise in bullying prevention at an event they organized with the school district, called "Back Off, Bully." Before the event, the first author met with the CAPA-MC leaders to identify the problem, community needs, goals for the workshop, and collaboration aims. The leaders of CAPA-MC identified bullying as the target problem of interest in the community, including lack of clarity about the definition of bullying, how to report bullying to authorities, and how to work with schools to reduce bullying rates. After two working sessions, we decided to invite local Asian American parents to the event, where we presented data on the prevalence of bullying and reasons for bullying (particularly as it related to Asian American youth). To engage parents in the discussion, we developed vignettes featuring Asian American youth of varying ages who experience different types of bullying. These vignettes led to discussions with parents on how to better respond to bullying incidents. Parents were encouraged to express their viewpoints and also listen to other parents' perspectives. An online clicker system was implemented where parents choose among multichoice responses on their phone. The anonymous responses were tabulated and displayed for the group to see.

To capture the voices of community members, we also invited parents and youth to share their personal stories related to bullying, and how they responded to the incidents and lessons learned. Adolescents, parents, and young adults disclosed their own experiences of bullying. For example, being kicked or pushed on the playground, called racial slurs, and being harassed for having an accent and "slanted eyes." These impactful stories centered on the themes of ethnic and racial bullying in schools as well as experiences of reporting bullying incidents (e.g., to the school principal, to police). Additionally, older students shared insight with younger students about how to handle bullying in schools.

Moreover, leaders from the school districts shared about the procedures (e.g., the Bullying Report form) that parents and youth should use to report bullying. An Asian American school principal also shared his experience in handling bullying issues at his school. More than 100 parents and their youth attended the events alongside community leaders. Dinner was provided by a nonprofit organization for the speakers, leaders in the organizations, and staff who were involved in organizing the event to give them an opportunity to build rapport and get to know one other further. At the end of the event,

TABLE 14.1. Back Off! Antibullying Workshop Participant Feedback

	Strongly agree	Agree	Disagree
I have a better understanding of bullying after attending the workshop.	88% (*n* = 43)	12% (*n* = 6)	0
I have a better understanding of bullying reporting procedures after attending the workshop.	96% (*n* = 47)	4% (*n* = 2)	0
I am interested in learning additional techniques on how to handle bullying situations.	92% (*n* = 45)	8% (*n* = 4)	0

we collected evaluations using survey items and open-ended questions to help identify the needs of the participants (see Table 14.1). The responses were positive, suggesting that participants perceived the events as being informative and helpful. Participants suggested additional topics for future workshops, including workshops to build parenting skills and cross-cultural or cross-generational communication skills. However, parents were also concerned about whether, when they report the bullying to school officials, this will be in their child's educational record and have a negative impact on their child's college application.

DEVELOPING CULTURE-INFORMED INTERVENTION AND EVALUATION

On the basis of the feedback from the "Back Off, Bully" event, the university team in collaboration with the partners (CAPA-MC, the school district, and several leaders from the Chinese language schools) developed and implemented a 2-hour parenting workshop titled "Dos and Don'ts: Bullying Prevention for Asian American Parents." The purpose of this workshop was to disseminate evidence-based bullying prevention strategies to Asian American parents. The team elaborated on the bullying scenario vignettes using information from stories shared by other Asian American parents and community leaders. Before the workshop implementation, the research team met with Asian American leaders in the community to ensure the intervention is culturally responsive to the community's needs. School leaders at the Chinese language schools and other Asian American organizations (e.g., the Pan Asian health clinic) helped advertise the workshop to parents, facilitated the event (e.g., introducing us), and participated in the discussion by sharing their unique perspectives during the workshop. The community leaders' involvement was a tremendous asset allowing us to tailor the intervention to be culturally informed.

Additionally, we partnered with the school district's Parent Academy program, whose mission is to inform and empower families as advocates and partners in their children's education. We were able to present the workshop at local schools with a facilitator, translators (for parents who speak different

TABLE 14.2. Future Workshop Topics of Interest Based on Back Off! Antibullying Workshop

Topic	n
Building my parenting skills	65% (n = 32)
Helping my child explore career choices	57% (n = 28)
College application information	61% (n = 30)
Preventing drug/alcohol abuse	49% (n = 24)
Cross-cultural/cross-generational communication	65% (n = 32)

Asian languages), and a day care provider present (for parents with young children). In addition to presenting the workshop through Parent Academy at the school district, we also offered the workshop to parents at three different Chinese language schools on Saturdays. Chinese American parents (as well as some other East Asian parents) usually send their children to Chinese language schools to learn their native language and many stay at the school to wait for their children. This provided a good opportunity to meet parents where they are.

The content of the workshop included discussions on how to foster healthy ethnic–racial socialization (a protective factor against bullying victimization), how to teach children social skills through stories and role-plays, how to monitor internet access and use, and how to respond to children who disclose being bullied (e.g., show empathy, do not blame children for the bullying). Substantial time was built into the lesson to allow parents to share their experiences. Parents shared emotionally charged stories of their children being made fun of for bringing Asian food to school for lunch, for their Asian eyes, foreign accents, and so on. Parents also shared with the group how they handled bullying and discrimination. We hoped that the workshop would provide a context for immigrant parents to build their social support networks. Some parents formed an online support group through WeChat (an online platform commonly used in China) to share information and resources after the event.

At the end of the workshop, we collected data on parent satisfaction and recommendations for future workshops (see Tables 14.1, 14.2, and 14.3). In the

TABLE 14.3. Participant Satisfaction Ratings for the Intervention From the First Iteration of the Workshop

	Strongly agree	Agree	Disagree or strongly disagree
Attending this workshop was a valuable use of my time.	68% (n = 13)	32% (n = 6)	0
I will take what I learned at this workshop and use it at home with my child.	47% (n = 9)	53% (n = 10)	0
The presenter was clear and the information was easy for me to understand.	58% (n = 11)	42% (n = 8)	0

Note. These data were collected by the school district at the end of the workshop and shared with the research team.

feedback collected from the first session, parents requested more training on cyberbullying and how to monitor screen use. During the second iteration of the workshop, this information was integrated into the workshop content. The ratings were again very positive, suggesting the workshops were well received by Asian American parents.

Preventing Bullying of Sikh American Students

Sikh American students are frequent targets of bullying due to certain physical and religious markers (e.g., turban, uncut beard; Ahluwalia, 2011; Falcone, 2006). To specifically address bullying toward Sikh American communities, the third author, who is Sikh American herself, collaborated with members of the Sikh community and Sikh organizations over the past several years. First, she conducted a survey to gain a better understanding of the severity of bullying of Sikh American youth, including the prevalence and perceived reasons for the bullying, as well as mental health of and coping strategies used by the youth. The third author described the project to community members who then referred the research team to community leaders. These leaders included the principal of a Sikh weekend school and a leader of a Sikh Gurdwara (place of worship). Contact was also established with the Jakara Movement, a grassroots community-building Sikh organization, which provided information about different events being held for Sikh American adolescents in California.

With the help of these Sikh community organizations, survey data were collected from 202 Sikh American adolescents from 75 cities in California (54% male, age: $M = 14.19$ years, $SD = 1.86$). Results indicated that 76.4% of the Sikh American students experienced bullying victimization at school. Specifically, these adolescents reported at least one incident of physical (e.g., hurt me physically in some way, kicked me, punched me), verbal (e.g., called me names, swore at me, made fun of me because of my appearance) or relational (e.g., made other people not talk to me, tried to make my friends turn against me) victimization by a peer. Adolescents were also asked, "What group of students is most likely to be bullied at school?" and 43.7% reported that Asians or religious minorities were most likely to be bullied.

Additionally, results indicated that wearing a religious head covering is related to being perceived as a foreigner, which predicted greater victimization and adjustment difficulties. While speaking to Sikh youth and parents at community events, the third author was told that Sikh American youth are often called "terrorists" or "Osama Bin Laden's family" due to wearing a *patka* or turban or having long uncut hair. Youth also report experiencing physical violence, such as having rocks thrown at them or having their *patkas* or turbans touched or removed by peers.

Peer victimization and the "perpetual foreigner" stereotype (i.e., the stereotype of being perpetually foreign and therefore not truly "American") were significantly related to lower self-esteem and more depressive and anxiety symptoms (Atwal & Wang, 2019). High avoidant coping exacerbated the relationship between peer victimization and anxiety symptoms. Low enculturation (engaging in cultural and religious practices) also exacerbated the relationship between the perpetual foreigner stereotype and depressive symptoms (Do et al., 2019).

After data collection, the third author contacted the Sikh Coalition to share these research findings. She talked to the community development director at the Sikh Coalition, who responded with a high level of interest; she is also currently collaborating with the staff member at Sikh Coalition to work on disseminating the research findings. There are plans to further share these research findings with the community by e-mailing various Sikh organizations and asking for the content to be included in their presentations to schools and the community and be disseminated through the organizations' listservs. This project is ongoing, but the response we received from the community leaders has been very positive.

It is important to share research findings with the Sikh American community as well as the larger society (e.g., school system) to reduce bullying and improve the lives of Sikh American youth. Numerous organizations are focused on Sikh American issues, including the Sikh American Legal Defense and Education Fund, the Sikh Coalition, Jakara Movement, and United Sikhs. Researchers can share their findings by collaborating with these organizations. The Sikh Coalition also develops campaigns focused on incorporating Sikhism in state curriculum standards, preventing and ending school bullying, and revising textbooks to include accurate Sikh content. On their website, they ask for individuals to report school bullying to the Sikh Coalition's legal team, to organize a Sikh Awareness Presentation at your child's school, and to share the Sikhism Educator's Guide with teachers and administrators (https://www.sikhcoalition.org). The Sikh Coalition has many accessible resources for the public and can be used by individuals, schools, and organizations. Individuals can also request guest presentations to promote awareness about bullying in their own communities. These organizations work hard to increase awareness of and knowledge about Sikh Americans and welcome individuals to contact them at any time with any information or concerns. For example, the Sikh Coalition supported CNN's episode of *United Shades of America* with Kamau Bell in 2019. This episode was the first hour-long cable episode exclusively focused on the Sikh American community.

DISCUSSION

The integrative risk and resilience model (Suárez-Orozco et al., 2018) suggests that individual (e.g., cognitive resources, social–emotional resources), microsystems (e.g., schools, families, neighborhood), political and social contexts (e.g., national immigration policies, attitudes toward migrants), and global forces all contribute to immigrant-origin students' adjustment. All of these factors contribute to Asian American students' experiences with bullying and discrimination. Most Asian American children live with at least one immigrant parent; immigrant parents tend to lack knowledge about U.S. school systems and have difficulty advocating for their children at school. For researchers and clinicians who work with communities, it is imperative to share research findings with the Asian American community and local schools. To do so, researchers need to initially establish connections and relationships with the community. This can be accomplished by attending events at community organizations, religious places, such as temples, Gurdwaras (Sikh places of worship), and Asian churches. An important consideration during this initial stage is to be cognizant, respectful, and open to learning cultural norms. For example, when entering a Sikh religious place of worship, all individuals are asked to cover their heads and remove their shoes. It is important to respect the norms of the setting while sharing information.

Additionally, it is important to "understand the cultural norms and behaviors of families as well as the language differences that exist between and even within cultures" (Leiber-Miller, 2012, p. 13). For educators to communicate with families effectively and serve as effective cultural advocates for families and students, researchers and clinicians must also consider ecological variables that impact Asian American youth and families, reflect on their own assumptions or preconceived notions about a student or family, consider acculturation and its effects on families and students, understand that a negative response to acculturation can lead to maladaptive cultural characteristics, and when in doubt, communicate respectfully, clearly, and thoroughly (Guerrero & Leung, 2008). To develop culturally responsive interventions for Asian Americans, it is also important to include voices from parents and community leaders during the development, reiteration (modification), and evaluation of the intervention.

Additionally, schools play a crucial role in bullying prevention given the substantial time that youth spend in the classroom. Multi-tiered systems of support (MTSS) is a systemic approach for schools to build more inclusive communities that can be an effective way to prevent bullying at school. MTSS is an evidence-based framework that integrates academic and behavior instruction and intervention and utilizes data-based problem-solving to improve outcomes for all students (Batsche, 2014). School-wide positive behavior support is an example of a specific framework that "provides an infrastructure that can support and maintain inclusive practices demonstrated to be effective for improving outcomes for all students" (Freeman et al., 2006, p. 15). In addition, systemic implementation of social and emotional learning (SEL) can also help build more inclusive communities, by fostering caring and equitable learning environments. The Collaborative for Academic, Social, and Emotional Learning (CASEL) identified the five core competencies of SEL as self-awareness, self-management, social awareness, relationship skills, and responsible decision making. In a systemic approach, these competencies are infused into different aspects of students' school experience. By implementing SEL, individual cultural assets that students bring to their schools can be promoted. To accomplish this, schools should implement equitable SEL practices that promote understanding, examine biases, address the impact of racism, build cross-cultural relationships, and create inclusive school communities (CASEL, 2020). By improving inclusivity and school climate through SEL, schools can also improve their bullying prevention efforts. Embedding bullying prevention programs into SEL frameworks fosters inclusive, warm, and respectful school climates that minimize the occurrence of bullying behaviors (CASEL, 2009).

Furthermore, to prevent bullying, researchers and clinicians need to work with schools and foster partnerships among school, family, and community to support students from diverse populations. Clinicians should collaborate with school staff members to promote awareness about bullying through school assemblies, parent information nights, and other modalities (such as the Parent Academy program, as we discussed). Moreover, school staff could also promote awareness of Asian American culture (e.g., during Asian American heritage month) so that Asian American students feel that they are an integral and respected part of the school community. Schools must make cultural modifications to their current ways of working with families, including "making home visits, respect for parents' cultural style, respect for parent gender roles, finding community services, using the school as a resource, and providing follow-up" (Behring et al., 2000, p. 363). Asian American students, including Sikh Americans, who have experienced marginalization, may be more vulnerable to stressors. Researchers and clinicians should encourage educators to understand the effect of stressors and trauma on Asian American students' mental health and functioning, be sensitive to family stressors (including acculturative stress), understand cultural views regarding mental health, and encourage families to access community resources (National Association of School Psychologists, 2016). Only when researchers, clinicians, schools, families, and communities work together, can we reduce bullying of Asian American students.

REFERENCES

Ahluwalia, M. K. (2011). Holding my breath: The experience of being Sikh after 9/11. *Traumatology, 17*(3), 41–46. https://doi.org/10.1177/1534765611421962

Ahuja, K. (2014, November 18). *Strengthening the AAPI community through new bullying prevention efforts.* Obama Whitehouse Archives. https://www.whitehouse.gov/blog/2014/11/18/strengthening-aapi-community-through-new-bullying-prevention-efforts

Asian American Legal Defense and Education Fund. (2013). *One step forward, half a step back: A status report on bias-based bullying of Asian American students in New York city schools.* Issuelab. https://www.issuelab.org/resource/one-step-forward-half-a-step-back-a-status-report-on-bias-based-bullying-of-asian-american-students-in-new-york-city-schools.html

Atwal, K., & Wang, C. (2019). Religious head covering, being perceived as foreigners, victimization, and adjustment among Sikh American adolescents. *School Psychology, 34*(2), 233–243. https://doi.org/10.1037/spq0000301

Bajaj, M., Ghaffar-Kucher, A., & Desai, K. (2016). Brown bodies and xenophobic bullying in US schools: Critical analysis and strategies for action. *Harvard Educational Review, 86*(4), 481–505. https://doi.org/10.17763/1943-5045-86.4.481

Baker, Ö. E., & Tanrikulu, İ. (2010). Psychological consequences of cyber bullying experiences among Turkish secondary school children. *Procedia: Social and Behavioral Sciences, 2*(2), 2771–2776. https://doi.org/10.1016/j.sbspro.2010.03.413

Batsche, G. (2014). Multi-tiered systems of support for inclusive schools. In J. McLeskey, N. L. Waldron, F. Spooner, & B. Algozzine (Eds.), *Handbook of effective inclusive schools: Research and practice* (pp. 183–196). Routledge. https://doi.org/10.4324/9780203102930.ch14

Behring, S. T., Cabello, B., Kushida, D., & Murguia, A. (2000). Cultural modifications to current school-based consultation approaches reported by culturally diverse beginning consultants. *School Psychology Review, 29*(3), 354–367. https://www.tandfonline.com/doi/abs/10.1080/02796015.2000.12086020

CASEL. (2009). *Social and emotional learning and bullying prevention.* https://www.casel.org/wp-content/uploads/2016/01/3_SEL_and_Bullying_Prevention_2009.pdf

CASEL. (2020). *What is social and emotional learning? CASEL Guide to SEL.* https://schoolguide.casel.org/what-is-sel/what-is-sel/

Child Trends. (2018). *Key facts about immigrant children.* https://www.childtrends.org/?indicators=immigrant-children

Costello, M. R. (2016). *Teaching the 2016 election. The Trump effect: The impact of the presidential campaign on our nation's schools.* Southern Poverty Law Center. https://www.splcenter.org/sites/default/files/splc_the_trump_effect.pdf

Crepeau-Hobson, F., & Leech, N. L. (2016). Peer victimization and suicidal behaviors among high school youth. *Journal of School Violence, 15*(3), 302–321. https://doi.org/10.1080/15388220.2014.996717

Davis, J. P., Dumas, T. M., Merrin, G. J., Espelage, D. L., Tan, K., Madden, D., & Hong, J. S. (2018). Examining the pathways between bully victimization, depression, academic achievement, and problematic drinking in adolescence. *Psychology of Addictive Behaviors, 32*(6), 605–616. https://doi.org/10.1037/adb0000394

Dempsey, A. G., Sulkowski, M. L., Nichols, R., & Storch, E. A. (2009). Differences between peer victimization in cyber and physical settings and associated psycho-social adjustment in early adolescence. *Psychology in the Schools, 46*(10), 962–972. https://doi.org/10.1002/pits.20437

Do, K. A., Wang, C., & Atwal, K. (2019). Peer victimization and the perpetual foreigner stereotype on Sikh American adolescents' mental health outcomes: The moderating effects of coping and behavior enculturation. *Asian American Journal of Psychology, 10*(2), 131–140. https://doi.org/10.1037/aap0000132

Falcone, J. (2006). Seeking recognition: Patriotism, power and politics in Sikh American discourse in the immediate aftermath of 9/11. *Diaspora, 15*(1), 89–119. https://doi.org/10.1353/dsp.0.0030

Fisher, C. B., Wallace, S. A., & Fenton, R. E. (2000). Discrimination distress during adolescence. *Journal of Youth and Adolescence, 29*(6), 679–695. https://doi.org/10.1023/A:1026455906512

Fredstrom, B. K., Adams, R. E., & Gilman, R. (2011). Electronic and school-based victimization: Unique contexts for adjustment difficulties during adolescence. *Journal of Youth and Adolescence, 40*(4), 405–415. https://doi.org/10.1007/s10964-010-9569-7

Freeman, R., Eber, L., Anderson, C., Irvin, L., Horner, R., Bounds, M., & Dunlap, G. (2006). Building inclusive school cultures using school-wide positive behavior support: Designing effective individual support systems for students with significant disabilities. *Research and Practice for Persons with Severe Disabilities, 31*(1), 4–17. https://doi.org/10.2511/rpsd.31.1.4

Goebert, D., Else, I., Matsu, C., Chung-Do, J., & Chang, J. Y. (2011). The impact of cyberbullying on substance use and mental health in a multiethnic sample. *Maternal and Child Health Journal, 15*(8), 1282–1286. https://doi.org/10.1007/s10995-010-0672-x

Greene, M. L., Way, N., & Pahl, K. (2006). Trajectories of perceived adult and peer discrimination among Black, Latino, and Asian American adolescents: Patterns and psychological correlates. *Developmental Psychology, 42*(2), 218–236. https://doi.org/10.1037/0012-1649.42.2.218

Guerrero, C., & Leung, B. (2008). Communicating effectively with culturally and linguistically diverse families. *Communique, 36*(8). https://www.nasponline.org/publications/periodicals/communique/issues/volume-36-issue-8

Hoglund, W. L. G., & Hosan, N. E. (2013). The context of ethnicity: Peer victimization and adjustment problems in early adolescence. *The Journal of Early Adolescence, 33*(5), 585–609. https://doi.org/10.1177/0272431612451925

Juvonen, J., Wang, Y., & Espinoza, G. (2011). Bullying experiences and compromised academic performance across middle school grades. *The Journal of Early Adolescence, 31*(1), 152–173. https://doi.org/10.1177/0272431610379415

Koo, D. J., Peguero, A. A., & Shekarkhar, Z. (2012). Gender, immigration, and school victimization. *Victims & Offenders, 7*(1), 77–96. https://doi.org/10.1080/15564886.2011.629773

Leiber-Miller, R. (2012, January). Families as partners: Making the connection. *The School Social Worker: Principal Leadership. 2012*, 12–16.

López, G., Ruiz, N. G., & Patten, E. (2017). *Key facts about Asian Americans, a diverse and growing population*. Pew Research Center. Fact Tank: News in the Numbers. http://www.pewresearch.org/fact-tank/2017/09/08/key-facts-about-asian-americans/

Ma, G. X., Toubbeh, J. I., Su, X., & Edwards, R. L. (2004). ATECAR: An Asian American community-based participatory research model on tobacco and cancer control. *Health Promotion Practice, 5*(4), 382–394. https://doi.org/10.1177/1524839903260146

Maynard, B. R., Vaughn, M. G., Salas-Wright, C. P., & Vaughn, S. (2016). Bullying victimization among school-aged immigrant youth in the United States. *The Journal of Adolescent Health, 58*(3), 337–344. https://doi.org/10.1016/j.jadohealth.2015.11.013

McKenney, K. S., Pepler, D., Craig, W., & Connolly, J. (2006). Peer victimization and psychosocial adjustment: The experiences of Canadian immigrant youth. *Electronic Journal of Research in Educational Psychology, 9*(4), 239–264.

Nakamoto, J., & Schwartz, D. (2010). Is peer victimization associated with academic achievement? A meta-analytic review. *Social Development, 19*(2), 221–242. https://doi.org/10.1111/j.1467-9507.2009.00539.x

Nansel, T. J., Overpeck, M., Pilla, R. S., Ruan, W. J., Simons-Morton, B., & Scheidt, P. (2001). Bullying behaviors among U.S. youth: Prevalence and association with psychological adjustment. *JAMA, 285*, 2094–2100. https://jamanetwork.com/journals/jama/fullarticle/193774

Nastasi, B. K. (2017). A transcultural approach to systems-level consultation. In C. Hatzichristou & S. Rosenfield (Eds.), *The international handbook of consultation in educational settings* (pp. 97–114). Routledge. https://doi.org/10.4324/9781315795188-6

National Association of School Psychologists. (2016). *Supporting marginalized students in stressful times: Tips for educators* [Handout]. https://www.nasponline.org/resources-and-publications/resources-and-podcasts/diversity/social-justice/supporting-marginalized-students-in-stressful-times-tips-for-educators

Nishina, A. (2012). Microcontextual characteristics of peer victimization experiences and adolescents' daily well-being. *Journal of Youth and Adolescence, 41*(2), 191–201. https://doi.org/10.1007/s10964-011-9669-z

Olweus, D. (1999). Sweden. In P. K. Smith, Y. Morita, J. Junger-Tas, D. Olweus, R. Catalano, & P. Slee (Eds.), *The nature of school bullying: A cross-national perspective* (pp. 7–27). Routledge.

Peguero, A. A. (2009). Victimizing the children of immigrants: Latino and Asian American student victimization. *Youth & Society, 41*(2), 186–208. https://doi.org/10.1177/0044118X09333646

Peguero, A. A., & Williams, L. M. (2013). Racial and ethnic stereotypes and bullying victimization. *Youth & Society, 45*(4), 545–564. https://doi.org/10.1177/0044118X11424757

Pyke, K., & Dang, T. (2003). "FOB" and "whitewashed": Identity and internalized racism among second generation Asian Americans. *Qualitative Sociology, 26*(2), 147–172. https://doi.org/10.1023/A:1022957011866

Qin, D. B., Way, N., & Rana, M. (2008). The "model minority" and their discontent: Examining peer discrimination and harassment of Chinese American immigrant youth. *New Directions for Child and Adolescent Development, 2008,* 27–42. https://doi.org/10.1002/cd.221

Romero, A. J., Gonzalez, H., & Smith, B. A. (2015). Qualitative exploration of adolescent discrimination: Experiences and responses of Mexican-American parents and teens. *Journal of Child and Family Studies, 24*(6), 1531–1543. https://doi.org/10.1007/s10826-014-9957-9

Rosenbloom, S. R., & Way, N. (2004). Experiences of discrimination among African American, Asian American, and Latino adolescents in an urban high school. *Youth & Society, 35*(4), 420–451. https://doi.org/10.1177/0044118X03261479

Scherr, T. G., & Larson, J. (2010). Bullying dynamics associated with race, ethnicity, and immigration status. In S. R. Jimerson, S. M. Swearer, & D. L. Espelage (Eds.), *Handbook of bullying in schools: An international perspective* (pp. 223–234). Routledge.

Shea, M., Wang, C., Shi, W., Gonzalez, V., & Espelage, D. (2016). Parents and teachers' perspectives on school bullying among elementary school-aged Asian and Latino immigrant children. *Asian American Journal of Psychology, 7*(2), 83–96. https://doi.org/10.1037/aap0000047

Shin, J. Y., D'Antonio, E., Son, H., Kim, S.-A., & Park, Y. (2011). Bullying and discrimination experiences among Korean-American adolescents. *Journal of Adolescence, 34*(5), 873–883. https://doi.org/10.1016/j.adolescence.2011.01.004

The Sikh Coalition. (2010). *Sikh coalition Bay Area civil rights report 2010.* https://www.sikhcoalition.org/wp-content/uploads/2016/11/2010-Bay-Area-Civil-Rights-Report.pdf

The Sikh Coalition. (2014). *"Go home terrorist": A report on bullying against Sikh American school children.* https://www.sikhcoalition.org/documents/pdf/go-home-terrorist.pdf

Spriggs, A. L., Iannotti, R. J., Nansel, T. R., & Haynie, D. L. (2007). Adolescent bullying involvement and perceived family, peer and school relations: Commonalities and differences across race/ethnicity. *Journal of Adolescent Health, 41*(3), 283–293. https://doi.org/10.1016/j.jadohealth.2007.04.009

Suárez-Orozco, C., Motti-Stefanidi, F., Marks, A., & Katsiaficas, D. (2018). An integrative risk and resilience model for understanding the adaptation of immigrant-origin children and youth. *American Psychologist, 73*(6), 781–796. https://doi.org/10.1037/amp0000265

Sulkowski, M. L., Bauman, S., Wright, S., Nixon, C., & Davis, S. (2014). Peer victimization in youth from immigrant and non-immigrant US families. *School Psychology International, 35*(6), 649–669. https://doi.org/10.1177/0143034314554968

United Sikhs. (2010). *United Sikhs bullying prevention initiative.* http://www.unitedsikhs.org/docs/UNITED-SIKHS-Bullying-Prevention.pdf

U.S. Department of Education. (2011). *Student reports of bullying and cyber-bullying: Results from the 2009 School Crime Supplement to the National Crime Victimization Survey.* http://nces.ed.gov/pubs2011/2011336.pdf

Vergara, G. A., Stewart, J. G., Cosby, E. A., Lincoln, S. H., & Auerbach, R. P. (2019). Non-suicidal self-injury and suicide in depressed adolescents: Impact of peer victimization and bullying. *Journal of Affective Disorders, 245,* 744–749. https://doi.org/10.1016/j.jad.2018.11.084

Wang, C., Wang, W., Zheng, L., & Atwal, K. (2016). Bullying prevention as a social justice issue: Implications with Asian American elementary school students. *School Psychology Forum, 10*(3), 251–264.

Zych, I., Farrington, D. P., & Ttofi, M. M. (2019). Protective factors against bullying and cyberbullying: A systematic review of meta-analyses. *Aggression and Violent Behavior, 45*(2), 4–19. https://doi.org/10.1016/j.avb.2018.06.008

15

Toward a Liberatory Practice

Shifting the Ideological Premise of Trauma Work With Immigrants

Lara Sheehi and Leilani Salvo Crane

*She has undisguised contempt for America and its people, this should worry you . . .
Ilhan Omar is living proof that the way we practice immigration has become dangerous
to this country. A system designed to strengthen America is instead undermining it. Some
of the people we try our hardest to help, have come to hate us passionately. Maybe that's
our fault for asking too little of immigrants. We are self-confident enough to never make
them assimilate, so they never feel fully American. Or maybe the problem is deeper than
that. Maybe we're importing people from places whose values are simply antithetical
to ours . . . there is a problem. Whatever the cause, this is unsustainable. No country can
import a large number of people who hate it and expect to survive. . . . So be grateful for
Ilhan Omar; as annoying as she is, she is a living fire alarm. A warning to the rest of us:
we better change our immigration system immediately, or else.*

TUCKER CARLSON, *TUCKER CARLSON TONIGHT*, JULY 10, 2019

As psychoanalytic clinicians interested in how all things are multidetermined as well as the way language can be used to work against and through surface process, we call attention to the more insidious communication in Carlson's tirade. While we acknowledge that Carlson represents an extreme, we also contend that he could not come to exist, nor would his words find traction, should the systemic configuration not allow it. The communiqué belies an ideological assumption, a "truth" of sorts, that reflects the underbelly of anti-immigrant sentiment in the United States and represents a fundamentally raw, undefended exposé of the current sociopolitical terrain. That is, while he

https://doi.org/10.1037/0000214-016
Trauma and Racial Minority Immigrants: Turmoil, Uncertainty, and Resistance,
P. Tummala-Narra (Editor)

panders to a right-wing, extremist base, we believe he also harnesses the conscious and unconscious racist and, therefore, fundamentally anti-immigrant, attitudes that birthed the United States. Indeed, in discussing President Obama's 2014 speech on immigration where he claimed that providing safe haven for immigrants is an integral part of the United States social fabric, Chavez-Dueñas et al. (2019) reminded us that

> While it is factually accurate to say that the United States has a long history of immigrants coming to its borders, this phrase renders invisible the contributions and experiences of Native American and African populations who were colonized, enslaved, and oppressed. The phrase also hides the experiences of violence, racism, and ethnic oppression faced by many immigrant populations (e.g., people of Middle East and North African descent, Asian/Pacific Islanders, individuals of Latin American descent). (p. 50)

We view this acknowledgment as an ethical imperative that undergirds the clinical and assessment work in which we both engage.

In this chapter, we challenge some key ideological principles in the field, with attention to trauma work in general, and with immigrant populations in specific. These ideological principles include Eurocentric premises of trauma, diagnostic categories, and treatment options and approaches (Duran & Duran, 1995; Duran et al., 2008; Root, 1992). We also offer recommendations of how we can begin to decenter these "common sense" (Hollander, 2010) ideological constructs, relying heavily on liberation psychology principles as well as the tremendous existing body of work by indigenous scholars. Finally, we offer clinical vignettes to provide experiential texture to the recommendations provided. We conclude by offering hope for potential aggregate outcomes of what we believe is an imperative shift in our practice and techniques.

We contend that an ethical and attuned practice with immigrant populations cannot happen without an ideological shift in the theoretical and technical basis of how we function as clinicians. This necessarily includes locating our own selves, as clinicians, but also as a whole profession, within a sociopolitical history that accounts for intersectional (Crenshaw, 1989) experience within oppressive systems. Historical and geographical specificity is also key. To this end, at the time of writing, we locate ourselves on occupied Pamunkey and Lenape land, respectively, as well as within a particularly tumultuous and violent political landscape in which immigration plays a central role. Indeed, while we currently live in the onslaught of hyperethnonationalist anti-immigrant rhetoric, the legal bedrock for this reality, dubbed "crimmigration" (Stumpf, 2006), was set half a century ago—what Burstow (2003) referred to as a process of naming who makes a "legitimate" immigrant or refugee.

Our analysis, therefore, exists against the backdrop of seminal legislative acts[1] that had the effect of criminalizing immigrants and adding to what

---

[1]See The Immigration and Nationality Act of 1965, Immigration Reform and Control Act (IRCA), and Illegal Immigration Reform and Immigrant Responsibility Act (IIRIRA), as noted in Chavez-Dueñas et al., 2019, p. 52.

scholars and clinicians have warned are deleterious psychological effects (Comas-Díaz, 2007; Furman et al., 2015; Tummala-Narra, 2014). These legislative acts culminated in the Criminal Alien Program (CAP) and the formation of the Immigration and Customs Enforcement (ICE) agency, which works to "purposefully . . . instill fear in immigrants; in other words, to terrorize, to make them voluntarily deport themselves to their countries of origin" (Chavez-Dueñas et al., 2019, p. 53). The Congressional Research Service has identified at least 219 immigration bills in 2019 alone.[2] Furman et al. (2015) warned, "by criminalizing immigrant populations, the structural inequities in various societies minimize, as immigrants become pathologized and criminalized" (p. 815).

With an increase in immigrant arrests, there has also been an increase in hate crimes against immigrants (Costello, 2016). Perhaps more difficult to digest, however, is our own implication as a field: How may we be complicit in continued aggressions against immigrant populations, even if unconsciously? This is especially important to consider when we are alerted to how, for example, clinical assessments of undocumented youth by providers working for the Office of Refugee Resettlement are being abused by the current administration to shore up detention orders (Nilson, 2018).

PSYCHOLOGICAL EFFECTS OF IMMIGRATION

The psychological stress inherent to immigration is augmented by a reality-based anxiety regarding anti-immigrant sentiment, even when migration has been done "legally."[3] Hernandez-Wolfe et al. (2015) alerted us to the possibility that immigrant communities face "extreme hardship" (p. 155) when they relocate to the United States. This is particularly true of the squalor found in the current-day inhumane detention centers in the United States (Office of the Inspector General, 2019).[4]

The effects of these various experiences and immigration stress include symptoms that mimic what is clinically expected in the wake of trauma, and scholars have warned of a communal effect (Lopez & Minushkin, 2008). Further, scholars have underscored the threat to one's identity coherence and sense of belonging under race-specific immigration stress (Ainslie et al., 2013; Tummala-Narra, 2014). Research indicates that posttraumatic stress disorder (PTSD) symptoms are more acute in individuals who have experienced discrimination (Lowe et al., 2019) and corroborates findings that discrimination

---

[2]Found online (https://projects.propublica.org/represent/bills/category/immigration?page=1)

[3]We do not endorse the xenophobic use of legality, especially regarding persons exercising their rights for freedom of travel and movement, as well as seeking refuge; please see Aliverti (2012), for a reading of how "legality" was introduced in immigration discourse with the ideological purpose of criminalization.

[4]Full redacted report can be found online (https://int.nyt.com/data/documenthelper/1358-ig-report-migrant-detention/2dd9d40be6a6b0cd3619/optimized/full.pdf#page=1)

itself, including both subtle and overt forms, can be traumatizing (Broman et al., 2000; Carter, 2007; Lowe et al., 2019). This is why Burstow (2003) reminded us, "Trauma is inherently political" (p. 1306).

We will discuss how our field as a whole, and as an ideological practice (Duran & Duran, 1995; Duran et al., 2008; Harlem, 2009), has tended to split off the inherently sociopolitical backdrop of trauma and therefore silo off its etiology exclusively in the psychic realm. We discuss the basis of this ideological misattunement, so as to further advocate for a shift of ideology toward a more sensitive, attuned, and, ultimately, liberatory practice with immigrant communities.

The Ideology of Misattuned Care

If Fanon was writing in 1961 about the "muscular" (i.e., felt on a cellular level) memory and dreams of the colonizer by the colonized, and Erickson (1995) spoke of community "tissues" being cumulatively torn under the stress of trauma, how have the overwhelming structures of the mental health field—to include psychology, counseling, and psychiatry—largely eschewed a historically specific, cultural, and sociopolitical understanding of trauma in favor of an individually based "point-in-time" theoretical construct? Further, how does one justify ethically attuned care if one does not take into account social, political, and systemic oppressions in the wake of even the American Psychological Association's (APA's; 2017) call to include intersectionality in our thinking and practice and encouragement to "challenge systems of oppression"?

That this split is ideologically based (e.g., in contrast to lack of knowledge) has been documented for decades by Braveheart-Jordan and DeBruyn (1995), Duran and Duran (1995), Duran et al. (1998), and Gone (2007). Indeed, these scholars have long advocated for a historically rooted understanding of trauma with specific focus on the deleterious (and ongoing) effects of colonization on indigenous peoples. Burstow (2003), in recounting feminist contributions to the trauma literature, modeled what feminists have advocated for, that is, "the significance of social location [in] trauma discourse" (p. 1295) by acknowledging how her own work was ensconced in a world

> in which women, the working class, Natives, people of color, Jews, lesbians and gays, and the disabled are routinely violated both in overt physical ways and in other ways inherent in systemic oppression and where the psychological effects of this violation are often passed down from generation to generation. (p. 1294)

Brown (2008) and Mattar (2011) called attention to how trauma work must attend to immigrant populations. The trauma literature, unfortunately, has tended to exclude nuanced and textured readings of how sociocultural, historical, and political dimensions contribute meaningfully to working with survivors. These scholars contended that, as a result, the ways in which these communities come to access healing that is linked to their specific identities and social positioning has been largely absent from the field. This is what

Burstow (2003), similarly contended when she underscored how "the political is not fully integrated" (p. 1294) in theories and practice related to trauma.

As such, it came to be that diagnoses overwhelmingly located social and structural issues within the individual and, by direct result, pathologized the traumatized (Burstow, 2003; Gilfus, 1999; Lewis, 1999; Root, 1992). Burstow (2003) warned that this, by default, would lead to unattuned clinical work and assessment because "the diagnoses are not sensitizing, nor could they be" (p. 1300). This supports the position that many scholars have taken, advocating that diagnostic labels and criteria are not "natural categories," but rather are constructed committee-based definitions (Abdullah & Brown, 2020; Kinderman, 2019; Woolfolk, 2001).

Reliance on these institutionally constructed categories is especially problematic when we account for the overwhelmingly Eurocentric properties of what constitutes "mainstream" evidence-based clinical work (Joseph, 2015), especially in the context of "what is considered to be normative and pathological" (Harlem, 2009). Harlem (2009) reminded us that "theorists, researchers, and practitioners must examine and recognize the Euro American values that underlie conceptions of health and pathology" (p. 398). Disavowing the ideological roots of the profession may cause clinicians to perpetuate various forms of injustice and institutional racism by imposing helping paradigms that are often incongruent with the worldviews, values, beliefs, and traditional practices that have been used to promote the psychological well-being of persons in diverse groups (Duran et al., 2008, p. 288).

Decentering Eurocentric Practices

We offer four overarching recommendations that we believe may work to decenter Eurocentric practices in work with racial minority immigrant communities and, ultimately, lead to an attuned care that advocates for their liberated and dignified existence. We organized these guidelines with an understanding that, due to the fluidity of sociopolitical status and context, they cannot, by default, be comprehensive in nature. We therefore also advocate for a multidimensional reading of these suggestions and, most important, for a humility and openness to learn and adjust practices, theory, and treatment based on input and guidance from the immigrant communities we serve.

We used liberation psychology (Freire, 1968; Martín-Baró, 1996) principles to guide our recommendations, the primary tenets of which stipulate that "healing entails an explicit focus on active resistance rather than solely reactionary resilience" (Chavez-Dueñas et al., 2019). More specifically, liberation psychology is interested in attending to the oppressive structures in which impoverished and disenfranchised people exist and in which their psyche is implicated. As such, our suggestions are primarily concerned with an understanding that oppression—specifically in context of the immigrant community—does not target merely the individual, but rather the collective, therefore requiring collective response; that clinicians are implicated in oppression and should integrate the social and historical in all practice decisions; that treatment and intervention should always be in service of self-determination; and, that clinicians should be explicit in their challenging of oppressive systems and structures, to include the field in which we practice and the theories and techniques we use.

We offer our suggestions in tandem with (as opposed to replacement of or in competition with) existing admirable frameworks, such as the HEART (Healing Ethno And Racial Trauma) framework[5] (Comas-Díaz et al., 2019; Chavez-Dueñas et al., 2019) and the multicultural orientation (MCO) framework.[6] We offer clinical vignettes in the following section to explicate what these recommendations may look like in practice.

1. Relinquish "Trauma" as Disorder

The movement away from trauma as an individual disorder, held and felt primarily in the individual realm, is key. While at first glance this may read as a provocative suggestion, various models exist, including those that reject a medically based understanding of trauma response and instead locate it in nonpathological terms, within a normative response to sustained historical oppression. For example, Brave Heart (2000) expanded on her previous work defining and documenting *historical trauma*. Gone (2013) described *historical trauma* as "complex"—to differ from Herman's (1992) definition of complex trauma—and "collective," as well as

> incorporating both the psychological and social sequelae of historical oppression, whereas PTSD—as a form of *psycho*pathology that is officially classified as a *mental* disorder so that it can be treated by *mental* health professionals—is largely confined to the psychology . . . of the individual. (p. 687, italics in original)

A move to understand trauma as sociopolitically based versus individually felt or experienced is important because it decenters the emphasis on pathology and, instead, acknowledges and normalizes social and psychological responses to structurally embedded violence and violations. This shift further advocates for a move away from what scholars have referred to as a damning "deficit model" that focuses on "the psychological at the expense of the political" (Burstow, 2003, p. 1311).

Understanding trauma, and especially PTSD, primarily through a medical model also creates the potential of missing relevant contextual information in a bid to adhere to criterion purity—that is, understanding the diagnosis as fitting within the strict frame of descriptive criteria. This is to what, for example, Palestinian clinicians objected to (Ghanadry-Hakim, September 9, 2018, personal communication) and what Dr. Samah Jabr, head of mental

---

[5] Please see Chavez-Dueñas et al. (2019) pp. 58–59 for a table detailing recommendations for the HEART framework.
[6] Please see Watkins et al. (2019) for a discussion related to how the MCO framework combines notions of "cultural humility," "cultural opportunities," and "cultural comfort."

health services in the Palestinian Territories, warned of when she referred to PTSD as a "Western construct," highlighting that for the Palestinian community, "there is no 'post' because the trauma is repetitive and ongoing and continuous" (Goldhill, 2019).[7]

Likewise, and in specific relation to immigration experience, Ainslie and colleagues (2013) suggested that when we refer to or conceptualize trauma-in-immigration as solely linked to the medicalized understanding of such phenomena, we risk losing sight of the *person* implicated in the diagnosis. Specifically, they highlighted that

> Immigration status has been understood as a social condition or environmental circumstance—*a context*—that, although at times may illuminate (or obscure) essential intrapsychic phenomena, is nonetheless held as conceptually distinct from, and clinically less important than, the *mind/person* embedded within it. (Ainslie et al., 2013, p. 664)

Our recommendation, then, of moving beyond trauma-as-disorder, to incorporate existing and historically organizing concepts of how trauma is a response to a "wound" or "wounding" (Burstow, 2003; Gone, 2007, 2013), has the effect of recentering the person—and specific to this chapter, the immigrant community—above the disorder or symptom profile. This decentering of the medical and individual and recentering of a communal, historical, and political understanding of trauma contribute to what Duran et al. (2008) referred to as a "relationship with the disorder instead of being the disorder" (p. 290). This relational possibility, in turn, creates liberatory potential by way of new narratives.

2. Validate Sociopolitical Reality and History

Lewis (1999) highlighted how the deficit model's emphasis on "restoring" trust and the illusory belief in a just and safe world is, at best, indicative of the elitism embedded in the ideological base of our practice. Burstow (2003) expanded on this ideological fallacy, stating,

> for the most part, people feel traumatized or wounded because they *have been* wounded. For the most part, traumatized people experience the world as dangerous not because they have been rendered inadequate by the trauma and, therefore, have an essentially distorted worldview. They so experience it because events or conditions precluded the editing out practices by which less traumatized people construct an essentially safe and benign world. (p. 1304)

The nonpathologized view of hyperalertness and hypervigilance as one of many responses to real and therefore, *not merely perceived*, effects of current-day, as well as past or ongoing, traumas is a central part of working with the immigrant population. That is, we must work to validate sociopolitical reality, but also history. Indeed, Foster (2001) reminded clinicians of the imperative of contextualizing history and politics in work with immigrants, with specific

---

[7]Full interview found online (https://qz.com/1521806/palestines-head-of-mental-health-services-says-ptsd-is-a-western-concept/)

attention to the ways that context influences internalized narratives of the immigration process and journey.

Validating reality and history may include acknowledging the limitations of "mainstream" treatment methods, especially under the crush of current violence against immigrants. Indeed, it would be arrogant to assume that our theories and practices adequately address the material conditions of the politically constructed human rights crisis in U.S. detention centers, for example. Validation also implies moving beyond the "symbolic" into the real (Tummala-Narra, 2014), and eschewing outdated or archaic notions of treatment-resistant individuals. Duran and colleagues (2008) indicated that this type of validation can only be done when practitioners become intimately aware of "various forms of cultural oppression" (p. 289), to include acquainting oneself with historical and current-day immigration trends, consequences, and "political empathy, that is, empathy that joins with the individual and the group on the basis of social location and oppression" (Burstow, 2003, p. 51).

Incorporating such validation practices into our approach to working with immigrants buffers against potential collusion with ideology. Duran and colleagues (2008) reminded us:

> Once historical honesty becomes an integral part of the counseling/healing ceremony session, the fields of counseling and psychology will themselves begin the long-needed healing process that enables counselors and therapists to realize new and untapped aspects of their psychological liberation. (p. 291)

3. Recognize and Acknowledge Systems of Oppression

If, as Burstow (2003) wrote, "radical trauma practice is necessarily based on an awareness of the centrality of oppression in the traumatizing of human beings, communities, and the earth itself" (p. 1310), then incorporating knowledge of systemic and structural oppression is intimately linked with attuned care in the immigrant community. Indeed, since immigrants are increasingly non-White and non-European (Ainslie et al., 2013; Chavez-Dueñas et al., 2019), "one cannot adequately theorize about the experience of immigration without including the dimensions of ethnicity and race" (Ainslie et al., 2013, p. 670). When we acknowledge ethnicity, race, gender, ability, and status as integral parts of the immigrant experience, we are remiss to ignore the structural constructs that culminate in exclusionary practices based on intersectional identities (Crenshaw, 1989).

Recognizing and acknowledging systems of oppression positions us well to, for example, perceive discrimination and offer support to Muslim immigrants or locate "discrimination symptoms . . . as psychological injuries that are situational and outside of the person's control" (Lowe et al., 2019, p. 121); name the importance of social location in the context of immigration (Comas-Díaz, 2016; Tummala-Narra, 2016); be attuned to racial melancholia—what Eng and Han (2000) located as a distinct type of sadness borne out of social and psychic conflicts of Asian Americans—as a social phenomenon versus a dispositional deficit; and, perhaps most important,

develop an ability to bear the anxiety of listening to the impact of social oppression on the client's life, and the uncertainty of the shifting nature of identity in
the context of trauma . . . [in order] to help the client negotiate the multiplicity
of his or her identity with the awareness that this negotiation may be a lifelong
process. (Tummala-Narra, 2016, p. 402)

Acknowledging structural and systemic oppression includes a commitment
to challenge their existence and ongoing deleterious effects. This is especially
important because, by design, oppressive systems and structures function to
create, sustain, and maintain trauma in service of the social order—what we
might understand psychologically as perpetual *disorder*.

4. Locate Ourselves Within Systems of Oppression

In studying how social workers might remain ethically driven in their service
for immigrant communities—particularly those in the inhumane detention
centers—Byers and Shapiro (2019) posited that "the presence of licensed
social workers can serve as a fig leaf, obscuring larger institutional neglect and
abuse" (p. 177). This evocative suggestion is also grounding and centering,
as it reminds us of a key liberation psychology principle: the imperative for
clinicians to examine the ways in which they are complicit in oppressive structures, perhaps unconsciously, by association, or with conscious well-meaning
intentions. Locating these effects in larger systems of oppression helps deindi-
vidualize blame, and rather, recenters a professional imperative to understand
how our practice, our theories, and our profession are constitutive of larger
sociopolitical power structures. This runs directly counter to models that might
inadvertently understand the clinical room or profession as existing outside of
or in opposition to these structures. It also helps recenter how we are implicated in the suffering of others (Layton, 2009). Duran and colleagues (2008)
further located us:

The various forms of psychological oppression that continue to be perpetuated
by many well-meaning and good-hearted counselors, psychologists, and social
workers are by-products of broader economic, political, religious, and social
mechanisms that have historically been used to colonize persons from diverse
groups and backgrounds in the United States. (p. 288)

On a practical level, locating ourselves within systems of oppression necessitates a self-examination, with particular focus on various privileges that are
inextricably linked to our social and cultural positions and identities. For
example, in her book, *Psychoanalytic Theory and Cultural Competence in Psychotherapy*, Tummala-Narra (2016) emphasized

the therapist's self-examination and attention to experiences of social oppression . . . [and] the importance of recognizing the client's indigenous narratives
of psychological distress and health, language use, expressions of distress, and
the cultural system of meaning in which they are rooted. (p. 403)

Likewise, Hernandez-Wolfe and colleagues (2015) suggested we expand our
notion of systems and adopt a global human rights perspective, to include

how immigrant communities as well as other countries view and understand U.S. politics and policy.

Locating ourselves also includes attending to the ways in which we counter the very systems we come to see ourselves existing within. That is, it does not suffice to merely name the system, but rather, "insofar as is feasible, it is critical that counselors take proactive measures so that they are not co-opted by organs of the state that traditionally traumatize our clients" (Burstow, 2003, p. 1316). This might mean objecting, for example, to working within systems that are fundamentally imbricated in unethical practices, such as international black sites, torture facilities, or immigrant detention centers. Oftentimes, clinicians are drawn to work within these sites to offer relief and support; however, we may come to consider this work as potentially lending credibility and structural soundness to inhumane and, under international law, illegal circumstances. This should not be read as a rejection of our objection to these sites, nor should it deter us from demanding ethical and imperative care to these communities. However, it grounds us in the reality that the only viable option for ethical and imperative care is to, in fact, dismantle rather than reform these very structures.

Clinical Vignettes

In presenting the following two vignettes, I (Dr. Crane) describe ways in which two immigrant patients, Lin and Joseph, and their families, have been traumatized by White supremacist systems of oppression in the United States.[8] Utilizing afforded privileges, I choose to resist the dictates of managed care by working in independent practice[9] and, therefore, shield my patients from potentially being pathologized by diagnoses related to trauma. In keeping with our first step, to relinquish "trauma" as a disorder, I was able to see and help them see how the sociopolitical realities of living as non-White immigrants in the United States exposed them relentlessly to traumatic situations.

---

[8]All case material has been altered to protect confidentiality.

[9]While it is beyond the scope of this chapter to discuss the large-scale implications of private versus community-based practice, in keeping with the points we outline above, we both acknowledge that the choice of practice setting is one that is imbricated in historic trends toward denying access to the most disenfranchised. Practicing with liberation in mind works against some of the access complications that are typically associated with private practice work. For example, we are active in networking with, and compiling and sharing resources of BIPOC (Black, Indigenous, People of Color) practitioners with our patients and their extended networks. We are both cognizant of the labor involved in this type of commitment and yet understand it within an ethical imperative of disrupting systems that perpetuate disorder. Namely, we contextualize it within a communal understanding of healing that helps work against potential "burnout" often connected with excessive unremunerated work. We also both commit to not turning away BIPOC patients who ask for our services, and are able to do so on an extensive sliding fee or "pay what you can" scale. Because we understand this is not feasible for all practitioners, especially those more junior to the field, we consciously make space for those with less means, so that our less financially established colleagues can build their practices.

Finally, I was transparent about my positionality as a second generation mixed Asian–White American who is also negatively impacted by U.S. systems of oppression while simultaneously holding privilege and power as a licensed psychologist. I made clear to Lin and Joseph that I used my power and privilege to provide safety in the treatment room and to increase their efforts toward safety and empowerment in the wider community.

Lin

At the time, Lin was a 24-year-old, cisgender, heterosexual graduate student from Vietnam. Arriving in the United States at age 14 to attend boarding school, Lin would be considered a "parachute kid" (Eng & Han, 2019; Zhou, 1998). Lin carries the double-edged weight of both expected achievement, coming from a family with the means to send her for a U.S.-based education and assimilation program, but also, daily experiences of racism. Lin was aware of the privilege of attending a U.S. high school, and commented on how it gave her access to U.S. higher education, and, subsequently, employment at a U.S.-based company. She was at that time in a 3-year master of architecture program, as well as in a new relationship with a White nonimmigrant man from the United States.

Lin began her clinical work with me when she was a junior in college, recommended for therapy by her advisor.

"My advisor thinks I'm depressed, so I should be in therapy."

I asked her why or how she was referred to me, specifically.

> They said you know Asian culture and work with bicultural students. I tried someone at the university counseling center, but they really didn't get where I was coming from. And they kept wanting me to take medication and do group therapy. I can't do group therapy, it's too scary.

When we began our work, Lin told me matter-of-factly, "I'm crazy. I smoke weed, do molly, hook up with all sorts of guys. I do what I want." She related to me that she was intent on becoming fully "Americanized," intent on fitting into U.S. majority culture seamlessly.

> When I got to boarding school, I felt like an outsider. Everybody knew I was FOB (Fresh Off the Boat) and treated me like a charity case or a disease. The program directors told us we shouldn't speak our home language or even speak to our families much if we wanted to become fully fluent. I know that my family is counting on me to succeed in America, so I owe them full success.

Lin barely admitted to experiencing homesickness, instead dedicating herself fully to being "as American as possible." As a result, she told me that she avoids Vietnamese music, food, social media, and people. "I just don't feel comfortable around Vietnamese."

My countertransference with Lin was deep sadness and dismay. As the daughter of an Asian immigrant, I longed for connection with my mother's Filipino culture. I could not imagine having grown up with it only to reject it all. However, I am a second-generation racial minority, born and raised in the United States. While intellectually understanding Lin's efforts, I frequently conceptualized her efforts as embodying racial erasure and internalized xeno-phobia. This was even more pronounced against the historical and political backdrop of U.S. imperial policy in Vietnam, the devastation wrought on the country that continued to be felt, and the various social and class alliances embedded in an identification with U.S. culture. Additionally, I recognized that her impressions of U.S. culture, learned from predominantly White instructors and White dominant popular culture were "colorblind," not attuned to matters of import to minority people, including, or perhaps specifically, herself.

Early in our work, Lin talked about an ex-boyfriend with whom she had had an "unsatisfying" relationship:

> He always texted me at night to come over. He had a demanding job that required him to travel on weekends and work long hours during the week. We would talk and watch movies and hook up. He never came to my place. Maybe he didn't want to meet my roommates because he was older. We never went out on proper dates. Sometimes he'd order in and we'd eat in bed or in front of the TV. I nearly broke up with him a few times because I sometimes felt he was just using me for sex. But he could be really tender and was really into Asian culture, so I felt like he cared for me.

Employing the second and third recommendations, validating sociopolitical reality and history and acknowledging systems of oppression, I asked Lin how she knew that her ex-boyfriend was "really into Asian culture." She said that he was into Asian martial arts and dated only Asian girls because he felt they were more caring than "American" girls. My "yellow fever" antennae went up, sensing the possibility of racial fetishization. As Lin recounted her dis-appointments with her ex-boyfriend, as well as with several Tinder dates, I perceived her experiences through the lens of exoticization, of being targeted for her being Asian, rather than for her particular personal qualities. Locating her experience in a systemic understanding of how bodies of color are often sexualized and objectified, as well as the ways in which misogyny can cloak itself in care, I queried Lin to learn about her awareness of and feelings about the phenomenon of yellow fever. I wondered with her what she knew of individuals targeting Asians for their looks and for the racial stereotypes they held about Asian women, specifically. Initially, Lin stated that she was aware of yellow fever and "okay" with being considered exotic.

Working with Lin's capitulation to exoticism and objectification was challenging, especially as my own traumatic history with these phenomena constitute my earliest memories as a *hapa*, mixed Asian and White, female. "She looks just like a little China doll," said a South Carolina gas station atten-dant. I began traveling with my father from Connecticut to Atlanta at the age of 18 months to visit my paternal grandmother. He took great pride in my being his "little China doll" and being mixed. "Half-breeds are best," he would often say. I learned much later that the reason he and I traveled alone to visit Grammy was that she was a profound racist who did not accept my mother as human. Until I was born, she considered my mother to be like a monkey. I grew up steeped in intrafamilial racism, as my father, too, was deeply racist. Yet he prized me as an exotic product and praised me for my otherness.

In this, and other ways, I grew to internalize my exotic objectification. These are the parts of Lin to which I was responding.

When I am asked about my specialties of practice or areas of expertise, I often state, "Resisting racism, resisting oppression." I find that this is a short-hand way of stating that I take a feminist and liberatory stance with my patients of color, those with disabilities, those who are gender nonconforming, and those who lie outside the confines of cisheteronormativity. Given that my practice is predominantly with people of color, "resisting oppression" describes a main focus of my work.

Locating myself within U.S. systems of oppression with Lin, I acknowledged and shared experiences of being the target of yellow fever and queried her in such a way that she was able to view those experiences critically, rather than immediately feeling flattered or positive about them. That is, we opened up alternate possibilities of feeling and experience. Additionally, as I introduced themes of systemic oppression and White supremacy in U.S. culture (corresponding with Recommendations 2 and 3), Lin developed a framework for locating her discomfort with some of her boyfriend's White-centric views and actions. After describing and discussing White fragility, she began to imagine how she could have confronted her ex-boyfriend's "White blindness" and lack of appreciation for her race-based pain. She stated that she wanted him to understand the pain she experienced when his friends told racist jokes, or when she experienced racial attacks on the street. With these discussions came more nuanced memories that starkly juxtaposed the woman intent on "being American":

> I told him that some guy just yelled at me, "Go back to where you came from, ya chink!" and he just told me to ignore it. I had to lock myself in the bathroom because I was sobbing so hard I couldn't catch a breath. He didn't even try to understand! How can I be with him if he can't even try? If he can't even back me up?

Lin was able to eventually articulate that she broke up with her boyfriend because her experience with him was "screaming into the wind." She also began to seek more Asian spaces and gatherings, especially political groups on campus. Most recently, she began dating a Chinese medical student, feeling that he understood her experiences better and was therefore more supportive. This development, however, brought different complications as she knew she could never tell her parents.

> Even though they sent me here for education and opportunity, they are pretty traditional. They expect me to marry a Vietnamese man. Even a White American would be okay. But my cousin married a Chinese man and she was basically kicked out of the family. I don't want that to happen to me, but I've really fallen hard.

Caught between worlds and cultures, Lin struggled to position herself in a way that felt good to her. Conditioned by her parents to avoid Chinese "oppressors" due to the long history of Chinese occupation and colonization of Vietnam, Lin reported feeling some shame that she'd fallen for a Chinese man.

She described herself as "caught between worlds." With my active encouragement, as well as my challenges to her internalized racism and exoticism,
Lin began to choose for herself how and with whom she wanted to be. After
more than a decade of striving to be "as American as possible," Lin tearfully
shared that she was ready to be herself,

> whoever that may be. I want to be a strong woman, like you. A woman who
> takes no shit from White people, who stands up for herself, and who fights the
> power. I feel like you are giving me my voice.

Acknowledging Lin's resilience, I frequently reminded her that she was the
one doing the work, that she was the one finding her voice and choosing how
to be in the world. I found I must be ever-vigilant to the power I had in our
relationship, so that I did not reenact the abuses of power perpetrated in
the nation outside of our shared treatment room (in correspondence with
Recommendation 4). I did not want her to feel dictated to, overpowered, or
colonized by my U.S.-born self.

Joseph

Joseph was the 30-year-old, cisgender, heterosexual son of Mexican migrants.
Born in the United States, he would be considered second generation and
holds a certain degree of privilege and security in his status as a U.S. citizen.
Joseph was identified as gifted in elementary school and, since that time, was
mentored by several teachers and chosen to participate in a program that guides
children from "underserved communities" to academic success, including
college or university graduation. Joseph cited "certainty" as a guiding principle
in his love for math; he majored in computer science and was employed by a
major U.S.-based tech company. He entered treatment after several incidents
challenged his sense of safety and self.

"What's the first thing a police officer asks when he pulls you over?"
Joseph asked me.

I answered, "License and registration?"

"Right?! That's what they ask most people. You know what the cop asked
me? 'Where'd you get that car?'"

Joseph reported that he drove a 5-year-old Lexus, "nothing super-charged
or tricked out. Just a nice, reliable commuter car that also happens to be fun
to drive. Plus, it's a four-door and I can drive my mom and sisters around in
it." Joseph expressed rage at the officer's assumption that he had stolen the
car, or somehow obtained it illegally rather than earning it through his own
hard work. Yet, he also expressed fear about being pulled over "for being
brown." Joseph recalled his childhood in Texas, where people in his community were routinely pulled over "for being Mexican," for driving older cars,
or for carrying brown people. "I saw it over and over again. I mean, even
my White friends saw and knew what was happening!" Moreover, Joseph
witnessed countless raids by ICE officials, *"la migra,"* in which building sites
were targeted by immigration officials hunting for undocumented workers.

Most of the construction in Texas, heck most of the landscaping, nannying, house cleaning, and senior care is done by Mexicans! The employers know that they can pay Mexicans less than American workers and that the undocumented workers won't complain. These workers have no protections whatsoever—no sick time, no health insurance, no paid time off—and they know they can be deported at any time. Especially now. I mean, one of my uncles was hauled off just the other month—and he left a wife and two children behind. I'm really worried for some of my little cousins—their moms aren't U.S. citizens either, and I worry about their moms being deported and then who's going to take care of the little ones? My mom already takes care of two of my sisters' kids.

Joseph's world is not like that of most of his coworkers. His U.S.-born White colleagues, most of whom assumed from preschool that college and careers were in their futures, expressed disbelief that he could be targeted by police for "driving while brown" or while Mexican. As he described his experience, I reflected on the terror I experienced listening to my brothers—who were also targeted for being brown men—sharing experiences of being targeted by the police or by White coworkers and managers. The ideological basis of their assumptions was clear to Joseph and experienced as particularly ignorant of the historical realities of the indigenous Mexican community in what is now considered Texas—historically occupied land.

I didn't think my coworkers were racist, for the most part. But the fact that they didn't believe me or believed it was because of a legitimate traffic violation— I mean, what the—? With my uncle being deported, me getting pulled over, and now hearing about more neighbors being deported—I'm having nightmares. I mean, my father isn't a citizen and I wake up in the middle of the night sweating, worrying that he's going to be caught up in a raid. My mind races all the time, wondering who's next. I can't eat, I can barely sleep, and I'm having these experiences where I feel like I'm not in reality.

Working with Joseph meant more than giving him grounding exercises and referring him for medication evaluation. Joseph's trauma responses arose from both past and current, chronic traumatic exposures (in keeping with recommendation 2). As Nadal (2018) explained,

When people face discrimination in their lives that is (a) intense, (b) extensive and enduring, (c) threatening to one's sense of safety, and (d) causal of symptoms that are aligned with PTSD (e.g., avoidance, dissociation), their experiences might be labeled as *traumatic discrimination*. (p. 13)

Moreover,

Treatment may focus on changing the client's cognitive or behavioral reactions to discrimination, or exploring and analyzing the reasons the client is having such a negative reaction to discrimination. In other words, although people who experience PTSD are taught that external reasons are the causes for their mental illness, people who face discrimination are taught that internal reasons are why they are suffering. (Nadal, 2018, p. 13)

Joseph's symptoms related directly to past and current experiences of terror—terror of loss and dislocation, terror of family separation, terror of losing friends and neighbors to deportation. As I listened to him, I could not help but reflect on how after the 2016 elections, all of my patients of color—immigrants, U.S.-born minorities, and international sojourners—reported increased anxiety, depression, and in some cases, suicidality, for the first time. I also reflected on my own anxieties spiking around worries about my own undocumented relatives (in keeping with Recommendation 4). As I wrote this, I worried that I might be endangering them by even mentioning their existence. Would *la migra* track them down and deport them because of my words?

As with Lin, employing Recommendation 2, I validated Joseph's reality, both current and historical, as well as his fears. Emphasizing the undue resilience it took to achieve financial stability as the son of immigrants, I worked with him to find safety, identify White allies, and identify safe spaces where he could calm himself and feel supported. Working with someone like Joseph meant acknowledging the lack of safety embodied in his non-White appearance. Working with Joseph meant acknowledging the chronicity and ongoing reality of threats to him and his people. Working with Joseph meant helping him mourn the homes, communities, and cultures he or his parents or various relatives left behind. Working with Joseph meant helping him to navigate a society that actively and sometimes violently rejected him, even when he acted "legally." Most important, working with Joseph meant acknowledging and stating these realities—reflecting back to him that these systems of oppression indeed exist, and that his responses to them are expected given the current political climate, generational exposure to systemic inequities and violence, and continued disenfranchisement (Recommendations 1, 2, 3).

CONCLUSION

This chapter's aim is to advocate for an ideological shift in the way our profession and practice approach trauma work with immigrant communities. Central to this ideological shift is our ability to (a) relinquish trauma as a disorder, (b) validate sociopolitical reality and history, (c) recognize and acknowledge systems of oppression, and (d) locate ourselves within systems of oppression.

Taking these steps both as individual practitioners, but also, systemically, as a field, will contribute to what Freire (1968) termed *conscientization*, that is, a change in consciousness via radical transformation brought about by deconstructing life experiences of oppressed people. Applying this concept to treatment, assessment, and intervention with the immigrant population, in tandem with existing models of communal containment (Duran et al., 2008) and special attention to "epistemological hybridity" (Duran et al., 2008)—what Comas-Díaz (2016) also referred to as a combination of psychotherapy, group counseling, and community methods to ethnopolitical interventions—creates the foundation for liberation-grounded work with immigrant communities. It also works toward materializing psychology as a "sanctuary discipline" (Chavez-Dueñas et al., 2019).

REFERENCES

Abdullah, T., & Brown, T. L. (2020). Diagnostic labeling and mental illness stigma among Black Americans: An experimental vignette study. *Stigma and Health, 5*(1), 11–21. https://doi.org/10.1037/sah0000162

Ainslie, R. C., Tummala-Narra, P., Harlem, A., Barbanel, L., & Ruth, R. (2013). Contemporary psychoanalytic views on the experience of immigration. *Psychoanalytic Psychology, 30*(4), 663–679. https://doi.org/10.1037/a0034588

Aliverti, A. (2012). Making people criminal: The role of the criminal law in immigration enforcement. *Theoretical Criminology, 16*(4), 417–434. https://doi.org/10.1177/1362480612449779

American Psychological Association. (2017). *Multicultural Guidelines: An ecological approach to context, identity, and intersectionality.* http://www.apa.org/about/policy/multicultural-guidelines.pdf

Brave Heart, M. Y. H. (2000). *Wakiksuyapi:* Carrying the historical trauma of the Lakota. *Tulane Studies in Social Welfare, 2000,* 245–266. http://citeseerx.ist.psu.edu/viewdoc/download?doi=10.1.1.452.6309&rep=rep1&type=pdf

Braveheart-Jordan, M. Y. H., & DeBruyn, L. (1995). So she may walk in balance: Integrating the impact of historical trauma in the treatment of Native American Indian Women. In J. Adelman & G. Enguidanos (Eds.), *Haworth innovations in feminist studies. Racism in the lives of women: Testimony, theory, and guides to antiracist practice* (pp. 345–368). Harrington Park Press/Haworth Press.

Broman, C. L., Mavaddat, R., & Hsu, S. (2000). The experience and consequences of perceived racial discrimination: A study of African Americans. *The Journal of Black Psychology, 26*(2), 165–180. https://doi.org/10.1177/0095798400026002003

Brown, L. (2008). *Cultural competence in trauma therapy: Beyond the flashback.* American Psychological Association. https://doi.org/10.1037/11752-000

Burstow, B. (2003). Toward a radical understanding of trauma and trauma work. *Violence Against Women, 9*(11), 1293–1317. https://doi.org/10.1177/1077801203255555

Byers, D. S., & Shapiro, J. R. (2019). Renewing the ethics of care for social work under the Trump administration. *Social Work, 64*(2), 175–180. https://doi.org/10.1093/sw/swz008

Carter, R. T. (2007). Racism and psychological and emotional injury: Recognizing and assessing race-based traumatic stress. *The Counseling Psychologist, 35*(1), 13–105. https://doi.org/10.1177/0011000006292033

Chavez-Dueñas, N. Y., Adames, H. Y., Perez-Chavez, J. G., & Salas, S. P. (2019). Healing ethno-racial trauma in Latinx immigrant communities: Cultivating hope, resistance, and action. *American Psychologist, 74*(1), 49–62. https://doi.org/10.1037/amp0000289

Comas-Díaz, L. (2007). Ethnopolitical psychology: Healing and transformation. In E. Aldarondo (Ed.), *Advancing social justice through clinical practice* (pp. 91–118). Lawrence Erlbaum Associates.

Comas-Díaz, L. (2016). Racial trauma recovery: A race informed therapeutic approach to racial wounds. In A. Alvarez, C. Liang, & H. A. Neville (Eds.), *The cost of racism for people of color: Contextualizing experiences of discrimination* (pp. 133–162). American Psychological Association. https://doi.org/10.1037/14852-012

Comas-Díaz, L., Hall, G. N., & Neville, H. A. (2019). Racial trauma: Theory, research, and healing: Introduction to the special issue. *American Psychologist, 74*(1), 1–5. https://doi.org/10.1037/amp0000442

Costello, M. R. (2016). *Teaching the 2016 election. The Trump effect: The impact of the presidential campaign on our nation's schools.* Southern Poverty Law Center. https://www.splcenter.org/sites/default/files/splc_the_trump_effect.pdf

Crenshaw, K. (1989). Demarginalizing the intersection of race and sex: A Black feminist critique of antidiscrimination doctrine, feminist theory, and antiracist politics.

University of Chicago Legal Forum, 1898(1), 139–167. https://chicagounbound.uchicago.edu/cgi/viewcontent.cgi?article=1052&context=uclf

Duran, E., & Duran, B. (1995). *Native American postcolonial psychology*. State University of New York.

Duran, E., Duran, B., Brave Heart, M. Y. H., & Yellow Horse-Davis, S. (1998). Healing the American Indian soul wound. In Y. Danieli (Ed.), *International handbook of multigenerational legacies of trauma* (pp. 341–354). Plenum. https://doi.org/10.1007/978-1-4757-5567-1_22

Duran, E., Firehammer, J., & Gonzalez, J. (2008). Liberation psychology as the path toward healing cultural soul wounds. *Journal of Counseling and Development, 86*(3), 288–295. https://doi.org/10.1002/j.1556-6678.2008.tb00511.x

Eng, D. L., & Han, S. (2000). A dialogue on racial melancholia. *Psychoanalytic Dialogues, 10*(4), 667–700. https://doi.org/10.1080/10481881009348576

Eng, D. L., & Han, S. (2019). *Racial melancholia, racial dissociation: On the social and psychic lives of Asian Americans*. Duke University Press.

Erickson, K. (1995). Notes on trauma and community. In C. Caruth (Ed.), *Trauma: Explorations in memory* (pp. 183–199). Johns Hopkins University Press.

Fanon, F. (1961). *The wretched of the Earth*. Grove Press.

Foster, R. P. (2001). When immigration is trauma: Guidelines for the individual and family clinician. *American Journal of Orthopsychiatry, 71*(2), 153–170. https://doi.org/10.1037/0002-9432.71.2.153

Freire, P. (1968). *Pedagogy of the oppressed*. Seabury.

Furman, R., Sanchez, M., Ackerman, A., & Ung, T. (2015). The immigration detention center as a transnational problem: Implications for international social work. *International Social Work, 58*(6), 813–818. https://doi.org/10.1177/0020872813500803

Gilfus, M. (1999). The price of the ticket: A survivor-centered appraisal of trauma theory. *Violence Against Women, 5*(11), 1238–1257. https://doi.org/10.1177/10778012990050011002

Goldhill, O. (2019, January 13). *Palestine's head of mental health services says PTSD is a Western concept*. Quartz. https://qz.com/1521806/palestines-head-of-mental-health-services-says-ptsd-is-a-western-concept/

Gone, J. P. (2007). "We never was happy living like a Whiteman": Mental health disparities and the postcolonial predicament in American Indian communities. *American Journal of Community Psychology, 40*(3–4), 290–300. https://doi.org/10.1007/s10464-007-9136-x

Gone, J. P. (2013). Redressing First Nations historical trauma: Theorizing mechanisms for indigenous culture as mental health treatment. *Transcultural Psychiatry, 50*(5), 683–706. https://doi.org/10.1177/1363461513487669

Harlem, A. (2009). Thinking through others: Cultural psychology and the psychoanalytic treatment of immigrants. *Psychoanalysis, Culture & Society, 14*(3), 273–288. https://doi.org/10.1057/pcs.2009.12

Herman, J. (1992). *Trauma and recovery*. Basic books.

Hernandez-Wolfe, P., Killian, K., Engstrom, D., & Gangsei, D. (2015). Vicarious resilience, vicarious trauma, and awareness of equity in trauma work. *Journal of Humanistic Psychology, 55*(2), 153–172. https://doi.org/10.1177/0022167814534322

Hollander, N. C. (2010). Anti-Muslim prejudice and the psychic use of the ethnic other. *International Journal of Applied Psychoanalytic Studies, 7*(1), 73–84. https://doi.org/10.1002/aps.193

Joseph, A. J. (2015). The necessity of an attention to Eurocentrism and colonial technologies: An addition to critical mental health literature. *Disability & Society, 30*(7), 1021–1041. https://doi.org/10.1080/09687599.2015.1067187

Kinderman, P. (2019). *A manifesto for mental health: Why we need a revolution in mental health care*. Palgrave Macmillan. https://doi.org/10.1007/978-3-030-24386-9

Layton, L. (2009). Who's responsible? Our mutual implication in each other's suffering. *Psychoanalytic Dialogues, 19*(2), 105–120. https://doi.org/10.1080/10481880902779695

Lewis, T. (1999). *Living beside: Performing normal after incest memories return.* McGilligan Books.

Lopez, M. H., & Minushkin, S. (2008). *2008 National survey of Latinos: Hispanics see their situation in U.S. deteriorating: Oppose key immigrant enforcement measures.* https://www.pewresearch.org/hispanic/2008/09/18/2008-national-survey-of-latinos-hispanics-see-their-situation-in-us-deteriorating-oppose-key-immigration-enforcement-measures/

Lowe, S. R., Tineo, P., Bonumwezi, J. L., & Bailey, E. J. (2019). The trauma of discrimination: Posttraumatic stress in Muslim American college students. *Traumatology, 25*(2), 115–123. https://doi.org/10.1037/trm0000197

Martín-Baró, I. (1996). Toward a liberation psychology. (A. Aron, Trans.) In A. Aron & S. Corne (Eds.), *Writings for a liberation psychology.* Harvard University Press.

Mattar, S. (2011). Educating and training the next generations of traumatologists: Development of cultural competencies. *Psychological Trauma: Theory, Research, Practice, and Policy, 3*(3), 258–265. https://doi.org/10.1037/a0024477

Nadal, K. L. (2018). *Microaggressions and traumatic stress: Theory, research, and clinical care.* American Psychological Association. https://doi.org/10.1037/0000073-000

Nilson, E. (2018). *Kids who cross the border meet with therapists and social workers. What they say can be used against them.* Vox. https://www.vox.com/policy-and-politics/2018/6/18/17449150/family-separation-policy-immigration-dhs-orr-health-records-undocumented-kids

Office of the Inspector General. (2019). *Management alert—DHS needs to address dangerous overcrowding and prolonged detention of children and adults in Rio Grande Valley (Redacted).* Department of Homeland Security. https://int.nyt.com/data/documenthelper/1358-ig-report-migrant-detention/2dd9d40be6a6b0cd3619/optimized/full.pdf#page=1

Root, M. (1992). Restructuring the impact of trauma on the personality. In L. Brown & M. Ballour (Eds.), *Personality and Psychopathology* (pp. 108–118). Guilford Press.

Stumpf, J. (2006). The crimmigration crisis: Immigrants, crime, and sovereign power. *The American University Law Review, 56*(2), 367–419. https://digitalcommons.wcl.american.edu/cgi/viewcontent.cgi?article=1274&context=aulr

Tummala-Narra, P. (2014). Cultural identity in the context of trauma and immigration from a psychoanalytic perspective. *Psychoanalytic Psychology, 31*(3), 396–409. https://doi.org/10.1037/a0036539

Tummala-Narra, P. (2016). *Psychoanalytic theory and cultural competence in psychotherapy.* American Psychological Association. https://doi.org/10.1037/14800-000

Watkins Jr., C. E., Hook, J. N., Owen, J., DeBlaere, C., Davis, D. E., & Van Tongeren, D. R. (2019). Multicultural orientation in psychotherapy supervision: Cultural humility, cultural comfort, and cultural opportunities. *American Journal of Psychotherapy, 72*(2), 38–46. https://doi.org/10.1176/appi.psychotherapy.20180040

Woolfolk, R. (2001). The concept of mental illness: An analysis of four pivotal issues. *Journal of Mind and Behavior, 22*(2), 161–187.

Zhou, M. (1998). "Parachute kids" in Southern California: The educational experience of Chinese children in transnational families. *Educational Policy, 12*(6), 682–704. https://doi.org/10.1177/0895904898012006005

16

Human Rights, Policy, and Legal Interventions

Diya Kallivayalil and Robert P. Marlin

Of all the forms of inequality, injustice in health is the most shocking and inhuman.
—DR. MARTIN LUTHER KING, JR., SPEECH TO THE MEDICAL COMMITTEE
FOR HUMAN RIGHTS, 1966 (GALARNEAU, 2018)

In this chapter, we argue for the value of a human rights frame for psychologists in all aspects of their work—research, practice, teaching, and training. There appear to be no studies that have directly examined how much training in human rights occurs in graduate or postgraduate training programs, but a 2014 study surveyed respondents from 20 psychology graduate programs about their training in military ethics and the Geneva conventions, and the vast majority (73.6%) reported receiving less than one hour of training in their programs. Only a third of respondents correctly answered basic questions regarding the Geneva Conventions. The authors concluded,

> Since a large number of psychologists will be military-involved at some point in their careers, the issue of dual loyalties should be part of the curriculum in every psychology training program. Such curricula should address the obligations imposed by the Geneva Conventions and other international codes. (Boyd et al., 2014, p. 623)

In the available American Psychological Association (APA) professional competency benchmarks, there is no reference to competency in the human rights literature apart from a general reference to going beyond APA's (2017)

https://doi.org/10.1037/0000214-017
Trauma and Racial Minority Immigrants: Turmoil, Uncertainty, and Resistance,
P. Tummala-Narra (Editor)

Ethical Principles of Psychologists and Code of Conduct (hereinafter, Ethics Code): "Demonstrates advanced knowledge and application of the APA Ethical Principles and Code of Conduct and *other* relevant ethical, legal and professional standards and guidelines" (APA, 2012, p. 3). There are several practice and training settings that provide care to individuals who have been subjected to torture and other human rights violations. However, these programs are seen as electives or specialty settings, rather than as a centerpiece of education and professional development. As a result, there is limited knowledge of treating torture survivors, the role of psychological evaluations of those seeking immigration relief, of human rights statutes of particular relevance to psychology and our Ethics Code and human rights advocacy. These are essential skills and knowledge for those working in mental health, particularly with vulnerable immigrant racial minority populations. This is a growing population that greater numbers of psychologists are increasingly exposed to, both in training and practice. This is of particular relevance and urgency given the current political climate with the Trump Administration's xenophobic and anti-immigration rhetoric and policies that have led to documented harm and human rights violations (Human Rights Watch, 2018, 2019; Linton et al., 2017; Wood, 2018).

In this chapter, we (a) discuss human rights principles and connect them with our Ethics Code; (b) discuss human rights statutes of particular relevance to vulnerable immigrant racial minority population; (c) provide both an individual and a programmatic case example; and (d) provide recommendations for practice, research, and training.

HOW CAN PSYCHOLOGISTS AND MENTAL HEALTH CARE PROVIDERS ENDORSE A MORE EXPLICIT HUMAN RIGHTS FRAME, AND HOW IS THIS COMPATIBLE WITH OUR ETHICS CODE?

We use the Universal Declaration of Human Rights (United Nations, 1948) as a starting point for a common understanding of human rights and argue that the principles of human rights are compatible with ethical codes for psychologists. Hagenaars (2016) argued that psychologists have a particular professional and scientific responsibility to uphold human rights due to our expertise in human behavior and relationships and our mission to promote human welfare. As Hagenaars outlined, psychologists have a professional obligation to (a) promote awareness of human rights and risks of their violation, (b) prevent human rights violations, and (c) alleviate their effects when they occur.

Psychologists' intervention and/or activism on behalf of human rights is based largely in psychological science and its ability to demonstrate the negative impact of violations of human rights. However, it is important to note that morality and humanity can also be the basis of a human rights claim by psychologists, particularly in areas where traditional scientific research is impractical or unethical (EFPA Board of Human Rights and Psychology, 2015).

Hagenaars (2016) argued that the "do no harm" clause in most professional ethical codes refer to the respect for the dignity of persons explicitly referred to in the UDHR and, therefore, ethical codes should be in concert with the UDHR. Ethical principles are generally based on four foundations: respect for autonomy, nonmaleficence, beneficence, and social justice (Beauchamp & Childress, 2001). Further, in the current APA Ethics Code, Principle E explicitly refers to "respect for rights and dignity" (APA, 2017). These principles are grounded in the idea that, due to the power inherent in our work and our professional status, we have a certain power to prevent harm and also a particular capacity to inflict harm. Further, although ethical standards require us to "do no harm," Hagenaars referred to the EFPA 2015 guidelines in arguing the general principles outlined in the Ethics Code are also *aspirational* and speak to our commitment to justice, fairness, inclusion, and humanity.

Another important relationship between a human rights framework and our profession of psychology is that our Ethics Code may require us to go beyond the current "local" law to protect our obligation to patients, research participants, and others with whom we work, and to prevent violations that are then defended by the so-called Nuremberg defense (Buitenweg, 2007). The International Covenant on Civil and Political Rights (ICCPR; United Nations General Assembly [UNGA], 1966a) identified *liberty rights*, which are protection from the state's intervening in individual liberty and economic, social, and cultural rights. It also outlines the so-called debt obligation of the state to stand up for its citizens (United Nations, Treaty Series, Vol. 999, p. 171). This is of particular relevance for human rights violations, as they often occur under the guise of or in the context of legal authority. A human rights framework is in accord with our Ethics Code by holding us to international human rights standards. This is of particular importance for working with vulnerable immigrants in our current political climate as "local" laws and policies have led to human rights violations and fall short of international standards (Human Rights Watch, 2019; Woodman et al., 2019).

Although fairness and inclusion are fundamental human rights, psychologists are also frequently called upon to document and speak to human rights *violations.* This is especially relevant when people's identities are the basis of mistreatment, exploitation, persecution, and discrimination. Injustices and inequities are often based on or the result of violations of those with less access to power and whose identities are "other" or dehumanized—such as lesbian, gay, bisexual, transgender, queer or questioning, and intersex (LGBTQI) individuals, women, children, racial, ethnic, and religious minorities, intellectually or physically disabled people, and psychiatric patients. It is our role as psychologists to examine and understand the mechanisms for this and then attempt to use whatever mechanisms are available to us (research, clinical care, advocacy, and so on) to vigorously safeguard human rights and use psychological science to influence change. It is also incumbent on us to document the ill effects of a practice or policy and, in so doing, advocate and call attention to these violations such as we see with racial minority immigrant populations today (as well as many others).

As an example of how to incorporate human rights principles into our professional ethics codes, Steinert (2017) attempted to reconcile ethics in psychiatry as it pertains to decisions about coercive treatment with the United Nations Convention on the Rights of Persons with Disabilities (UNCRPD). Steinert noted that people are generally not forced to take medicine for diabetes or cancer, even if the likely result is disability or death. The UNCRPD does not attend to impaired capacity or refer to mental disability specifically, but Articles 12 (*equal recognition before the law*), 14 (*liberty and security of the person*), and 15 (*freedom from torture and inhuman or degrading treatment or punishment*) are potentially relevant to coercive psychiatric treatment. Steinert attempted to reconcile these perspectives by referring to four ethical principles: respect for autonomy, nonmaleficence, beneficence, and justice. She argued that coercive treatment can be justified only when a patient's capacity to consent is substantially impaired by the illness and poses a danger to health or life and cannot be prevented by less intrusive means. In this case, withholding treatment can violate the principle of *justice*. In the case of danger to others, interventions that temporarily restrict freedom can be seen as necessary to prevent long-term social exclusion and loss of freedom, which can harm psychosocial health (beneficence, nonmaleficence). Withholding treatment can also cause harm, as it can lead to the patient being potentially detained in a criminal justice setting (nonmaleficence), which can justify coercive treatment. She also argued that significant efforts should be made to support patients' informed decisions, thereby supporting *autonomy*.

The psychology Ethics Code similarly outlines various principles in working with racial minority immigrants such as Principle E: Respect for People's Rights and Dignity, which contains the following language:

> Psychologists respect the dignity and worth of all people, and the rights of individuals to privacy, confidentiality, and self-determination. Psychologists are aware that special safeguards may be necessary to protect the rights and welfare of persons or communities whose vulnerabilities impair autonomous decision making. (APA, 2017)

Principle D: Justice says, "Psychologists exercise reasonable judgment and take precautions to ensure that their potential biases, the boundaries of their competence, and the limitations of their expertise do not lead to or condone unjust practices" (APA, 2017).

Many psychologists do not receive training in working with immigrant populations and even less specialized training in working with them under conditions of duress, when they may not have rights such as consent or confidentiality. Yet, many graduate students and trainees in clinical settings are drawn to working with these populations. We believe that some barriers to implementing more training and knowledge of human rights principles reflect a lack of knowledge of how to directly integrate them into our day to day work, "othering" of human rights and immigration issues as "special interest" rather than a field deeply rooted in a large body of work, and/or limiting the understanding of human rights in our work as restricted to helping people with asylum cases. Further, examination of biases with regards to issues of immigration is less common than other issues such as racism or sexism. Human rights principles and statutes are of uncommon relevance in the current political era of documented human rights violations and discrimination against racial minority immigrant patients, from death and solitary confinement in ICE custody, forced separation of families, ongoing disruption of already marginalized communities due to vitriolic rhetoric and threats of raids and violence, and increased uncertainty and distress for asylum seekers and refugees (Borque, 2019, Oglesby, 2018; UNICEF, 2016; Woodman et al., 2019). As illustrated below, we believe that drawing clear links between our practice and human rights materials will provide a framework for psychologists and other health care providers to integrate these principles into their daily work.

Human Rights Statutes of Particular Relevance to Vulnerable Immigrant Populations

In this spirit, we outline two important human rights statutes of particular relevance to working with vulnerable racial minority immigrant populations, whether in teaching, research, or clinical work, in order to provide some examples of how a human rights frame can be integrated into ethical codes of practice.

Article 7 of the ICCPR (Preventing Torture and Mitigating the Impact of Human Rights Violations)

Relevant International Legal Standards. The right to be free from torture is firmly established under international law. The UDHR, ICCPR, and the Convention Against Torture and Other Cruel, Inhuman or Degrading Treatment or Punishment (CAT, 1984) all expressly prohibit torture. Similarly, several regional instruments establish the right to be free from torture, such as the American Convention on Human Rights (OAS, 1969), the African Charter on Human and Peoples' Rights (OAU, 1981), and the European Convention for the Protection of Human Rights and Fundamental Freedoms (Council of Europe, 1950). Common Article 3 of the Geneva Convention states,

> the following acts are and shall remain prohibited at any time and in any place whatsoever . . . violence to life and person, in particular murder of all kinds, mutilation, cruel treatment and torture; . . . outrages upon personal dignity, in particular humiliating and degrading treatment. (International Committee of the Red Cross, 1949, p. 92)

According to Article 7 of the ICCPR, "No one is to be subjected to torture or to cruel, inhuman or degrading treatment or punishment. In particular, no one shall be subjected without his free consent to medical or scientific experimentation" (UNGA, 1966a). Despite these statutes, torture is endemic and practiced systematically and generally with impunity in various countries and settings around the world (Amnesty International, 2010, 2014;

Furtmayr & Frewer, 2010) and affects vulnerable immigrants in particular, either in their country of origin or in the process of migration or displacement. Huminuik (2017) argued that mental health professionals can play a positive role in the fight against torture by developing competencies to assess torture's psychological sequelae: "High quality psychological evidence can help to substantiate allegations of torture, thereby increasing the likelihood of success in civil, administrative and criminal proceedings" (p. 2) and that as part of building these competencies, mental health professionals must gain knowledge of forensic assessment of torture, as well as the relevant legal and sociopolitical contexts in which it occurs.

Relevant Ethical Codes Regarding Preventing and Intervening in Torture. The Istanbul Protocol (IP), officially known as the *Manual on the Effective Investigation and Documentation of Torture and Other Cruel, Inhuman or Degrading Treatment or Punishment* (2004), was developed by the office of the United Nations High Commissioner for Human Rights (UNHCR) in consultation with human rights organizations and represents a comprehensive set of guidelines for physicians and psychologists investigating and documenting allegations of torture, as well as clear statements on health care ethics. It brings together human rights principles and ethical considerations that can guide psychologists to both intervene in cases of human rights violations and understand their ethical obligations. As stated in the IP, "This manual was developed to enable States to address one of the most fundamental concerns in protecting individuals from torture—effective documentation" (OHCHR, 2004, p. 1). The IP goes on to list its various uses and functions, which are of particular interest and relevance to clinicians:

> Such documentation brings evidence of torture and ill-treatment to light so that perpetrators may be held accountable for their actions and the interests of justice may be served. The documentation methods contained in this manual are also applicable to other contexts, including human rights investigations and monitoring, political asylum evaluations, the defense of individuals who "confess" to crimes during torture, and needs assessments for the care of torture victims, among others. In the case of health professionals who are coerced into neglect, misrepresentation, or falsification of evidence of torture, this manual also provides an international point of reference for health professionals and adjudicators alike. (OHCHR, 2004, p. 1)

Further, the IP reinforces the ethical obligations of clinicians to treat and act in the best interests of patients for whom they have a duty to care, particularly in settings with the possibility or high likelihood of coercion such as prisons and locked psychiatric settings. The guidelines further emphasize that health professionals have a moral duty to protect the physical and mental health of detainees or those incarcerated by emphasizing that the only ethical relationship between prisoners and health professionals is one designed to evaluate, protect, and improve their health: "They are specifically prohibited from using medical knowledge and skills in any manner that contravenes international statements of individual rights" (OHCHR, 2004, p. 12). Health professionals also have a duty to support colleagues who speak out against human rights violations, currently referred to explicitly in Principle B: Fidelity and Responsibility of the psychology Ethics Code (APA, 2017). It is important also to recognize that the IP represents "minimum" standards in evaluation standards and health care ethics. The guidelines also explicitly state that it is a particularly heinous violation of health care ethics to participate, actively or passively, in torture, including

> evaluating an individual's capacity to withstand ill-treatment; being present at, supervising or inflicting maltreatment; providing professional knowledge or individuals' personal health information to torturers; and intentionally neglecting evidence and falsifying reports, such as autopsy reports and death certificates. (OHCHR, 2004, p. 12)

The IP also addresses issues regarding the duty to provide compassionate care, informed consent, confidentiality, and health professionals with dual obligations, and should be required reading for health professionals working with racial minority immigrants in general and with currently vulnerable immigrant populations who are vulnerable to torture, coercion, and maltreatment, such as detainees in ICE solitary confinement, migrant children in detention, and vulnerable research subjects (Woodman et al., 2019).

Article 15 of the ICESCR (Ensuring Equal Access to Scientific Advancement and Its Benefits)

Relevant International Legal Standards. Article 15 of the International Covenant on Economic, Social and Cultural Rights (ICESCR; UNGA, 1966b) recognizes the right of everyone (a) to take part in cultural life and (b) to enjoy the benefits of scientific progress and its applications. Article 15 goes on to say that the covenant

> Recognizes the responsibility of governments to respect, protect, fulfill and promote the right of everyone to "enjoy the benefits of scientific progress and its applications," take steps for the "conservation, the development and the diffusion of science," respect "freedom indispensable for scientific research," and encourage and develop "international contacts and cooperation" in science. (UNGA, 1966b)

Further, Article 12(1) of the ICESCR recognizes "the right of everyone to the enjoyment of the highest attainable standard of physical and mental health" (UNGA, 1966b).

In reference to psychology and mental health, this refers to our obligations to ensure equity, nondiscrimination, and inclusion in research participation, clinical service delivery, and teaching and training, as well as use of and interpretation of psychological research and findings. This calls upon psychologists to pay closer attention to demonstrated disparities in each of these areas, particularly as it relates to vulnerable immigrants and other marginalized groups (Betancourt, 2006; Ku & Matani, 2001).

Article 15 also states, "The States Parties to the present Covenant undertake to respect the freedom indispensable for scientific research and creative activity" (UNGA, 1966b). This last statement explicitly draws attention to the importance of intellectual freedom and the ability to collaborate across countries, including for psychologists currently at risk in various countries around the world. Article 15 emphasizes the importance of *monitoring*, both of academic freedom and other forms of human rights violations, as a human rights obligation of professional associations and states, which is of uncommon relevance to racial minority faculty and students. A recent report by Scholars at Risk details increased geopoliticized restrictions on travel, including scientific or academic travel, threats to institutional autonomy, and personal attacks on academics under the guise of rooting out "political bias" on university campuses (Scholars at Risk, 2018).

Relevant Ethical Codes and Considerations. In our current Ethics Code, Principle D: (Justice) is most closely related to Article 15 protections and aspirations, stating

> Psychologists recognize that fairness and justice entitle all persons to access to and benefit from the contributions of psychology and to equal quality in the processes, procedures, and services being conducted by psychologists. Psychologists exercise reasonable judgment and take precautions to ensure that their potential biases, the boundaries of their competence, and the limitations of their expertise do not lead to or condone unjust practices. (APA, 2017)

This principle has several important implications for psychologists to work to ensure equity, particularly in the context of caring for or working with vulnerable immigrant populations given the substantial data on disparities. This includes who is included in research studies. Another ethical issue to bring to bear is psychologists' "boundaries of competence"—few training programs and clinical settings offer training in working with vulnerable immigrants, people of color, LGBTQI individuals, or victims of human rights violations, often relegating this training to specialty fellowships that only a very small number of psychologists participate in. Psychologists have a role to play in training and to advocate for training that prepares psychologists for a complex world and to be advocates for human rights. Education and training must also include, based on both our Ethics Code and human rights statutes like Article 15, encouragement for psychologists to follow our ethical code to report violations when we see them occurring. We can also use our profession's influence to pressure governments and states to uphold human rights and dignity by holding them accountable to their obligations to respect, protect, and fulfill human rights obligations. Some examples include scientific freedom, the negative impact on mental health of current "legal" policies such as detention of children, solitary confinement, and demonstrated and severe disparities such as documented high rates of homicide and disappearances of Native American women and girls (Krishnan, 2016).

The Right to Health

In 1979, the U.S. Department of Health, Education, and Welfare (the predecessor to the Department of Health and Human Services) issued the *Belmont*

Report: Ethical Principles and Guidelines for the Protection of Human Subjects of Research (United States, 1979). This was in response to earlier atrocities committed by Nazi physicians against concentration camp inmates and civilians and the more recently acknowledged, decades-long abuse of poor African American sharecroppers in rural Alabama by U.S. Public Health Service researchers (Centers for Disease Control and Prevention [CDC], n.d.; Shuster, 1997). Since its publication 40 years ago, the Belmont Report has served as the foundation for the ethical treatment of research study subjects, outlining their rights and the obligations of medical and behavioral researchers, as well as forming the basis of all subsequent federal regulations and policy in this area. So, while human research subjects have rights delineated by this document and enshrined in U.S. federal regulation and policy, there is no equivalent policy, regulation, or legislation that codifies the right to health in the United States.

In 1948, the World Health Organization (WHO) was established as an agency of the UN, itself a response to the horrors of World War II. The WHO constitution clearly lays out health as a fundamental human right, and this is also outlined in the ICESCR, which the UN adopted two decades later (UNGA, 1966b; WHO, 1948). The United States is a signatory to the UN Charter, as well as the ICESCR. However, despite this, the U.S. government has never ratified the Covenant (MacNaughton & McGill, 2012). So, the federal government has never affirmed the right to health. In the current context of the COVID-19 pandemic, we are already seeing the impact of institutional failures and built-in structural inequities that are resulting in a startling disproportionate burden of both death and disease on individuals from racial and ethnic minority groups and the extreme vulnerability of incarcerated individuals, particularly detained immigrants (CDC, 2020).

It has historically fallen to nongovernmental organizations and actors to promulgate and invoke the right to health for the U.S. population. Launched in 1964, the Medical Committee for Human Rights was composed of health care professionals who wanted to support civil rights workers in Mississippi during "Freedom Summer" and included physicians, nurses, social workers, and psychologists (Dittmer, 2014). There, they witnessed the poor health of rural African Americans and their lack of access to health care. Under the direction of Dr. H. Jack Geiger and grounded in the understanding of health as a human right, the organization launched the first two community health centers in the United States: the Delta Health Center in rural Mound Bayou, Mississippi, and the Columbia Point Health Center in urban Dorchester, Massachusetts. These were not just physician offices transplanted to underserved areas. Rather, they were comprehensive, community-based organizations that provided access to food, nutrition education, housing assistance, environmental interventions, community organizing, and health care training opportunities overseen by the community itself, in addition to health care services (Massachusetts League of Community Health Centers, 2019). This model of community-oriented primary care replicated that created by Drs. Sidney and Emily Kark in South Africa in the 1940s and 1950s (Susser, 1993; Yach & Tollman, 1993). Geiger studied their model of care as a medical student and brought this knowledge back to the United States (Geiger, 1993; Hawkins, 2015).

Geiger witnessed and then harnessed the power of clinicians to help communities realize the right to health. Two decades later, he and a number of colleagues formed Physicians for Human Rights (PHR) in order to advocate against human rights abuses around the world. One of these colleagues was Dr. Robert Lawrence, then chief of medicine at Cambridge Hospital in Cambridge, Massachusetts, a safety net hospital and teaching affiliate of Harvard Medical School (PHR, n.d.). Dr. Lawrence imparted his concern over human rights abuses to his faculty and trainees at Cambridge Hospital, and there they developed methods for clinicians to evaluate the sequelae of human rights abuses later adopted by PHR and disseminated globally (R.S. Lawrence, personal communication, November 20, 2017; R.J. Pels, personal communication, August 29, 2017). Cambridge Hospital had been established in the early part of the 20th century to care for indigent residents of the city, and it continued to provide care for poor immigrants and asylum seekers, among others, in recognition of the right to health (Cambridge Health Alliance, 2017). At the same time, Dr. Judith Herman and colleagues in Cambridge Hospital's Department of Psychiatry were developing methods to treat survivors of trauma, including domestic violence (Herman, 1992).

In 2005, the Coordinated Care Program for Political Violence Survivors (CCPPVS) was launched at Cambridge Health Alliance (CHA), the now expanded Cambridge Hospital. An increasing number of asylum seekers with histories of trauma were seeking care at CHA, throughout the greater Boston area, and across the United States. Building upon the previous work done in the Departments of Medicine and Psychiatry, the program offered them medical and psychological care. Even though medical and mental health services existed at CHA to address these respective needs, they had not previously worked together closely. However, these patients with complex medical and psychological needs also had complicated legal, housing, and employment needs that directly impinged upon their clinical needs.

There was no way to effectively address one of these areas without addressing the others. The Greater Boston area enjoyed a relative wealth of free and pro bono immigration legal services, as well as other resources for immigrant political violence survivors, but CCPPVS now began to bring these together with clinical services in order to address the needs of these patients more holistically. Unlike the community health centers in Mound Bayou or Columbia Point, they could not offer all of the needed services for these patients in one physical space. So, CCPPVS created an integrated network of services physically located at different organizations, but linked by close electronic, telephonic, and, when possible, in-person communication.

Initially, the CCPPVS team consisted of staff physicians and psychologists at CHA, as well as staff attorneys and social workers at partnering organizations. However, mental health trainees in psychology and psychiatry soon expressed a strong interest in learning how to care for and advocate on behalf of political violence survivors/victims of human rights abuses. Especially for the psychology trainees, they had not had any formal, academic exposure to human rights training or the care and evaluation of patients who had experienced human rights abuses in their doctoral programs. In order to address this training need, a group of psychology, psychiatry, and internal medicine faculty created a dedicated seminar for trainees to learn about these patients and their needs. The focus was case-based and included immigration attorneys, legal scholars, human rights researchers and advocates, in addition to clinical faculty. Trainees worked through issues for actual patients they were caring for, rather than simply learning about abstract human rights theories (Hannibal & Lawrence, 1996). They worked on evaluations and documentation that often made the difference in their patients being able to remain in the United States, rather than being deported to face further trauma, torture, and/or death. In so doing, psychology trainees also developed a human rights frame within which to situate all of their patients and their clinical work. The seminar also served as a space for trainees to discuss their own reactions to cases involving extreme suffering and, thereby, avoid secondary trauma.

The role of psychological evaluations for those seeking immigration relief in the United States took on even greater significance with the passage of the Illegal Immigration Reform and Immigrant Responsibility Act (IIRIRA) by the U.S. Congress in 1996. This law mandated that any person applying for asylum in the United States had to do so within 1 year of entering the country, whether they were aware of this requirement or not. This is referred to as the "one-year bar" or "one-year filing deadline" (Xiao, 2017). Asylum seekers would only be allowed to file for immigration relief after the 1-year deadline if they could demonstrate the existence of an "extraordinary circumstance" that made this impossible (Harris, 2016). One such allowable circumstance is mental illness or mental disability, including those resulting from torture or other trauma (Harris, 2016). When Cambridge Hospital physicians initially developed guidelines for clinicians to evaluate asylum seekers, the majority of requests were for physical (medical) evaluations of scars or other sequelae of torture (R.S. Lawrence, personal communication, November 20, 2017). Decades later, after torturers had adopted techniques designed not to leave any physical marks, the number of asylum seekers with scars or other physical evidence of torture declined. At the same time, research clearly demonstrated that those asylum seekers who had a forensic evaluation had a much higher likelihood of having their asylum request granted (Lustig et al., 2008). These factors together meant that the number of psychological evaluations requested by attorneys in asylum cases rose significantly. At the same time, the complexity of the mental health sequelae among asylum seekers had also increased.

The following case exemplifies these issues and the role of psychologists in supporting such claims:

M.S. was man in his 30s from Eastern Africa who had been referred by his attorneys.[1] He had grown up in a refugee camp there and then lost multiple

---

[1] All case material has been altered to protect confidentiality.

family members in an ongoing ethnic conflict. He was forcibly conscripted and subsequently tortured. M.S. eventually fled to the United States where he sought asylum, leaving his remaining family members behind. He was initially held in immigration detention, which exacerbated his symptoms, but his attorneys were able to have him released on bond. When he initially presented for care, he was suffering from chronic posttraumatic stress disorder and major depressive disorder and was unable to discuss his experiences of trauma, his family, or his country of origin without dissociating. His attorneys knew that if M.S. were returned to his country of origin, he would be subject to further torture and would not be able to access the trauma-informed psychological care that he needed. They therefore argued against his return (*refoulement*) under the CAT and for his need to remain in the United States to receive care for his ongoing mental health symptoms under Article 15 of the ICESCR (OHCHR, 1984; UNGA, 1966b). They sought documentation of his symptoms and diagnoses from the psychologist treating him in the form of an affidavit she produced as part of a process commonly referred to as an "asylum evaluation" and based on the Istanbul Protocol (OHCHR, 2004). Such an effort is a human rights intervention that any psychologist can undertake.

Historically, asylum evaluations were completed independently of clinical care and evaluators generally had no ongoing relationship with the asylum seeker. In the case of M.S., his symptoms made it impossible for him to discuss his history of trauma with either his own attorneys or a psychological evaluator, let alone an immigration judge or a government attorney. He was referred for treatment with a psychologist at a community-based outpatient clinic, who focused on his current symptoms and function rather than his previous trauma. Through ongoing psychotherapy, she was able to document for the court that he was unable to engage in his own immigration legal case due to the severity of his previous trauma and the continuing burden of his chronic symptoms. On this basis, his immigration attorneys were able to successfully argue that he should not have to participate in his own legal case and he was granted asylum without ever having to testify (see Sherman-Stokes, 2016, 2017).

By receiving services at a safety net institution, M.S. was not only able to access general care, but trauma-informed mental health care at an institution that specializes in the development and provision of such care. This is in keeping with Article 15 of the ICESCR, which upholds the right to "enjoy the benefits of scientific progress and its applications" (UNGA, 1966b). Safety net institutions have a special obligation to provide access to such care, as this is where the vast majority of vulnerable immigrants, including asylum seekers and refugees, access health care services in the United States. Moreover, the principle of health care equity calls for such patients to be able to access these specific services wherever they receive care. The notion of equal access to health care requires that all patients be able to access the same services, but for the human rights of vulnerable immigrants delineated in the UDHR, ICESCR, and CAT to be upheld, they need to be able to access services that meet their specific needs. This is the principle of health equity. Currently, such services may only exist at dedicated treatment centers, but they should not be limited to such settings. Trauma related to human rights violations is widespread, and its treatment cannot be left to only a small subset of clinicians. All psychology students should be trained in the care of such patients, as well as the advocacy tools to ensure that their human rights related to such health needs are upheld.

Postdoctoral psychology fellows working with CCPPVS regularly take on such cases for both ongoing care and evaluation for immigration cases. Under the supervision of staff clinicians, they approach such patients from a case-based learning perspective, acquiring both skills and knowledge not available in their academic programs. Fellows also learn how health care administration, clinical care, and advocacy can all employ a human rights frame. They see CCPPVS assist incoming patients in obtaining health care coverage and access to health care, navigating and accompanying them through an often byzantine process that is especially confusing and potentially distressing for those who have suffered severe trauma, are unfamiliar with U.S. health care, and often fearful of involvement with any government entity. They work with program partners who approach legal and other community-based services from a rights-based perspective and participate in pressuring government to uphold human rights. And they work with supervising clinicians who model care that is grounded in the right to health. In all of these ways, human rights are at the core of their training.

CONCLUSION

In our current national context, human rights broadly and refugees and immigrants specifically seem to be under constant threat. In fact, the ideals they represent and these populations on the whole have been at risk in the United States for decades. It is up to psychologists, along with other health care professionals, to advocate for the observance of human rights in order to protect these populations. We have attempted to provide psychologists with a human rights frame with which they can approach everyday issues in clinical practice, research, and teaching, and which is compatible with professional ethical codes for psychologists. By building collaborations with community-based organizations focusing on the needs of refugees and immigrants and utilizing the core human rights statutes outlined here, psychologists can meet their responsibility to uphold the human rights of these vulnerable populations.

REFERENCES

American Psychological Association. (2012). *Competency initiatives in professional psychology.* https://www.apa.org/ed/graduate/competency
American Psychological Association. (2017). *Ethical principles of psychologists and code of conduct* (2002, Amended June 1, 2010, and January 1, 2017). http://www.apa.org/ethics/code/index.aspx

Amnesty International. (2010). *Amnesty International report 2010: The state of the world's human rights.* https://www.amnesty.org/en/documents/pol10/001/2010/en/

Amnesty International. (2014). *Torture in 2014: 30 years of broken promises.* http://www.amnestyusa.org/sites/default/files/act400042014en.pdf

Beauchamp, T. L., & Childress, J. F. (2001). *Principles of biomedical ethics.* Oxford University Press.

Betancourt, J. R. (2006). Eliminating racial and ethnic disparities in health care: What is the role of academic medicine? *Academic Medicine, 81*(9), 788–792. https://doi.org/10.1097/00001888-200609000-00004

Borque, S. (2019). *Sleeping in an ice box: Report describes dire health conditions at border detention centers.* Fronteras. https://fronterasdesk.org/content/1172176/sleeping-ice-box-report-describes-dire-health-conditions-border-detention-centers

Boyd, J. W., LoCicero, A., Malowney, M., Aldis, R., & Marlin, R. P. (2014). Failing ethics 101: Psychologists, the U.S. military establishment, and human rights. *International Journal of Health Services, 44*(3), 615–625. https://doi.org/10.2190/HS.44.3.j

Buitenweg, R. (2007). *Human rights, human plights in a global village.* Clarity Press.

Cambridge Health Alliance. (2017). *Cambridge Health Alliance: 2017 Academic overview.* Harvard Medical School.

Centers for Disease Control and Prevention. (n.d.). *U.S. Public Health Service syphilis study at Tuskegee: The Tuskegee timeline.* https://www.cdc.gov/tuskegee/timeline.htm

Centers for Disease Control and Prevention. (2020). *COVID-19 in racial and ethnic minority groups.* https://www.cdc.gov/coronavirus/2019-ncov/need-extra-precautions/racial-ethnic-minorities.html

Council of Europe, European Convention for the Protection of Human Rights and Fundamental Freedoms, as amended by Protocols Nos. 11 and 14, 4 November 1950, ETS 5. https://www.refworld.org/docid/3ae6b3b04.html

Dittmer, J. (2014). The medical committee for human rights. *Virtual Mentor, 16*(9), 745–748. https://doi.org/10.1001/virtualmentor.2014.16.09.mhst1-1409

EFPA Board Human Rights and Psychology. (2015). Psychology matters in human rights—Human rights matter in psychology. *EFPA policy and action in the area of human rights and psychology.* http://human-rights.efpa.eu/introduction/policy-paper/

Furtmayr, H., & Frewer, A. (2010). Documentation of torture and the *Istanbul Protocol*: Applied medical ethics. *Medicine, Health Care, and Philosophy, 13*(3), 279–286. https://doi.org/10.1007/s11019-010-9248-1

Galarneau, C. (2018). Getting King's words right. *Journal of Health Care for the Poor and Underserved, 29*(1), 5–8. https://doi.org/10.1353/hpu.2018.0001

Geiger, H. J. (1993). Community-oriented primary care: The legacy of Sidney Kark. *American Journal of Public Health, 83*(7), 946–947. https://doi.org/10.2105/AJPH.83.7.946

Hagenaars, P. (2016). Towards a human rights based and oriented psychology. *Psychology and Developing Societies, 28*(2), 183–202. https://doi.org/10.1177/0971333616657170

Hannibal, K., & Lawrence, R. S. (1996). The health professional as human rights promoter: Ten years of Physicians for Human Rights (USA). *Health and Human Rights, 2*(1), 110–127. https://doi.org/10.2307/4065238

Harris, L. M. (2016). *The one-year bar to asylum in the age of the immigration court backlog.* Retrieved from https://ssrn.com/abstract=2833404

Hawkins, D. (2015). Jack Geiger: Our founding father and so much more. *Community Health Forum,* Spring 2015, 16–18.

Herman, J. L. (1992). *Trauma and recovery: The aftermath of violence.* Basic Books.

Human Rights Watch. (2018). *Code red: The fatal consequences of dangerously substandard medical care in immigration detention.* https://www.hrw.org/report/2018/06/20/code-red/fatal-consequences-dangerously-substandard-medical-care-immigration

Human Rights Watch. (2019). *US: Suit over indefinite detention of children amicus brief supports plantiffs'* [sic] *challenge to new rules.* https://www.hrw.org/news/2019/09/03/us-suit-over-indefinite-detention-children

Huminuik, K. (2017). Special competencies for psychological assessment of torture survivors. *Transcultural Psychiatry, 54*(2), 239–259. https://doi.org/10.1177/1363461516675561

International Committee of the Red Cross. (1949). *Geneva Convention Relative to the Protection of Civilian Persons in Time of War (Fourth Geneva Convention).* https://www.refworld.org/docid/3ae6b36d2.html

Krishnan, M. (2016, August 3). *Here's what the missing and murdered indigenous women inquiry is missing.* Vice News. https://www.vice.com/en_ca/article/bn3b98/heres-what-the-missing-and-murdered-indigenous-women-inquiry-is-missing

Ku, L., & Matani, S. (2001). Left out: Immigrants' access to health care and insurance. *Health Affairs, 20*(1), 247–256. https://doi.org/10.1377/hlthaff.20.1.247

Linton, J. M., Griffin, M., Shapiro, A. J., & Council on Community Pediatrics. (2017). Detention of immigrant children. *Pediatrics, 139*(5), e20170483. https://doi.org/10.1542/peds.2017-0483

Lustig, S. L., Kureshi, S., Delucchi, K. L., Iacopino, V., & Morse, S. C. (2008). Asylum grant rates following medical evaluations of maltreatment among political asylum applicants in the United States. *Journal of Immigrant and Minority Health, 10*(1), 7–15. https://doi.org/10.1007/s10903-007-9056-8

MacNaughton, G., & McGill, M. (2012). Economic and social rights in the United States: Implementation without ratification. *Northeastern University Law Journal, 4*(2), 365–406. https://papers.ssrn.com/sol3/papers.cfm?abstract_id=2054736

Massachusetts League of Community Health Centers. (2019). *History of community health centers.* http://www.massleague.org/CHC/History.php

Oglesby, E. (2018). *How immigration raids inflict trauma on communities.* Citylab. https://www.citylab.com/equity/2018/06/immigration-customs-enforcement-ice-raids-community-impact/563039/

Organization of African Unity (OAU). (1981). African Charter on Human and Peoples' Rights ("Banjul Charter"), 27 June 1981, CAB/LEG/67/3 rev. 5, 21 I.L.M. 58 (1982). https://www.refworld.org/docid/3ae6b3630.html

Organization of American States (OAS). (1969). American Convention on Human Rights ("Pact of San Jose"), Costa Rica, 22 November 1969. https://www.refworld.org/docid/3ae6b36510.html

Physicians for Human Rights. (n.d.). *Our history.* https://phr.org/about/history/

Scholars at Risk. (2018). *Free to think 2018.* https://www.scholarsatrisk.org/wp-content/uploads/2018/10/Free-to-Think-2018.pdf

Sherman-Stokes, S. (2016). Sufficiently safeguarded? Competency evaluations of mentally ill respondents in removal proceedings. *The Hastings Law Journal, 67*(4), 1023–1066. https://repository.uchastings.edu/hastings_law_journal/vol67/iss4/3/

Sherman-Stokes, S. (2017). No restoration, no rehabilitation: Shadow detention of mentally incompetent noncitizens. *Villanova Law Review, 62*(4), 787–827. https://digitalcommons.law.villanova.edu/vlr/vol62/iss4/5

Shuster, E. (1997). Fifty years later: The significance of the Nuremberg Code. *The New England Journal of Medicine, 337*(20), 1436–1440. https://doi.org/10.1056/NEJM199711133372006

Steinert, T. (2017). Ethics of coercive treatment and misuse of psychiatry. *Psychiatric Services, 68*(3), 291–294. https://doi.org/10.1176/appi.ps.201600066

Susser, M. (1993). A South African odyssey in community health: A memoir of the impact of the teachings of Sidney Kark. *American Journal of Public Health, 83*(7), 1039–1042. https://doi.org/10.2105/AJPH.83.7.1039

UNICEF. (2016). *Uprooted: The growing crisis for refugee and migrant children.*

United Nations. (1948). *Universal declaration of human rights* (UDHR) [General Assembly Resolution 217 A]. https://www.un.org/en/universal-declaration-human-rights/

United Nations General Assembly. (1966a). *International covenant on civil and political rights. United Nations, Treaty Series, 999,* p. 171. https://www.refworld.org/docid/3ae6b3aa0.html

United Nations General Assembly. (1966b). *International covenant on economic, social and cultural rights. United Nations, Treaty Series, 993,* p. 3. https://www.refworld.org/docid/3ae6b36c0.html

United Nations Office of the High Commissioner for Human Rights (OHCHR). (1984). *Convention against torture and other cruel, inhuman or degrading treatment or punishment.* https://www.ohchr.org/en/professionalinterest/pages/cat.aspx

United Nations Office of the High Commissioner for Human Rights (OHCHR). (2004). *Manual on the effective investigation and documentation of torture and other cruel, inhuman or degrading treatment or punishment ("Istanbul Protocol").* https://www.refworld.org/docid/4638aca62.html

United States. (1979). *The Belmont report: Ethical principles and guidelines for the protection of human subjects of research.* The National Commission for the Protection of Human Subjects of Biomedical and Behavioral Research. https://www.hhs.gov/ohrp/regulations-and-policy/belmont-report/read-the-belmont-report/index.html

Wood, L. C. N. (2018). Impact of punitive immigration policies, parent–child separation and child detention on the mental health and development of children. *BMJ Paediatrics Open, 2*(1), e000338. https://doi.org/10.1136/bmjpo-2018-000338

Woodman, S., Kehoe, K., Saleh, M., & Rappleye, H. (2019). *Thousands of immigrants suffer in U.S. solitary confinement.* International Consortium of Investigative Journalists. https://www.icij.org/investigations/solitary-voices/thousands-of-immigrants-suffer-in-us-solitary-confinement/

World Health Organization. (1948). *Constitution.* https://www.who.int/about/who-we-are/constitution

Xiao, R. (2017). Refuge from time: How the one-year filing deadline unfairly frustrates valid asylum claims. *North Carolina Law Review, 95*(2), 523–552. https://scholarship.law.unc.edu/nclr/vol95/iss2/6

Yach, D., & Tollman, S. M. (1993). Public health initiatives in South Africa in the 1940s and 1950s: Lessons for a post-apartheid era. *American Journal of Public Health, 83*(7), 1043–1050. https://doi.org/10.2105/AJPH.83.7.1043

Afterword

Looking to the Future

Pratyusha Tummala-Narra

Traumatic stress among immigrants has a long-standing history in the United States and across the globe. However, to date, little attention has been directed toward examining traumatic experiences among racial minority immigrants in the United States. This volume takes an important step in engaging with various facets of violence and trauma in the context of immigration. The authors explore how the broader socioecological context of immigration shapes traumatic stress among racial minority immigrants, including a sense of uncertainty about the future. They emphasize the ways in which historical and ongoing sociopolitical trauma impacts individuals and communities in unique ways based on various social position factors, such as gender, race, religion, sexual orientation, social class, and authorization/documentation status (American Psychological Association, 2012; García Coll & Marks, 2012). They also describe the distinct ways that subgroups of immigrants, such as youth, survivors of trafficking, and LGBTQ people, are affected by xenophobia, racism, and multiple forms of marginalization.

Importantly, the authors explore how racial minority immigrants cope with traumatic stress and resist oppression. They highlight that resilience is both contextual and culturally embedded and therefore should be approached with consideration for how conceptualizations of resilience may vary for immigrants based on sociocultural background and social location. Taken together, the chapters underscore the complexity of the traumatic experiences of racial minority immigrants and call for psychologists and other mental health

https://doi.org/10.1037/0000214-018
Trauma and Racial Minority Immigrants: Turmoil, Uncertainty, and Resistance,
P. Tummala-Narra (Editor)

professionals to expand theory, research, and practice that reflect this complexity. In this brief concluding chapter, I explore some key issues that require further inquiry in future research, scholarship, practice, and education in the area of trauma and immigration.

First, it is important to recognize that the study of immigration experience encompasses historical traumas; ongoing exposure to xenophobia, racism, and intersectional discrimination; and crisis states, such as deportation and abrupt shifts in policies. At the present time, within the mental health professions, there are, in fact, structural pressures that guide conceptualizations of what constitutes trauma. For example, it continues to be the case that racial trauma is not officially considered a precipitant to posttraumatic stress disorder in psychiatric classification systems, yet there is ample empirical and clinical evidence indicating that both blatant and subtle forms of racism are associated with negative mental health outcomes, such as depression, anxiety, substance abuse, and suicidality, within different racial and ethnic groups in the United States. This evidence is in no way reflected in the *Diagnostic and Statistical Manual of Mental Disorders* (5th ed.; American Psychiatric Association, 2013) or the *International Statistical Classification of Diseases and Related Health Problems* (11th ed.; World Health Organization, 2019). It is also not reflected in many academic journals, even those focused on trauma, which focus more on biological issues related to posttraumatic stress than on ecological determinants of traumatic stress.

Divorcing empirical and clinical evidence from diagnostic categories serves not only to minimize the impact of sociopolitical trauma on immigrants' lives but also to limit access to culturally informed services and resources for coping with this trauma. Furthermore, as the authors of this volume have noted, such structural exclusion of sociopolitical trauma and decontextualized conceptualizations of trauma serve to locate the problem or disorder solely within individuals or communities rather than within the social structures and contextual realities that are, in fact, the source of violence and trauma. This is even more problematic during a public health crisis, such as COVID-19, or in the aftermath of an environmental disaster, both of which expose structural inequities that place many racial minorities at a disadvantage when securing safe and healthy lives. It is critical that psychologists and mental health professionals embrace the social context of trauma as foundational to an in-depth understanding of traumatic stress experienced by racial minority immigrants.

Second, we need to further consider the intergenerational impact of trauma faced by immigrants and their children. Research concerning the impact of trauma on immigrants and their families in the premigration, transit, and postmigration contexts is scarce, even though there is strong evidence for the intergenerational transmission of traumatic stress within the broader complex trauma literature (Herman, 1992). Intergenerational trauma can have important implications for the process of acculturation, family dynamics, mental health, identity, and resilience (Tummala-Narra, 2016). Psychologists can engage in research and theory development that extend and modify existing conceptualizations of attachment in the context of trauma and immigration. For example, we need to develop deeper understandings of the impact of race-based violence, deportations, and family separations on children and adolescents and of the long-term consequences of these collective traumas on subsequent generations. We can also examine the impact of historical events such as the terrorist attacks of 9/11 on mental health, identity, and relational life among racial minority immigrant children, adolescents, and young adults who have grown up primarily in a post-9/11 era. This type of research can be helpful in better understanding generational differences in experiences of sociopolitical trauma within immigrant families and communities. Relatedly, it is important to learn more about how the Trump effect (Zimbardo & Sword, 2017) is experienced by racial minority immigrants across different age and generation lines and how they are coping with stress related to xenophobia and uncertainty in immigration policy (e.g., Deferred Action for Childhood Arrivals [DACA] and Temporary Protected Status [TPS]).

Third, I recommend a closer examination of how historical and ongoing trauma related to Native American genocide and African slavery in the United States is connected with xenophobia, racism, and anti-immigrant violence (e.g., incarceration of Japanese Americans). This analysis would require that White people engage in learning about and reconnecting with their own family histories of migration to the United States and recognizing privileges accorded to them through the American racial hierarchy. What I am suggesting here is that we engage researchers, practitioners, and educators from all racial backgrounds in dialogue, empirical inquiry, and theory development regarding social oppression in its varied forms such that it no longer remains a sole problem located in and contained by people of color. Research and theory concerning racial minority immigrants should not only compose a specialized area but also should be integrated within mainstream psychological research, practice, and training. In other words, the study of immigrants' experiences should not be marginalized from mainstream models of development, psychopathology, resilience, and psychotherapy (and other interventions).

Fourth, the authors in this volume speak clearly to the importance of recognizing heterogeneity among immigrants, with regard to factors such as identity, social locations, types of traumatic exposure, acculturation, and authorization/documentation status. Understanding the complexity of racial minority immigrants' traumatic experiences requires further attention to intersectional aspects of identity, oppression, and resilience. As mentioned previously, future research and theory can expand knowledge concerning subgroups of racial minority immigrants. Specifically, we need to explore the psychological consequences of sociocultural oppression occurring on an ongoing basis and during crisis states, such as COVID-19, when subgroups of racial minorities are vulnerable to illness, death of loved ones, loss of economic resources and employment, and racism and stereotyping. With escalating threats to safety due to climate change, further inquiry into the impact of climate change and natural and environmental disasters on the lives of racial minorities will be especially important in the future. To gain more accurate and comprehensive conceptualizations of racial minority immigrants' experiences, we need evidence from multiple sources, such as quantitative, qualitative, mixed methods, and clinical case studies, and we need multiple theoretical lenses.

Fifth, I want to emphasize the importance of resistance by psychologists and other mental health professionals to oppressive policies, within their own professions and/or in broader society, that further marginalize racial minority immigrants. By working with researchers across disciplines such as public health, climate science, and economics and with policymakers, we can develop and propose policies that more effectively address the needs of racial minority immigrants amidst crises such as COVID-19 and climate change. This research is especially critical for vulnerable subgroups, including but not limited to individuals who are undocumented, coping with unsafe living conditions, and/or living in poverty. Psychologists and mental health professionals can serve in advocacy roles within schools, hospitals, outpatient mental health centers and clinics, home-based and community-based services, colleges and universities, community-based organizations, detention facilities, prisons, legal settings, and academic and professional organizations, all settings in which we can guide and implement culturally informed interventions and practices that respect human rights and the dignity of immigrants who are coping with collective and interpersonal violence. We can also collaborate with communities more directly (e.g., with parents, schools, community centers, religious centers, law enforcement) to develop interventions that are empowering to individuals and communities in ways that respect their sociocultural contexts and values. Resisting oppressive policies entails implementing training for graduate students and psychologists at all stages of their careers, focused on the concerns of racial minority immigrants and on culturally informed conceptualizations and practices.

Finally, we can conduct research in collaboration with immigrant communities who can directly benefit from the process and/or the outcome of the research. For example, research concerning racial trauma experienced by immigrant adolescents in a school can translate to school-based interventions that facilitate dialogue about prejudice and racism and are aimed to challenge stereotypes and race-based bullying. A study focused on sexual violence can result in a productive dialogue within communities in which sexual violence is typically a stigmatized topic. Such dialogue can facilitate understanding of sexual trauma and provide access to help for survivors. It is especially important that we continue to find ways to bridge research and practice such that evidence from empirical studies and clinical practice together inform approaches to trauma experienced by racial minority immigrants.

In conclusion, this volume underscores the pervasive effects of trauma experienced by racial minority immigrants. It behooves all of us to engage in ongoing inquiry and dialogue regarding traumatic stress in a way that recognizes and respects immigrants' perspectives. While we face an uncertain future with regard to local, state, and federal policies on immigration, psychologists have a tremendous opportunity to expand knowledge, implement culturally informed practices, and advocate for basic rights and dignity of immigrants.

REFERENCES

American Psychiatric Association. (2013). *Diagnostic and statistical manual of mental disorders* (5th ed.). https://doi.org/10.1176/appi.books.9780890425596

American Psychological Association Presidential Task Force on Immigration. (2012). *Presidential Task Force on Immigration Report: Crossroads: The psychology of immigration in the new century.* https://www.apa.org/topics/immigration/executive-summary.pdf

García Coll, C., & Marks, A. K. (Eds.). (2012). *The immigrant paradox in children and adolescents: Is becoming American a developmental risk?* American Psychological Association. https://doi.org/10.1037/13094-000

Herman, J. L. (1992). *Trauma and recovery.* Basic Books.

Tummala-Narra, P. (2016). *Psychoanalytic theory and cultural competence in psychotherapy.* American Psychological Association. https://doi.org/10.1037/14800-000

World Health Organization. (2019). *International statistical classification of diseases and related health problems* (11th ed.). https://icd.who.int/

Zimbardo, P., & Sword, R. (2017). Unbridled and extreme present hedonism. In B. X. Lee (Ed.), *The dangerous case of Donald Trump* (pp. 25–50). St. Martin's Press.

INDEX

ABOUT THE EDITOR

Pratyusha (Usha) Tummala-Narra, PhD, is a professor of counseling, developmental and educational psychology at Boston College. She is also in independent practice in Cambridge, Massachusetts. Her research and scholarship focus on immigration, trauma, race, and cultural competence and psychoanalytic psychotherapy. She has served as the chair of the Multicultural Concerns Committee and member-at-large on the Board of Directors for American Psychological Association (APA) Division 39 (Society for Psychoanalysis and Psychoanalytic Psychology) and as a member of the APA Committee on Ethnic Minority Affairs, the APA Presidential Task Force on Immigration, and the APA Task Force on Revising the Multicultural Guidelines. Dr. Tummala-Narra is an associate editor of the *Asian American Journal of Psychology*, an associate editor of *Psychoanalytic Dialogues*, and psychotherapy editor of the *Journal of Humanistic Psychology*. She is a Fellow of the American Psychological Association and of APA Division 39 and Division 45 (Society for the Psychological Study of Culture, Ethnicity and Race). She is the author of *Psychoanalytic Theory and Cultural Competence in Psychotherapy*, published by APA Books in 2016.